Sports Medicine and Sports Injury

Sports Medicine and Sports Injury

Edited by **Pablo De Souza**

hayle
medical

New York

Published by Hayle Medical,
30 West, 37th Street, Suite 612,
New York, NY 10018, USA
www.haylemedical.com

Sports Medicine and Sports Injury
Edited by Pablo De Souza

© 2015 Hayle Medical

International Standard Book Number: 978-1-63241-358-1 (Hardback)

Printed in the United States of America.

Contents

Preface   VII

Part 1   Physiology of Sports Medicine   1

Chapter 1   **Measurement and Physiological Relevance of the Maximal Lipid Oxidation Rate During Exercise (LIPOXmax)**   3
Jean-Frédéric Brun, Emmanuelle Varlet-Marie, Ahmed Jérôme Romain and Jacques Mercier

Chapter 2   **Physical Activity Measures in Children – Which Method to Use?**   41
Juliette Hussey

Chapter 3   **Glutamine and Glutamate Reference Intervals as a Clinical Tool to Detect Training Intolerance During Training and Overtraining**   53
Rodrigo Hohl, Lázaro Alessandro Soares Nunes, Rafael Alkmin Reis, René Brenzikofer, Rodrigo Perroni Ferraresso, Foued Salmen Spindola and Denise Vaz Macedo

Chapter 4   **Applicability of the Reference Interval and Reference Change Value of Hematological and Biochemical Biomarkers to Sport Science**   77
Lázaro Alessandro Soares Nunes, Fernanda Lorenzi Lazarim, René Brenzikofer and Denise Vaz Macedo

Chapter 5   **Eccentric Exercise, Muscle Damage and Oxidative Stress**   99
Athanasios Z. Jamurtas and Ioannis G. Fatouros

Chapter 6   **Body Mass Bias in Exercise Physiology**   117
Paul M. Vanderburgh

Chapter 7   **Aging in Women Athletes**   131
             Monica C. Serra, Shawna L. McMillin and Alice S. Ryan

Chapter 8   **Physical Activity,**
             Physical Fitness and Metabolic Syndrome   145
             Xiaolin Yang

Chapter 9   **Exercise and the Immune System – Focusing on**
             the Effect of Exercise on Neutrophil Functions   171
             Baruch Wolach

Part 2   **Medical Issues in Sports Medicine**   185

Chapter 10   **Comparison of Seminal Superoxide**
             Dismutase (SOD) Activity Between Elite
             Athletes, Active and Non Active Men   187
             Bakhtyar Tartibian, Behzad Hajizadeh Maleki,
             Asghar Abbasi, Mehdi Eghbali, Siamak Asri-Rezaei and
             Hinnak Northoff

Chapter 11   **Effects of Exercise on the Airways**   197
             Maria R. Bonsignore, Nicola Scichilone, Laura Chimenti,
             Roberta Santagata, Daniele Zangla and Giuseppe Morici

Chapter 12   **Aquatic Sports Dermatoses:**
             Clinical Presentation and Treatment Guidelines   223
             Jonathan S. Leventhal and Brook E. Tlougan

Chapter 13   **Evaluation of Neural Networks to Identify Types**
             of Activity Among Children Using Accelerometers,
             Global Positioning Systems and Heart Rate Monitors   245
             Francisca Galindo-Garre and Sanne I. de Vries

Chapter 14   **The Involvement of Brain Monoamines in**
             the Onset of Hyperthermic Central Fatigue   257
             Cândido C. Coimbra, Danusa D. Soares and Laura H. R. Leite

Chapter 15   **The Application of Medical Infrared**
             Thermography in Sports Medicine   289
             Carolin Hildebrandt, Karlheinz Zeilberger,
             Edward Francis John Ring and Christian Raschner

             Permissions

             List of Contributors

Preface

I am honored to present to you this unique book which encompasses the most up-to-date data in the field. I was extremely pleased to get this opportunity of editing the work of experts from across the globe. I have also written papers in this field and researched the various aspects revolving around the progress of the discipline. I have tried to unify my knowledge along with that of stalwarts from every corner of the world, to produce a text which not only benefits the readers but also facilitates the growth of the field.

This book is dedicated to the recent findings and emerging concepts of sports medicine. For the last several years, sports medication has been a growing discipline in USA and Western Europe. Immense strides have been made in comprehending the fundamental functioning of work outs, power utilization and the mechanisms of sports damage. Furthermore, a development in minimally invasive surgeries and physical rehabilitation has led to athletes returning to their respective sport quickly after injuries. This book presents some latest information from experts on the physiology of work out and sports routine, and updates on medical disorders treated in athletes.

Finally, I would like to thank all the contributing authors for their valuable time and contributions. This book would not have been possible without their efforts. I would also like to thank my friends and family for their constant support.

Editor

Part 1

Physiology of Sports Medicine

Measurement and Physiological Relevance of the Maximal Lipid Oxidation Rate During Exercise (LIPOXmax)

Jean-Frédéric Brun[1], Emmanuelle Varlet-Marie[2],
Ahmed Jérôme Romain[3] and Jacques Mercier[1]
*[1]U1046, INSERM, Université de Montpellier 1,
Université de Montpellier 2, Montpellier, CHRU Montpellier,
Département de Physiologie Clinique, Montpellier,
[2]Laboratoire Performance Santé Altitude, Sciences et Techniques des Activités
Physiques et Sportives, Université de Perpignan Via Domitia,
[3]Laboratoire EA4556 Epsylon, Dynamique des Capacités Humaines et
des Conduites de Santé (Montpellier)
France*

1. Introduction

The intensity of exercise that elicits a maximal oxidation of lipids has been termed LIPOXmax, FATOXmax or FATmax. The three acronyms refer to three original protocols of exercise calorimetry which have been proposed almost simultaneously and it is thus interesting to maintain the three names in this review in order to avoid confusion. The difference among the three protocols is presented in table 1. Since our team has developed the technique called LIPOXmax (Perez-Martin et al., 2001; Brun et al., 2009b;) this acronym will be more employed in this chapter, keeping in mind that LIPOXmax, FATOXmax or FATmax represent obviously the same physiological concept.

As will be reviewed in this paper, the measurement of LIPOXmax by graded exercise calorimetry is a reproducible measurement, although modifiable by several physiological conditions (training, previous exercise or meal). Its measurement closely predicts what will be oxidized over 45-60 min of low to medium intensity training performed at the corresponding intensity. It might be a marker of metabolic fitness, and is tightly correlated to mitochondrial function. LIPOXmax is related to catecholamine status and the growth-hormone IGF-I axis, and occurs in athletes below the lactate and the ventilatory threshold (on the average around 40% VO_{2max}). Its changes are related to alterations in muscular levels of citrate synthase, and to the mitochondrial ability to oxidize fatty acids. A meta-analysis shows that training at this level is efficient in sedentary subjects for reducing fat mass, sparing fat-free mass, increasing the ability to oxidize lipids during exercise, reducing blood glucose and Hba_{1c} in type 2 diabetes, and decreasing circulating cholesterol. In athletes, various profiles are observed, with a high ability to oxidize lipids in endurance-trained athletes and in some samples of athletes trained for sprint or intermittent exercise a profile showing a predominant use of carbohydrates.

acronym	FATOXmax	FATmax	LIPOXmax	SIN model
initial publication	Dériaz et al., 2001	Achten et al., 2002, 2003, 2004; Jeukendrup, 2003; Venables et al., 2005	Perez-Martin et al., 2001; Brun et al., 2009b;	Chenevière et al., 2009b
Duration of steps	5-6 min (until steady state)	3 min	6 min	5 min
Calculation	Visual determination	Visual determination	Power intensity at which the derivative of the curve of lipid oxidation versus power is equal to zero (eg, top of the bell-shaped curve)	This model includes three independent variables (dilatation, symmetry, and translation). This SIN model has been reported to allow a more accurate calculation of Fatmin/LIPOXzero
Expression of results	% of maximal oxygen uptake (%VO_{2max} MFO in kJ.min-1	% of maximal oxygen uptake (%VO_{2max}) MFO in g. min-1	usually % of theoretical maximal power; also % extrapolated maximal oxygen uptake (%VO_{2max} ACSM)] or % maximal oxygen uptake (%VO_{2max}) determined by a previous test	Fatmax, MFO, dilatation, symmetry and translation

Table 1. Definition of LIPOXmax, FATOXmax or FATmax.

2. The physiological basis for measuring lipid oxidation during exercise

2.1 Balance of substrate oxidation during exercise: The "crossover concept"

Pioneering studies (Zuntz et al., 1901; Krogh et al., 1920; Christensen et al., 1939) have demonstrated that a mixture of carbohydrates and fat is used by the muscle as a fuel at rest and during exercise, and that the ratio between VCO_2 and VO_2 was a reflect of the relative proportion of lipids and CHO used for oxidation. It was clear already at this time that exercise intensity, exercise duration and prior diet modified this balance of substrates.

Recent studies have evidenced that quantitatively, the most important substrate oxidized at the level of the exercising muscle is glucose (Bergman et al., 1999; Friedlander et al., 2007). The maximal rate of CHO oxidation during exercise is about two fold higher than that of lipids (Sahlin et al., 2008). However, when substrate metabolism is assessed on the whole body, lipids remain a major source of fuel at rest and during exercise. At rest, lipids provide >50% of the energy requirements, and they remain an important source of energy during low to middle intensity exercise, while CHO become the main substrate at high intensity (>80% VO_2max) (Jeukendrup et al., 1998). As summarized in table 2, exercise may induce a significant amount of lipid oxidation by at least 4 mechanisms (Brun et al., 2011).

During the last quarter of the XXth century the literature became conflictual with several authors emphasizing the importance of carbohydrates and the others the importance of lipids. This controversy was actually clarified by the heuristic proposal of the "crossover concept" by George Brooks (Brooks et al., 1994). The "crossover concept" is an attempt to integrate the seemingly divergent effects of exercise intensity, nutritional status, gender, age and prior endurance training on the balance of carbohydrates and lipids used as a fuel during sustained exercise. It predicts that although an increase in exercise intensity results in a preferential use of CHO, endurance training shifts the balance of substrates during exercise toward a stronger reliance upon lipids (Fig.1).

The idea of developing a simple reliable exercise-test for assessing this balance of substrates thus emerged as a logical consequence of these fundamental studies (Perez-Martin et al.,

2001; Brun et al., 2007, 2011). Accordingly, several teams have developed this measurement and attempted to train patients at a level determined by this exploration, as reviewed below.

« CROSSOVER" CONCEPT

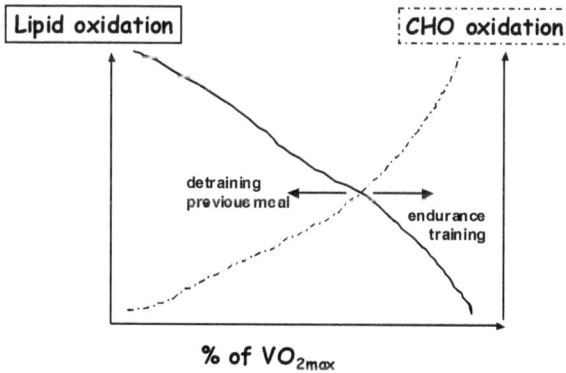

Fig. 1. The crossover concept: the balance of substrates at exercise is a function of exercise intensity, the proportion of lipids used for oxidation continuously decreasing when intensity increases, while CHO become the predominant fuel (>70%) above the "crossover point" (approximately 50% VO_{2max}, see text. This increase in CHO oxidation down-regulates lipid oxidation despite sustained lipolysis. Above the crossover point glycogen utilization scales exponentially. Endurance training, energy supply, overtraining, dietary manipulation and previous exercise modify this pattern. Most trained athletes exhibit a right-shift in this relationship.

a.	Muscular contractile activity by its own may use lipids as a source of energy.	During steady state exercise performed at low intensity, fat is oxidized at an almost constant rate (Bensimhon et al., 2006; Meyer et al., 2007), and there is an intensity of exercise that elicits the maximum oxidation of lipids termed *maximal fat oxidation rate* (MFO).
b.	Progressive rise in lipid oxidation with exercise duration	When exercise is heavy and prolonged enough to result in glycogen depletion, there is a shift toward lipids and their oxidation gradually increases (Ahlborg et al., 1974; Bergman et al., 1999; Watt et al.; 2003). This phenomenon is rather slow in mild to medium intensity exercise when the duration of this exercise does not exceed 1 hr.
c.	Compensatory rise in lipid oxidation after high intensity exercise	High intensity exercise oxidizes almost exclusively CHO but is frequently followed by a compensatory rise in lipid oxidation which compensates more or less for the lipids not oxidized during exercise (Folch et al., 2001; Melanson et al., 2002), but it is inconsistent and frequently quite low (Malatesta et al., 2009; Lazer et al., 2010), even more if exercise is discontinuous (Warren et al., 2009).
d.	Long term regular exercise may increase the ability to oxidize lipids at rest	Long term regular exercise may shift the balance of substrates oxidized over 24 hr toward oxidative use of higher quantities of lipids (Talanian et al., 2007). A training-induced increase in the ability to oxidize lipids over 24-hr is statistically a predictor of exercise-induced weight loss (Barwell et al., 2009).

Table 2. Effects of exercise on lipid oxidation: exercise may increase the oxidative use of lipids by at least 4 mechanisms (after Brun et al., 2011). According to Warren the most important and reliable of these mechanisms is the oxidation during exercise performed around the LIPOXmax or below. (Warren et al., 2009).

2.2 Mechanisms of substrate (fat vs CHO) selection during muscular activity

According to the data presented above, fat is the major energy supply for the muscle below 25% of VO_2max, since in this condition very few glycogen is employed as a source of energy (Romijn et al., 1993). Then, when exercise intensity increases, glycogen will rapidly become the predominant fuel. However, fat oxidation will still increase until the LIPOXmax/FATOXmax is reached. Above this level fat oxidation decreases. Interestingly, this decrease in fat oxidation coincides with lactate increase above baseline, as demonstrated in healthy adolescents during incremental cycling (Tolfrey et al., 2010).

The cellular mechanism of this decrease has been reviewed elsewhere (Sahlin et al., 2008) and is still incompletely understood. Theoretically, lipid supply by lipolysis, lipid entrance in muscle cell, lipid entrance in mitochondria, and mitochondrial fat processing may all be limiting steps. Experiments show that extracellular lipid supply is not limiting, since lipid oxidation decreases even if additional fat is provided to the cell. Limiting steps seem to be the entrance in mitochondria, governed by CPT-1, which can be inhibited by Malonyl-CoA and lactate (Starritt et al., 2000), and possibly downstream CPT-I other mitochondrial enzymes such as Acyl-CoA synthase and electron transport chain. All these steps are sensitive to the rate of CHO oxidation and thus a rise in CHO oxidation seems to depress lipid oxidation despite availability of fat and presence of all the enzymes of fat oxidation.

Experiments using intravenous infusion of labeled long-chain fatty acids in endurance-trained men cycling for 40 min at steady state at 50% of VO_2max clearly demonstrate that carbohydrate availability directly regulates fat oxidation during exercise. An increased glycolytic flux results in a direct inhibition of long-chain fatty acid oxidation (Coyle et al., 1997). Conversely, there is a wide body of evidence that glycogen depletion reverses this inhibition and thus increases fat oxidation, as observed during long duration glycogen-depleting exercise.

These processes are governed by cellular factors, that are under the influence of the central nervous system and circulating hormones (Ahlborg et al., 1974; Kiens & Richter, 1998; Kirvan et al., 1988; Thompson et al., 1998). Intracellular pathways have been reviewed elsewhere and this area of knowledge seems to be rapidly expanding. The activation of the AMPK (AMP-dependent kinase) pathway, together with a subsequent increase in the fatty acid oxidation, appear to constitute the main mechanism of action of these hormones in the regulation of lipid metabolism (Koulmann & Bigard, 2006). To summarize the main hormonal regulators of muscular lipid oxidation, epinephrine increases lipolysis (beta effect) and increases glucose oxidation in muscle (de Glisezinski et al., 2009). Norepinephrine increases lipid oxidation in muscle (Poehlman et al., 1994). Cortisol increases adipogenesis and lipolysis, and decreases non-insulin mediated glucose uptake. β-endorphin induces a lipolysis that can be blunted by naloxone (Richter et al., 1983, 1987). Growth hormone (GH) stimulates lipolysis and ketogenesis (Møller et al., 1990b). In the muscle and the liver, GH stimulates triglyceride uptake, by enhancing lipoprotein lipase expression, and its subsequent storage (Vijayakumar et al., 2010). GH also increases whole body lipid oxidation and nonoxidative glucose utilization and decreases glucose oxidation (Møller et al., 1990a). We have shown that GH-deficient individuals have a lower LIPOXmax and MFO that is restored after GH treatment (Brandou et al., 2006a). Dowstream GH, IGF-I that mediates many of the anabolic actions of growth hormone stimulates muscle protein synthesis, promotes glycogen storage and enhances lipolysis (Guha et al., 2009).

Interleukin-6 (IL-6) coming from the adipose tissue and the muscle acts as an energy sensor and thus activates AMP-activated kinase, resulting in enhanced glucose disposal, lipolysis and fat oxidation (Hoene et al., 2008). Adiponectin increases muscular lipid oxidation via phosphorylation of AMPK (Dick, 2009). Leptin increases muscle fat oxidation and decreases muscle fat uptake, thereby decreasing intramyocellular lipid stores (Dick, 2009).

Although the information on this issue remains limited, it is clear that the level of maximal oxidation of lipids is related to some of these hormonal regulators : norepinephrine, whose training induced changes are positively correlated to an improvement in LIPOXmax (Bordenave et al., 2008) and growth hormone, whose deficit decreases it, a defect that can be corrected by growth hormone replacement (Brandou et al., 2006a). Downstream GH, IGF-I has also been reported to be correlated to LIPOXmax in soccer players as shown on Fig 5 (Brun et al., 1999), reflecting either a parallel effect of training on muscle fuel partitioning or IGF-I release, or an action of IGF-I (or GH via IGF) on muscular lipid oxidation. Other endocrine axes are surely also involved but this issue is poorly known and remains to be studied.

3. Technical aspects of exercise graded calorimetry

3.1 Methodological aspects

As reminded above, the classic picture of Brooks and Mercier's "crossover concept" (Brooks & Mercier, 1994) has led to the development of an exercise-test suitable for routinely assessing this balance of substrates (Perez-Martin & Mercier, 2001; Brun et al., 2007). Based on our previous studies on calorimetry during long duration steady-state workloads (Manetta et al., 2002a, 2002b; Manetta et al., 2005) we developed a test (Perez-Martin et al., 2001) consisting of five 6-min submaximal steps, in which we assumed that a steady-state for gas exchanges was obtained during the 2 last minutes.

We proposed (Perez-Martin et al., 2001) a diagnostic test including four or five 6-minutes workloads, that may be followed by a series of fast increases in power intensity until the tolerable maximum under these conditions is reached. This final incremental part of the test can be avoided in very sedentary patients and the maximal level can be indirectly evaluated by the linear extrapolation according to the ACSM guidelines (VO$_2$max ACSM) (Aucouturier et al., 2009). The test is performed on an ergometric bicycle connected to an analyzer allowing the analysis of the gaseous exchange cycles by cycle. EKG monitoring and measurements of VO$_2$, VCO$_2$, and respiratory exchange ratio (RER) are performed during the test. After a period of 3 minutes at rest, and another period of initial warm-up at 20% of the predicted maximal power (PMP) for 3 minutes, the 6-min workloads set at approximately 30, 40, 50 and 60% of PMP are performed. The phase of recovery comprises two periods during which a monitoring of respiratory and cardiac parameters is maintained: active recovery at 20% of the PMP during 1 minute; passive recovery (ie, rest) during the 2 following minutes. At the end of each stage, during the fifth and sixth minutes, values of VO$_2$ and VCO$_2$ are recorded. These values are used the calculation of the respective rates of oxidation of carbohydrates and lipids by applying the classical stoichiometric equations of indirect calorimetry:

$$\text{Carbohydrates (mg/min)} = 4.585\ VCO_2 - 3.2255\ VO_2 \tag{1}$$

$$\text{Lipid Oxidation (mg/min)} = -1.7012\ VCO_2 + 1.6946\ VO_2 \tag{2}$$

These calculations are performed on values of the 5-6th minutes of each step, since at this CO_2 production from bicarbonate buffers compensating for the production of lactic acid becomes negligible. The increment in carbohydrate oxidation above basal values appears to be roughly a linear function of the developed power and the slope of this relation is calculated, providing the *glucidic cost of the watt* (Aloulou, 2002). The increase in lipid oxidation adopts the shape of a bell-shaped curve: after a peak, lipid oxidation decreases at the highest power intensities.

The exact mechanism of this reduction in the use of the lipids at the highest power intensities is actually imperfectly known: a reduction in lipolysis is likely to explain a part of it, together with a shift of metabolic pathways within the muscle fiber. The empirical formula of indirect calorimetry that gives the lipid oxidation rate is, as reminded above:

$$\text{Lipid oxidation (mg/min)} = -1.7 \, VCO_2 + 1.7 \, VO_2 \tag{3}$$

It is easy to deduce from this formula that the relation between power (P) and oxidation of lipids (Lox) displays a bell-shaped curve of the form:

$$\text{Lox} = A.P \, (1\text{-RER}) \tag{4}$$

The smoothing of this curve enables us to calculate the power intensity at which lipid oxidation becomes maximal, which is the point where the derivative of this curve becomes equal to zero. Therefore the LIPOXmax calculation is only an application of the classical empirical equation of lipid oxidation used in calorimetry.

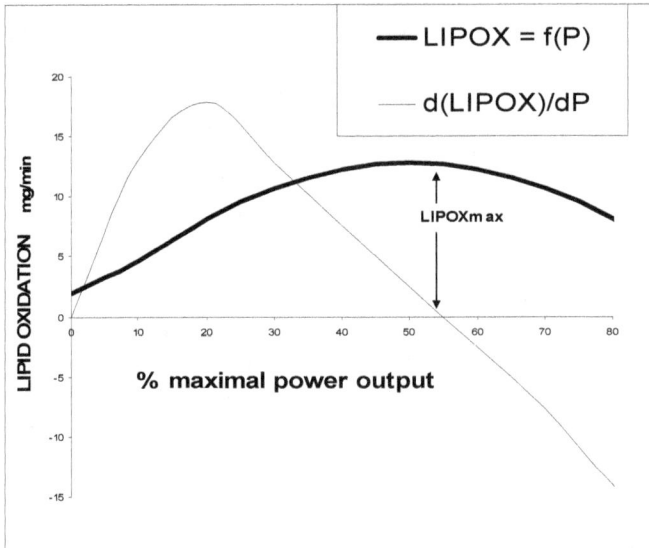

Fig. 2. Calculation of the LIPOXmax: The curve of lipid oxidation (mg/min) is given by the empirical formula of calorimetry Lipox = -1.7 VCO_2 + 1.7 VO_2. This curve Lipox = A.P (1-RER) (see text) can be derived and the point where its derivative equals zero is the top of the bell-shaped curve and thus represents the LIPOXmax. Actually in some subjects this is a broad zone and in others a narrow range of power intensities.

Recently a more sophisticated mathematical model (sine model, SIN) was proposed in order to describe fat oxidation kinetics as a function the relative exercise intensity [% of maximal oxygen uptake (%VO_{2max})] during graded exercise and to determine the exercise intensity elicits maximal fat oxidation and the intensity at which the fat oxidation becomes negligible. This model which will not be developed here includes three independent variables (dilatation, symmetry, and translation). This SIN model exhibits the same precision as other methods currently used in the determination of LIPOXmax and has been reported to allow a more accurate calculation of Fatmin/LIPOXzero (Chenevière et al., 2009b).

Actually, there is now a large body of literature to support the validity of such protocols of exercise calorimetry (Jeukendrup & Wallis, 2005). The theoretical concern was that, when exercise is performed above the lactate threshold, there is an extra CO_2 production which can be assumed to interfere with the calculations (MacRae et al., 1995). In fact, below 75% of the VO_{2max}, this increase in CO_2 has no measurable effect on calorimetric calculations (Romijn et al., 1992), so that these calculations predict closely oxidation rates measured by stable isotope labeling (Christmass et al., 1999). Clearly, even at high intensity exercise, respiratory gases are mostly the reflect of the balance of substrate oxidation.

A controversial issue appears to be: how to express the results. The crude power and/or heart rate at which lipid oxidation reaches its maximum is the most useful information if one aims at undertaking a targeted training procedure. The difficulty arises when units for reporting data in scientific studies are discussed. A percentage of the actual VO_{2max} is a logic solution, and was used by the team of A. Jeukendrup (Achten et al., 2002, 2003) but this requires to perform another exercise test designed for a precise measurement of VO_{2max}. Alternatively, in the initial protocol proposed by Perez-Martin (Perez-Martin & Mercier, 2001), after the four or five 6-min steps used for calorimetry, a rapid incremental protocol until the maximal level was proposed. However, after 24 or 30 min of exercise, subjects may be tired and unable to reach the actual maximum level which would thus be sometimes underestimated. In fact, in our team, we often express our results as a percentage of the theoretical maximal power calculated with Wasserman's equation. This method allows avoiding a maximal stress, which is sometimes perceived as very harmful by sedentary and obese individuals, and thus improves the acceptability of the test. Two French studies have challenged this approach. Aucouturier and coworkers (Aucouturier et al., 2009) report that a calculation of VO_{2max} according to the American College of Sports Medicine (ACSM) recommendations from submaximal VO_2 values provides a satisfactory evaluation of the actual VO_2max while theoretical VO_2max values given by Wasserman's equation are sometimes misleading in such subjects. These authors thus propose to express the LIPOXmax as a percentage of VO_2max ACSM. This approach was also employed by Lazzer (Lazzer et al., 2010). Michallet et al (Michallet et al., 2008) insisted on the fact that the theoretical design of the test with steps set at 20, 30, 40, 50 and 60% of theoretical maximal aerobic power can be inaccurate, and that a good protocol should include steps at a respiratory exchange ratio below and above 0.9, this value being that of the "crossover point". In a very recent study the team of E Bouhlel proposes an improvement that markedly increases the reproducibility and thus presumably the precision of the measurement : the authors propose a previous determination of the VO_2max with a maximal exercise test and then set the power intensity of the steps of the calorimetry according to this test (Gmada et al, 2011). This study has the interest to further demonstrate the precision and reproducibility of the method and to propose a protocol suitable for research purposes, but for the assessment of series of patients or athletes it is clearly necessary to rely upon a single test, ie, calorimetry if we want to measure te balance of substrates.

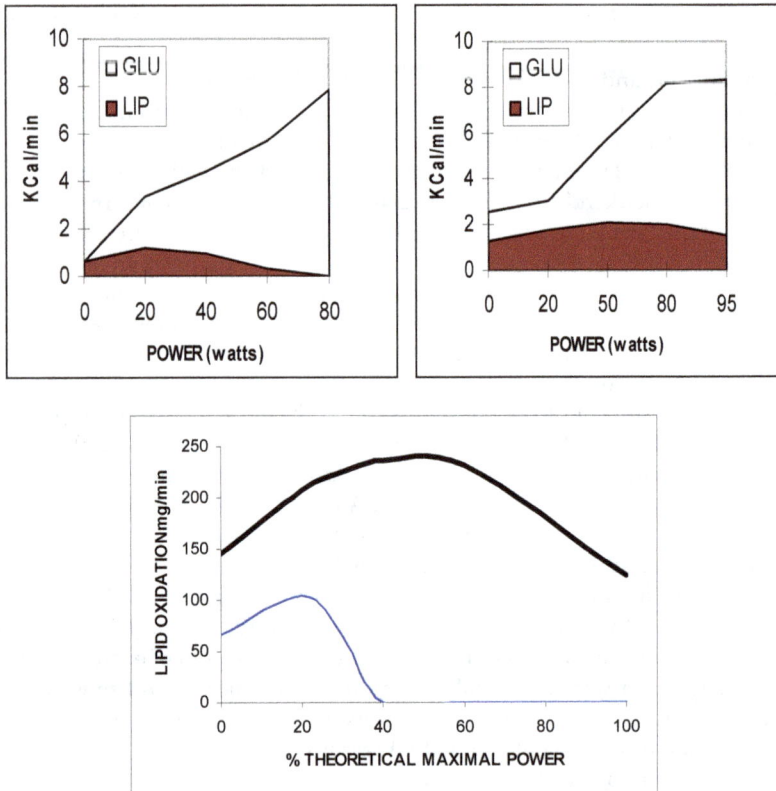

Fig. 3. Examples of individual exercise calorimetries: left; obese woman with "glucodependence" (ie, poor ability to oxidize lipids at exercise) with a peak of lipid oxidation at 135 mg/min located at a power intensity of 34 watts (40% % VO2max ACSM) ; right, overweight patient who oxidizes 235 mg/min of lipids at a LIPOXmax of 68 watts, (55% % VO2max ACSM.) In the last subject, the LIPOX zone is quite wide, indicating that lipids are oxidize over a wide range of exercise intensities. In the first subject it is restricted to a narrow area. The two curves of lipid oxidation are plotted together on the lower pannel, showing their difference in profile according to the theoretical maximal working capacity. Similar discrepancies can be found in athletes.

The maximal fat oxidation rate (MFO) has been expressed in mg/min (Perez-Martin & Mercier, 2001; Dumortier et al., 2002; Brandou et al., 2003, 2005, 2006a, 2006b), g/min (Achten et al., 2003; Achten & Jeukendrup, 2004; Jeukendrup, 2003), mg/min/kg body weight, mg/min/kg fat free mass, and more recently in mg/min/kg muscle mass (Lavault et al., 2011). Muscle can be evaluated from bioimpedance analysis with a validated equation (Janssen et al., 2000), and expression of MFO in mg/min/kg muscle offers at least two advantages: it helps to delineate the effects of training on muscle mass and on the ability of each kg of muscle to burn lipids; it provides an index which has been shown to be predictive of the effects of exercise on weight loss (Lavault et al., 2011) as indicated below. A MFO lower than 5 $mg.min^{-1}.kg^{-1}$ muscle mass predicts poor exercise induced weight loss while as a higher MFO value predicts more efficient exercise induced weight loss. MFO ranges on the average between 38 and 1073 mg/min and the boundary of the lowest quartile is 140 mg/min. The LIPOXmax occurs at a very variable level between 3.6 and 101.5% of P_{maxth} so that the boundary of the lowest quartile is 22% (ie, it is at 64.01% $\pm$ 0.52% of FC_{maxth} the boundary of the lowest quartile is 58%. Expressed in % of the reserve heart rate ie 44.5% of VO_2max. Thus targeting, on theoretical grounds, these values ± 5 % would be actually set at the LIPOXmax in only 30-40% of subjects, ie 60-70% of patients would not be trained at the expected level. The crossover point occurs on average at 32% of W_{maxth} so that the boundary of the lowest quartile is 23.4%. This corresponds to 45% of VO_2max (Brun et al., 2009b). Therefore, in an average French population, the LIPOXmax occurs around 30% of W_{maxth} ie 45% of VO_2max. In sedentary obese and diabetic patients, there is now considerable evidence that this level is more or less lowered and is sometimes extremely low. The point where there are no longer lipids oxidized (LIPOXzero or FATmax) is at 80% of P_{max} ie 85-90% of VO_2max (Brun et al, 2011c).

In addition as shown on Table 4, the LIPOXmax is shifted to lower intensities and the MFO is decreased in many situations referred as "glucodependence" (obesity, diabetes, sleep apnea... etc)

3.2 Physiological relevance of the balance of substrates at exercise as assessed with exercise calorimetry

During steady-state exercise at low intensity (LIPOXmax or below), lipid oxidation remains stable at the level predicted by exercise calorimetry over 45 min or more (Jean et al., 2007; Meyer et al., 2007).

When higher intensities are reached (60% VO_2max or more) there is a gradual increase in lipid oxidation when the duration of exercise increases. This enhanced fat oxidation results from a decrease in muscle glycogen content which diminishes the availability of CHO in the exercising muscle. For example, a 2hr exercise at 60% VO_2max induces a 77% reduction in muscle glycogen depletion (Thomson et al., 1979). The shift to lipids has been shown to occur when there is a reduction of 30-40% of glycogen stores (Kirwan et al, 1988).

Exercise calorimetry thus can be used as a basis for targeted training, as discussed below. On the other hand, the ability to oxidize lipids during exercise is likely to reflect a profile of "metabolic fitness" that is impaired in some diseases and improved by training, and which is correlated to muscle physiological status.

3.3 How short can be the steps of an exercise calorimetry?

The basic assumption that underlies exercise calorimetry is that blood lactate generation during exercise has minimal influence on RER after 3-4 minutes of exercise performed at a steady state. In this condition, the extra-CO_2 production from blood HCO_3^- buffers can indeed be regarded as negligible. One can calculate that even the fastest increase (approximately 2 $mmol^{-1}min^{-1}$) in blood lactate produces an increase of VCO_2 by only 3%. Indeed, if we assume that the volume of distribution of lactate is proportional by a factor of 100 $ml.kg^{-1}$ to body mass and thus represents approximately 8 L, this would mobilize 16 mmol HCO_3- and generate, over 6 min, roughly 1.8 CO_2 $l.min^{-1}$. Under these conditions,

VCO_2 would increase by less than 0.06 l.min^{-1}, *ie* roughly 3%. Thus, the increase in RER in these exercise conditions is almost completely explained by the balance between oxidized carbohydrates and lipids, independent of blood lactate. The validity of this calorimetric approach is further confirmed by a classical work of Romijn (Romijn et al., 1992) who showed in highly trained sportsmen that up to 80-85% VO_2max calorimetric calculations based on respiratory exchanges during exercise closely fit with much more sophisticated measurements using stable isotopes (MacRae et al., 1995). Concerning proteins, if one compares exercise bouts at 33 and 66% of VO_2max it can be demonstrated that their use for oxidation remains stable at the various levels of exercise, supporting the basal assumption that the balance of substrates may be interpreted in terms of respective percentage of oxidized fat and carbohydrates.

We have presented above our procedure based on 6-minutes workloads. However, other investigators (Achten et al., 2002) have simultaneously developed a procedure based on 3-minutes "ultra-short" workloads. This latter method has been validated by its promoters in athletes and healthy sedentary subjects (Achten et al., 2002, 2003). Actually, there was a paucity of data about its validity in very sedentary patients, in whom it usually takes more time to obtain a steady state of respiratory exchanges. We recently compared calorimetry data obtained with this procedure (2nd-3rd minutes) with the one presented above (5-6th minutes) and found that values measured during the 3 minutes steps are poorly correlated with values measured during the 6 minutes steps, due to an overestimation of steady state RER that can be as high as 0.35. This shift results in an average overestimation of carbohydrate oxidation of 15.8 mg/min (this difference can reach 1200 mg/min). Besides, lipid oxidations are poorly correlated between the two methods. Therefore, among very sedentary patients in whom these tests are used for targeting physical activity, 3-min steps appear too short to allow accurate calorimetric calculations. Our protocol based on 6-minutes workloads seems preferable (Bordenave et al., 2007).

As already developed above, Romijn (Romijn et al., 1992) compared, in highly trained endurance cyclists, calorimetric results and isotopic measurement during exercise tests up to 85% VO_2max and showed that at this level calorimetry is fully reliable. However, a look at the figures of this paper shows that the steady state of RER occurs after 4 min and is not obtained after 2 minutes. In addition, we recently showed that the estimate of lipid oxidation by this method during the 5th and 6th minutes of a 6 min step predicts fairly well the actual lipid oxidation rate that would be observed over 45 minutes performed at the same level (Fig.4). The mean difference between the predicted value and the measured value is only 4.51±8.7 mg/min (Jean et al., 2007). Meyer (Meyer et al., 2007) also reported that VO_2 used for fat oxidation after 6 min closely predicted fat oxidation measured between 30 and 40 min of a constant-load exercise performed at the same intensity. These two observations further support the use of the 6-min steps procedure rather than the 3-min steps procedure proposed by the team of Jeukendrup (Achten et al., 2002) that seems to be accurate mostly for sports medicine and exercise physiology but less reliable in sedentary subjects.

A recent study further addressed this issue in prepubertal children. Comparison of 10 min and 3 min steps showed that the 3 min procedure yielded a satisfactory assessment of the power intensity where the maximum was reached (55% VO_2peak) with 95% satisfactory limits of agreement ± 7% VO_2peak, but that the value of the lipid oxidation rate was less precisely assessed in this population with the 3 min procedure. The authors concluded that, in children, the 3 min procedure provides a valid estimation of the power intensity but was less precise for assessing the flow rate (Zakrzewski & Tolfrey, 2011).

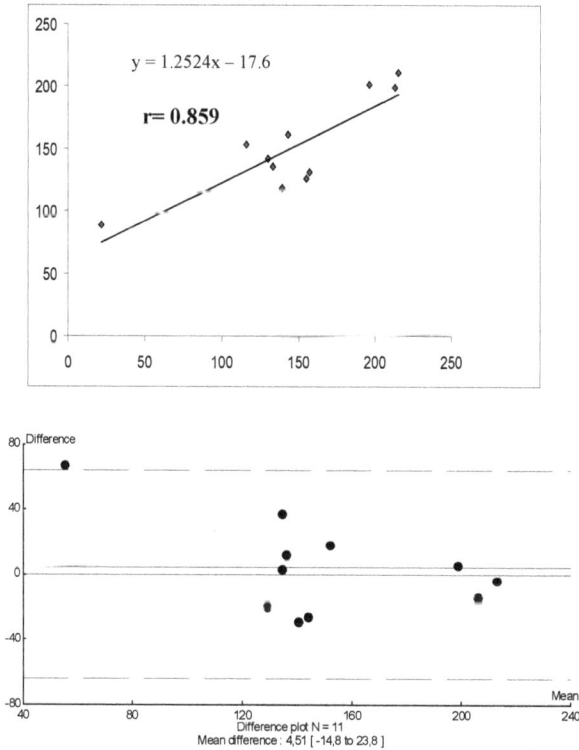

Fig. 4. Correlation and Bland-Altman plot showing the agreement between the measurement of MFO with LIPOXmax protocol and the average lipid oxidation rate maintained over 45 min during a steady state exercise set at this intensity level.

3.4 Factors of variation and reliability of LIPOXmax/FATmax

Initial studies on exercise calorimetry unanimously reported a fair reliability, which seems to be confirmed by daily clinical practice. The coefficient of variation (CV) for the LIPOXmax (at that time it was manually determined) was found to be 11.4% (Perez-Martin et al., 2001) and with Achten and Jeukendrup's procedure in 10 males tested three times it was 9.6% ie ±0.23 l/min (Achten et al., 2003). Similarly Michallet in 14 subjects aged 19-50 years found with the current LIPOXmax procedure a CV equal to 8.7%. The crossover point PCX appeared somewhat less reproducible with a CV of 17% (Michallet et al., 2006). However, Meyer investigating this methodology, reported variability as high as ±0.91 l/min that was supposed to be too wide (Meyer et al., 2009). Meyer's paper actually investigated the reproducibility in non-standardized conditions concerning recent exercise and food intake, two major modifiers of the balance of substrates, and therefore his conclusions are restricted to subjects tested in similarly non standardized conditions. More recently a careful methodological study proposing a more standardized approach based on prior determination of VO_{2max} by a maximal exercise test evidenced an even better reproducibility as low as 5.02% (Gmada et al, 2011). Therefore, on the whole, it is clear that the LIPOXmax is a fairly reproducible measurement, unless conditions of measure are not standardized for the major factors of variation such as exercise or prior meal (see Table 3). This last remark is important because, like all physiological parameters, the LIPOXmax can be acutely modified by several factors (see Table 4).

Author (reference)	Parameters of reproducibility	remarks
(Perez-Martin et al., 2001)	CV= 11.4%	Early LIPOXmax protocol, visual determination
(Achten et al., 2003)	CV= 9.6% ie ±0.23 l/min	FATmax protocol
(Michallet et al., 2006)	CV = 8.7%	Current LIPOXmax protocol
(Meyer et al., 2009)	Variability ±0.91 l/min	Not standardized for prior exercise and feeding
(Gmada et al, 2011)	CV= 5.02%	Standardized determination after prior maximal test to determine VO_{2max} markedly increases reproducibility of the LIPOXmax protocol

Table 3. reproducibility studies of the LIPOXmax/FATmax: reproducibility is fair unless patients are not fasting and not standardized for recent previous exercise, and reproducibility is even greater if the protocol is more standardized

4. LIPOXmax/FATmax in sports medicine

As reviewed below, most literature on the LIPOXmax/Fatmax deals with alterations of this parameter in patients and its potential interest for exercise targeting. However, there are some reports suggesting that this parameter has some interest in athletes.

Modifying factor	Effect	references
previous meal taken less than 3 hr before	decreased MFO and shifted LIPOXmax to a slightly lower intensity	Bergman & Brooks, 1999; Jeukendrup, 2003; Friedlander et al., 2007
high-fat diets in which more than 60% of the energy is derived from fat	decreases fat oxidation during exercise, even if the diet is consumed for only 2 to 3 days, due to reduced muscle glycogen stores	(Coyle et al., 2001).
previous exercise performed just before the exercise calorimetry	MFO slightly increased	(Chenevière et al., 2009a)
puberty	LIPOXmax and MFO are higher in prepubertal children and gradually decrease throughout puberty to reach adult values at the end of puberty	(Brandou et al, 2006b; Riddell et al., 2008 ; (Zakrzewski & Tolfrey, 2011b).
type of exercise	Higher during running than cycling in adults and in pre- to early pubertal children	(Achten et al., 2003; Zakrzewski & Tolfrey, 2011a).

Modifying factor	Effect	references
gender	Women oxidize slightly more lipids and on average their LIPOXmax occurs at higher power intensity This difference is confirmed in all studies but is actually quite moderate and has probably little relevance On the opposite, fat oxidation is higher in pre- to early pubertal boys compared with girls at similar relative (but not absolute) intensities	(Friedlander et al., 1998a, 1998b; Chenevière et al., 2011 ; Brun et al., 2009a ; Zakrzewski & Tolfrey, 2011b).
temperature	Shift to preferential CHO oxidation during exercise in hot environments. Reversal after acclimation and training.	Febbraio et al, 1994; del Coso et al, 2010
highly trained athletes	Most of them exhibit a markedly high ability to oxidize lipids during exercise but in some sports like soccer, a preferential use of CHO is observed	(Bergman & Brooks, 1999; Achten et al., 2003; Venables et al., 2005; González-Haro et al., 2007; Varlet-Marie et al., 2006).
Obesity and diabetes	LIPOXmax values markedly shifted to lower power intensities and MFO lowered.	(Perez-Martin et al., 2001; Sardinoux et al., 2009)
Metformin	increases fat oxidation during exercise and decrease its postexercise rise	(Malin et al., 2010).
type 2 diabetes	Lower ability to oxidize lipids when compared to subjects matched for body mass index (difference not found by others)	(Ghanassia et al., 2006; Mogensen et al., 2009)
type 1 diabetes	Lower ability to oxidize lipids	(Brun et al., 2008).
sleep apnea syndrome	Lower ability to oxidize lipids at exercise. Training improves both apnea-index and lipid oxidation at exercise	(Desplan et al., 2010).

Table 4. Factors of variation of LIPOXmax/FATmax

4.1 Endurance training improves the ability to oxidize fat during exercise

Over the 60-70 the literature is full of papers showing that endurance training allows fat to become the predominant substrate for endurance exercise, while other leading authors in that time emphasized the importance of CHO-derived energy stores for exercise performance (see review in Brooks & Mercier, 1994). According to the initial formulation of the crossover concept, it could be expected that endurance athletes would exhibit a profile of "lipid oxidizers" proportional to their fitness and the efficacy of their training. Most of the exercise calorimetry studies in athletes confirm this early statement. They show that on the average endurance-trained athletes oxidize more lipids. Data from cross-sectional and longitudinal studies have supported the notion that training reduces the reliance on CHO as an energy source, thereby increasing fat oxidation during submaximal exercise (Achten et al., 2004). In pre- to early pubertal children, brisk walking or slow running promotes higher fat oxidation (Zakrzewski & Tolfrey, 2011). A specific study on the effects of endurance training in women shows that endurance-trained women had a higher fat oxidation rate, but their peak values occur at a very similar intensity (56±3% VO$_2$max) compared with the untrained women (53±2% VO$_2$max) (Stisen et al., 2006). González-Haro and coworkers have fairly evidenced in high competitive level triathletes and cyclists various profiles of high lipid oxidation which differ among sports (González-Haro et al., 2007). However, the reason for the inter-individual variability of these parameters remains poorly understood (Achten & Jeukendrup, 2003, 2004; Brun et al., 2000; Jeukendrup & Wallis, 2005). Clearly, energetic pathways favorized by specific training programs may be markedly different among sports.

4.2 Endocrine correlates of this profile of high lipid oxidation
In soccer players relationships between the GH-IGF-I axis and the LIPOXmax were reported (Brun et al., 1999). These correlations are likely to reflect either a parallel effect of training on muscle fuel partitioning or IGF-I release, or an action of IGF-I (or GH via IGF) on muscular lipid oxidation (Fig. 5).

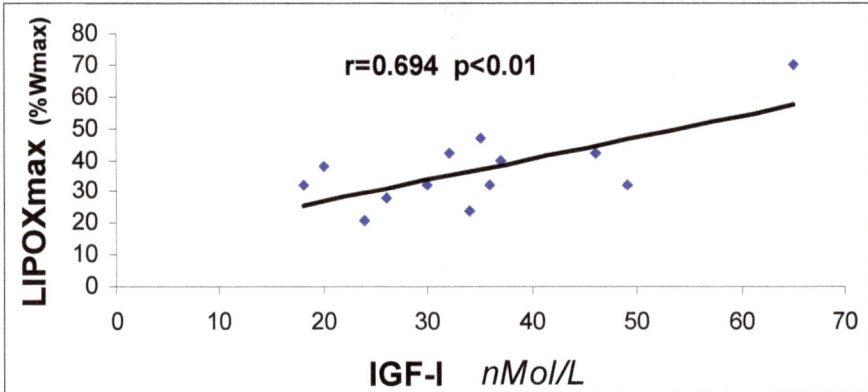

Fig. 5. Correlation between Insulin-like growth factor 1 (IGF-I) levels and the LIPOXmax in soccer players (Brun et al., 1999).

4.3 Are there 'glucodependent' sports
While low intensity training, as shown above, increases lipid oxidation, high intensity training has been reported to improve the ability to oxidize carbohydrates (Manetta et al., 2002a, 2002b).

Varlet-Marie et al (Varlet-Marie et al., 2006) described the profile of lipid oxidation in 90 trained athletes: 28 cyclists, 32 male soccer players, 19 male rugby players, 11 rugbywomen (national level in soccer and male rugby and regional level in cyclism and female rugby) and 41 healthy sedentary volunteers. All athletes had been involved in regular training for several years (>3 years), and trained 10.69 ± 0.9 hr/wk. The soccer team performed over the year a combination of endurance training under the form of interval training, strength training, speed training, skill and tactical training, in various proportions according to the period. Rugbymen and rugbywomen underwent an heavy training mostly based on strength training. The cyclists performed 14 hours of cycling (ie, about 450 km) per week during a nine-month training period. During the first month, training sessions were performed at low intensity with a specific target (below their ventilatory threshold: VT). During the other months, they added interval-training sessions to their endurance training, wherein they performed at high intensity with a specific target heart (above their VT).

When expressed as raw power values, the LIPOXmax and the crossover point ranked as follows: rugbymen > cyclists > male controls > rugbywomen > female controls > male soccer players (Figure 6).

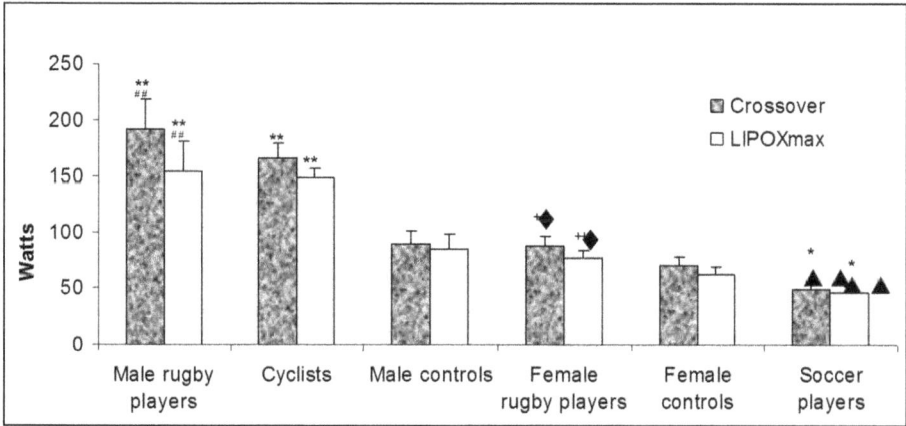

Fig. 6. Comparison of the power at which occur the crossover point and the LIPOXmax in control subjects and in various groups of athletes. *p<0.05; **p<0.0001 (male athletes vs. male control subjects); ##p<0.0001 (male rugby players vs. soccer players); ▲▲p<0.0001 (cyclists vs. soccer players); ⁺p<0.05 (female rugby players vs. female control subjects); ⁺⁺p<0.0001 (female rugby players vs. male rugby players)

When they were expressed as percentages of theoretical maximal power this ranking became: cyclists > rugbywomen > rugbymen > female controls > male controls > soccer players (Figure 7). Raw lipid oxidation rates at the level of the LIPOXmax ranked as follows (Figure 8): rugbymen > cyclists > rugbywomen > sedentary male controls > soccer. If lipid oxidation is expressed per kg of body weight this ranking becames: cyclists > rugbymen > rugbywomen > sedentary female controls > sedentary male controls > soccer players (Figure 9).

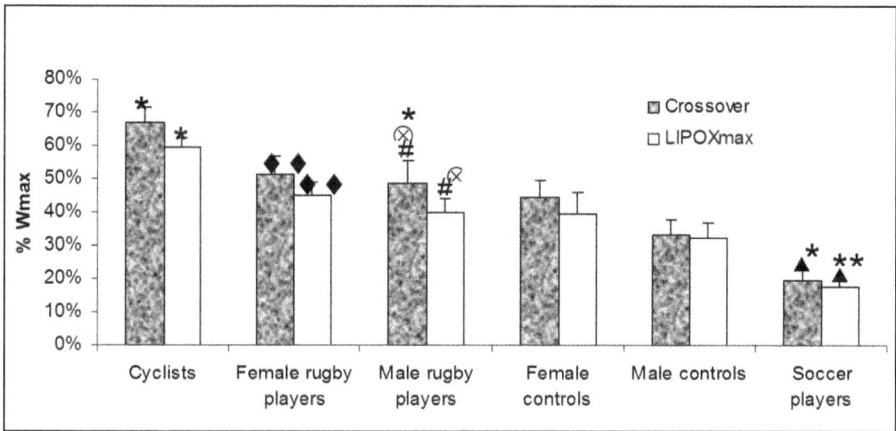

Fig. 7. Comparison of the crossover point and the LIPOXmax, expressed in % of Wmax, in control subjects and in various groups of athletes. *p<0.05; **p<0.0001 (male athletes vs. male control subjects); ##p<0.0001 (male rugby players vs. soccer players); ▲▲p<0.0001 (cyclists vs. soccer players); ⁺⁺p<0.0001 (female rugby players vs. female control subjects); ⊗p<0.05; ⊗⊗p<0.0001 (cyclists vs. male rugby players)

This study evidences markedly different patterns of balance of substrates among groups of athletes. Clearly, cycling and rugby are rather characterized by high rates of lipid oxidation which peaks at high exercise intensities, while in soccer there is an early predominance of CHO.

The finding of a high ability to oxidize lipids in athletes submitted to regular endurance training, like cyclists, is consistent with previous literature (Achten & Jeukendrup, 2003). By contrast, it is interesting to notice in soccer players, a pattern of "glucodependence" that implies a reduced reliance on lipids at exercise. Although in our study we can only present data on soccer, this pattern is likely to occur in several sports. Since exercise training at high intensity (Manetta et al., 2002a, 2002b) and intermittent exercise (Perez-Martin et al., 2000) both increase the ratio between CHO and fat used for oxidation during muscular activity, this pattern may reflect an adaptation of muscle metabolism to short repeated bouts of high intensity. Interestingly, such a "glucodependence" is also found in obesity (Perez-Martin et al., 2001) and type 2 diabetes (Blanc et al., 2000). In this case it can be rapidly reversed by a few weeks of targeted exercise training at the level of the LIPOXmax (Dumortier et al., 2002, 2003). Since physical inactivity rapidly shifts the balance of substrates at rest towards a lower ratio of lipid/CHO used for oxidation (Blanc et al., 2000) it can be assumed that sedentarity explains at least in part the glucodependence of these patients.

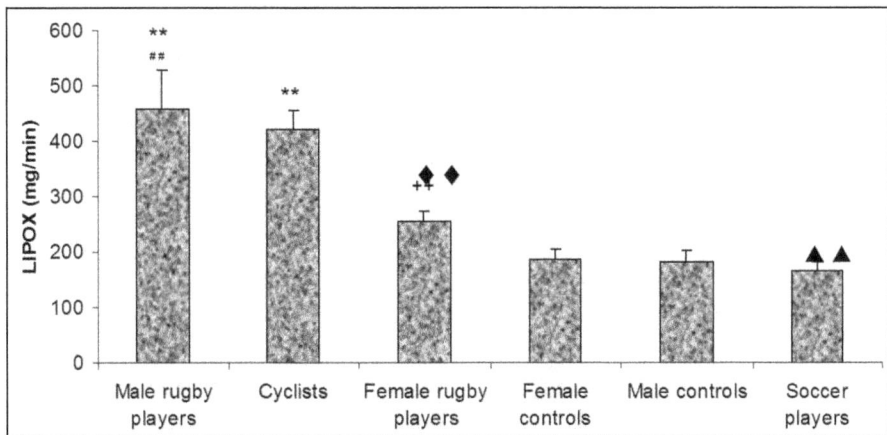

Fig. 8. Lipid oxidation rates in control subjects and in various groups of athletes, expressed in mg/min. **$p<0.0001$ (male athletes vs. male control subjects); ##$p<0.0001$ (male rugby players vs. soccer players); ▲▲$p<0.0001$ (cyclists vs. soccer players); ♦♦$p<0.0001$ (female rugby players vs. female control subjects); ++$p<0.0001$ (female rugby players vs. male rugby players)

4.4 Shifts in the balance of substrates during exercise with overtraining

According to the energy pathway mostly involved in a type of activity, training increases thus the ability to oxidize either lipids or CHO. This was clearly evidenced in a study conducted on competitive road cyclists in whom high intensity endurance training increased the ability to oxidize CHO above the ventilatory threshold, while at the end of the season most patients exhibited symptoms of overreaching associated with a reversal of this increase in CHO oxidation (Manetta et al., 2002a). By contrast overreaching in endurance athletes submitted to exercise calorimetry showed lowered ability to oxidize fat at low intensities, leading to the concept that training effects on the balance of substrates at exercise are reversed by overtraining (Aloulou et al, 2003). This issue remains poorly documented and requires more investigation.

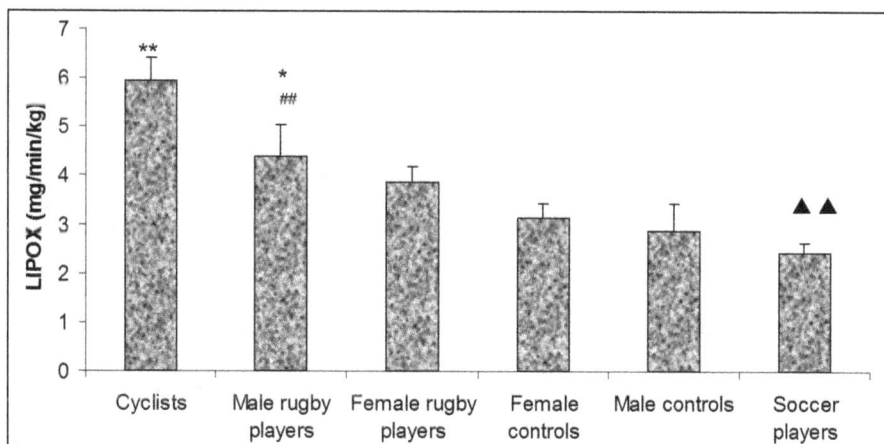

Fig. 9. Lipid oxidation rates in control subjects and in various groups of athletes, expressed in mg/min/kg of body weight.*p<0.05; ^^p<0.0001 (male athletes vs. male control subjects); ▲▲p<0.0001 (cyclists vs. soccer players); ##p<0.0001 (male rugby players vs. soccer players)

5. Interest of the LIPOXmax as a target for structured training in obesity and diabetes

5.1 Scientific background

It is now unanimously recognized that exercise is an efficient tool for : 1) preventing the onset of type 2 diabetes (Lindström et al., 2006; Kim et al., 2006); 2) improving blood glucose control (Marwick et al., 2009) and 3) preventing further weight regain in weight-reduced obese individuals (Bensimhon et al., 2006). Exercise is also beneficial for cardiovascular health, due to its positive effects on blood pressure (Pescatello et al., 2004; Pescatello, 2005), blood lipids (Kelley et al., 2006), inflammation (Fabre et al., 2002), blood viscosity (Brun et al., 2010b), mood (Krogh et al., 2010) and cognitive function (Fabre et al., 2002; Angevaren et al., 2008).

However the effects of exercise as a weight reducing procedure have been considered during many years as rather limited and almost negligible. It is beyond any doubt that regular exercise attenuates the metabolic drive to regain weight after long-term weight loss (MacLean et al, 2009). The interest of physical activity was thus mostly to prevent weight gain, to improve stabilization after slimming, and to reduce obesity-related co-morbidities but not to reduce weight by its own (Jakicic & Otto, 2005, 2006; Duclos et al., 2010).

This traditional view has been challenged by studies demonstrating that even without any change in diet, exercise alone may reduce body weight (Ross et al., 2000; Slentz et al., 2004). This has been further evidenced by a recent meta-analysis that concludes that exercise on its own improves the effects of a diet by on average 1.4 kg (Wu et al., 2009). It seems now well demonstrated that exercise considered alone can reduce body weight. The last American consensus (Donnelly et al., 2009) indicates that more than 250 min of weekly moderate-intensity physical activity is associated with clinically significant weight loss. Accordingly, lower weekly amounts of moderate-intensity exercise (between 150 and 250 min per week) is effective to prevent weight gain, but can provide only modest weight loss by their own. They can result in significant weight loss if associated to moderate diet restriction but, interestingly, not severe diet restriction.

The picture is thus slightly modified. Exercise appears nowadays as an effective means to reverse overweight, but its effects are shown to be very variable, sometimes impressive, but often poor. A major explanation for this heterogeneity is that exercise may induce marked compensatory changes in energy intake (King et al, 2008). Therefore exercise should be combined with a dietary approach based on correction of compensatory behaviors and errors (Bouchard et al, 1990; Caudwell, 2009). This approach is surely more logic than the traditional restriction which has some short-term efficiency but almost always result in a subsequent weight gain due to homeostatic mechanisms of fat mass preservation (MacLean, 2011).

What is the most important: duration or frequency? Chambliss (Chambliss, 2005) examined the effect of duration and frequency of exercise on weight loss and cardiorespiratory fitness in 201 previously sedentary, overweight women (Chambliss, 2005) over 12 months. He found a mean weight loss after 1 year was 8.9, 8.2, 6.3 and 7.0 kg, for the vigorous intensity/high duration, moderate intensity/high duration, moderate intensity/moderate duration, and vigorous intensity/moderate duration groups, respectively, but there was no effect of exercise duration or exercise intensity on changes in body weight or in BMI. Duration of exercise (at least 150 min/week in walking) was more important than vigorous versus moderate intensity in achieving these goals.

Most of the studies make little or no reference to the substrate (lipid or CHO) that is oxidized during exercise. However, there is a rationale to do so, as largely described above. Multiple studies have show that fatty acid handling and oxidation is impaired in skeletal muscle of obese, impaired glucose-tolerant, and T2D individuals (Blaak, 2004; Corpeleijn et al., 2008, 2009; Kelley et al., 1999; Mensink et al., 2001). This defect leads to propose exercise protocols aiming at restoring muscular ability to oxidize lipids. For this reason, LI protocols designed for oxidizing more lipids during exercise sessions were described by several authors (Blaak & Saris, 2002; Blaak, 2004) and were shown to improve both the ability to oxidize lipids and body composition (Schrauwen et al., 2002).

As shown on the meta-analysis of 12 LIPOXmax training studies, 3 or 4 weekly sessions of 45 min cycling at the LIPOXmax result in a weight loss of -2.25 % [confidence range -3.53 to -0.97] which is at least as efficient as the various protocols studied in the literature (Romain et al., 2010). Therefore, LIPOXmax training is one of the strategies that can be proposed to reduce body weight in obese subjects. A comparison with other more classical protocols remains to be done.

The issue of the exercise protocol that should be recommended for weight maintenance remains incompletely studied. Cross sectional studies show that weight maintenance is improved with physical activity > 250 min per week. However, no evidence from well-designed randomized controlled trials exists to judge the effectiveness of physical activity for the prevention of weight regain after weight loss (Donnelly et al., 2009). According to this consensus document, resistance training does not enhance weight loss but may increase fat-free mass and increase loss of fat mass and is associated with reductions in health risk. Existing evidence indicates that endurance PA or resistance training without weight loss improves health risk. There is no evidence that PA prevents or attenuates obesity-related detrimental changes (Donnelly et al., 2009).

5.2 Standardized vs personalized targeting?

There is an important discussion that underlies all the controversies about exercise prescription in chronic diseases. This is: should we use standard or personalized exercise prescriptions. Some current rules of prescription emphasize the need for taking into account the personal characteristics of each patient, but they are by essence "standardized", ie, they do not take into account the specific physiologic profile of each subject. All is based on the assumption that the most important mechanism underlying the metabolic effect of exercise is to generate an energy deficit, regardless of the actual quantity of lipids or CHO that have been oxidized (Strasser et al, 2007).

Such a standardized approach was used in pneumology and cardiology, before it was challenged by a new paradigm: the "individualization concept". Personalized targeting of exercise has been promoted in respiratory and cardiac chronic diseases and was shown to provide better results (Vallet et al., 1997). The "Hippocratic" concept of superiority of the individualized approach is taken into account by a number of practitioners and appears in national guidelines (Guidelines, 2005). However, some guidelines do not mention it, considering that evidence for counseling is not sufficient (Rochester, 2003).

In metabolic diseases, such a discussion about the "individualization concept" has not yet been initiated. Usual French recommendations for exercise in diabetes (Gautier et al, 1998; Gautier, 2004) do not take into account the individual metabolic background. Authors only indicate a broad zone of % VO_2max or heart rates assumed to be the most accurate.

Extending the individualization concept to obesity and diabetes raises the question of a specific individual target, and obviously the LIPOXmax/FATOXmax appears as a logic candidate for this purpose. Accordingly, several teams have undertaken the study of the metabolic effects of exercise training targeted at this level.

5.3 Targeting endurance exercise close to the LIPOXmax vs higher intensity levels

A topic which has generated a lot of discussion over the last decade is the selection of the optimal exercise protocol that could be used for the management of obesity and diabetes. Initially, low intensity endurance training (LI), as it was know to be the variety of exercise that oxidized the highest quantity of lipids, was logically proposed (Thompson et al., 1998). However, later focus was given on other kinds of exercise such high intensity endurance training (HI), resistance training (RT) and interval training (IT). All of them were evidenced to exert beneficial effects when applied to obese (Jakicic & Otto, 2005, 2006) and diabetic (Praet & van Loon, 2007, 2009) patients. On the whole, LI remains the easiest and the most widely evaluated procedure. It is also the best demonstrated as shown by a recent meta-analysis on exercise and diabetes that selected 34 from 645 papers. This paper confirmed that endurance exercise alone improves Hba1c (-0.6%), blood pressure, (-6.08 mmHg) , and triglycerides (-0.3 mmol/L), while RT has no effects demonstrable by meta-analysis on these parameters (Chudyk & Petrella, 2011).

An overlook at the rapidly expanding body of knowledge in the field of molecular biology of muscle shows that either LI, HI, RT or IT are able to improve muscular function and to be helpful for the correction of metabolic disturbances (Burgomaster et al. 2008). It is however important to emphasize that RT and ET act on separate and antagonistic intracellular pathways (Koulmann & Bigard, 2006), hence they are independant tools that cannot be expected to provide equivalent effects on muscle cells.

At the cellular level (Koulmann & Bigard, 2006) endurance training induces a set of regulatory adaptations that improve mitochondrial function and protein synthesis and overall, the enzymes for both CHO and fat oxidation are increased. As a result of these cellular adaptations, exercise training improves whole body lipid metabolism and carbohydrate tolerance, thus consisting in a fully recognized tool for reducing both blood lipids and glucose (see below).

As reminded above, most exercise physiology papers describe exercise protocols applied at a given percentage of maximal aerobic capacity without reference to exercise calorimetry. When exercise is performed at 40% VO_{2max} or below, it is likely to be performed in the LIPOXmax zone, but, since LIPOXmax is frequently much lower in obese subjects, a significant percentage of subjects are likely to exercise above this zone, in the range where lipid oxidation is close to zero and CHO almost becomes the exclusive energy source.

Therefore, LIPOX training represents a better defined exercise protocol, whose effects on lipid oxidation are predictable. Exercise performed above this zone results in more CHO oxidation. This CHO oxidation may be followed by some degree of fat oxidation after exercise but may frequently fail to induce this lipid oxidation rise. Although the energetic balance is assumed to result in both cases in a negative fat balance, these two types of exercise do not involve the same energetic pathways.

At the date of redaction of this article, there are several studies (or abstracts) published in peer-reviewed journals reporting the results of LIPOX training (table 4). Therefore, these effects of LIPOX training can now be well described on the basis of a recent meta-analysis (Romain et al., 2010) that included 16 studies shown in table 1, ie, 247 participants belonging to 5 different populations: obese teenagers, metabolic syndrome, HIV patients with lipodistrophy, type-2 diabetics, and psychiatric patients treated by neuroleptics. Study length ranged between 2 to 12 months. Weekly frequency of sessions ranged between 2 and 4. Preliminary results showed that LIPOXmax was shifted to a higher power intensity by 4.93 watts (95% confidence interval (CI) 4.74-5.13; p<0.0001). Weight decreased by -2.9 kg (95%CI: -4.1; -1.7; p<0.0001). Fat mass decreased by 1.7% (95% CI 1.82 – 1.64; p<0.0001), and waist circumference decreased by -4.9 cm [95%CI: -6.6; -3.2] (p<0.0001).

We have not included in this meta-analysis an interesting study by the team of A. Sartorio (Lazzer et al, 2011) that compared over three weeks energy-matched programs of low intensity (40% VO2max) and high intensity (60% VO2max) endurance, and showed that the exercise in the LIPOX zone was twice more efficient for fat loss. This protocol was not exactly targeted on the LIPOXmax but designed to train the subjects in this zone, and its results are in agreement with those pooled in the meta-analysis.

The results of these studies demonstrate the efficiency of training targeted at the LIPOXmax on weight loss, even over a short time period. In diabetics, HIV-infected patients, and psychiatric patients under neuroleptics, the efficiency of this procedure seems to be lower than in obesity or metabolic syndrome. As expected, the association with a diet improves the efficiency of this training. However, two thirds of the studies were without added diet and thus most of the weight-lowering effects of LIPOX training are likely to be due to the effects of exercise alone on energy balance and eating behavior. Therefore, it is clear that LIPOX training alone decreases body fat, even if no specific diet is applied. This effect is clearly and constantly evidenced in training protocols containing as few as 2 or 3 sessions per week. In fact, the number of sessions per week seems to improve the results and a dose-relationship can be postulated. However, this issue remains to be specifically investigated.

A crucial issue is that the extent of fat loss in response to exercise training varies quite widely among individuals (Snyder et al., 1997; King et al., 2008; Byrne et al., 2006), even when differences in compliance to the exercise program and energy intake are accounted for. In other terms, exercise is very efficient to lose weight in some individuals while in others it fails to induce weight loss and even more may induce weight gain. Focus on the specific profile of responders and nonresponders helps to understand this variability. It appears to be explained by two variables: eating behavior and fat oxidation.

A role for fat oxidation is suggested by recent studies. In sedentary premenopausal women, a 7-week endurance-type exercise training program reaching progressively to 5 x 60 minutes per week at 65% -80% of predicted maximum heart rate resulted in a mean change in fat mass for the group was -0.97 kg (range +2.1 to -5.3 kg). The strongest correlate of change in fat mass was exercise energy expenditure, as expected. However, the change in fasting RER correlated significantly with the residual for change in fat mass after adjusting for the effects of both exercise energy expenditure and change in energy intake. This means that training-induced increase in fat oxidation explains 7% of the variance of exercise-induced weight loss. In multiple regression analysis, exercise energy expenditure and change in fasting RER were the only statistically significant predictors of change in fat mass, together explaining 40.2% of the variance. Thus, fat loss in response to exercise training depends not only on exercise energy expenditure but also on exercise training-induced changes in RER at rest. Whether it is also the case for RER during exercise is suggested by recent studies (Lavault et al, 2011). This suggests that development of strategies to maximize exercise-induced fat loss may be useful for optimizing exercise-induced slimming (Barwell et al., 2009).

Another important issue in these exercise-based strategies would be to control changes in eating behavior (Bouchard et al, 1990). Muscular activity may induce a temporary postexercise anorexia, which is dose-dependent on the intensity and duration of the exercise (King et al, 1994; Westerterp-Plantenga et al, 1997). On the long term, the effect of exercise on eating behavior are complex and variable and largely explain the variability of weight loss responses. In fact, recent studies show that the effects of regular exercise on appetite regulation involves at least 2 processes: an increase in the overall (orexigenic) drive to eat and a concomitant increase in the satiating efficiency of a fixed meal (King et al, 2009). The former may be related to glycogen deficiency, which increases appetite (Melanson et al, 1999), so that exercise protocols that spare glycogen may avoid this increase in orexigenic drive (Hopkins et al, 2011). Exercise targeted at the LIPOXmax, due to its greater reliance on fat, is likely to spare more glycogen and thus to be less orexigenic than acute exercise that oxidizes mostly carbohydrates.

Clearly, exercise may be an efficient and safe technique to lose fat as shown by the results obtained in responders. The study of non responders suggests that focus on the two parameters explaining the lower efficacy of exercise (fat oxidation and eating behavior) may help to improve the results. Targeting on lipid oxidation during exercise may be a way to better control these two parameters. More studies are needed to verify this concept (Hopkins et al, 2011).

5.4 LIPOX training improves mitochondrial respiration and enzymes of lipid oxidation

Bordenave (Bordenave et al., 2008) described the effects of ten weeks of mild exercise training targeted at the LIPOXmax (45 min of cycling, twice a week). This training was not sufficient to significantly decrease weight, but it exhibited marked effects on whole body lipid oxidation and muscle oxidative capacities. Indeed, after training, the LIPOXmax was shifted to higher power intensity and the MFO was significantly increased compared with pre-training values (+51 mg.min-1). This study included biopsies and evidenced LIPOX training-induced improvements in mitochondrial respiration and citrate synthase activity. Changes in whole body lipid oxidation were associated with changes in parameters of muscle oxidation. In another study the 3-Hydroxyacyl-CoA dehydrogenase (HAD), an important enzyme that functions in mitochondrial fatty acid beta-oxidation by catalyzing the oxidation of straight chain 3-hydroxyacyl-CoAs, was studied in trained and untrained women. It was shown that HAD activity and fat oxidation rates were highly correlated indicating that training-induced adaptation in muscle fat oxidative capacity is an important factor for enhanced fat oxidation (Stisen et al., 2006).

5.5 Does LIPOX training increase REE and resting fat oxidation?
There is no study on the effects of LIPOX training on resting fat oxidation. Endurance training at higher levels yields conflicting results and it is likely that this effect is not constant with endurance protocols. A study by Van Aggel-Leijssen (Van Aggel-Leijssen et al., 2001) using a low-intensity exercise training program (40% VO$_2$max, ie the LIPOXmax zone) three times per week for 12 weeks showed that this variety of training increased the contribution of fat oxidation to total energy expenditure during exercise but failed to do so at rest in obese women (Van Aggel-Leijssen et al., 2001). However, another study may suggest an effect of endurance training in the LIPOXmax zone or below on resting fat oxidation. A very mild exercise consisting in an increase of regular physical activity equivalent to 45 min of walking 3 days/week induces some improvements in lipid metabolism such as an increase in skeletal muscle protein expression of PPARdelta and UCP3 in type 2 diabetic patients (Fritz et al., 2006), and improves lipid oxidation without changes in mitochondrial function in type 2 diabetes (Trenell et al., 2008). This protocol of walking an extra 45 min per day over an 8-week period is an insufficient stimulus to induce detectable mitochondrial biogenesis but demonstrates physical activity-induced enhancement of resting lipid oxidation, independently of intramuscular lipid levels. A specific study on LIPOXmax training and lipid oxidation at rest in obese and nonobese people remains to be done.

5.6 Low intensity training targeted at the LIPOXmax training improves inflammatory status
Low-grade systemic inflammation is suggested to play a role in the development of a variety of chronic diseases including obesity, diabetes and cancer. A number of studies suggest that in these diseases regular exercise has anti-inflammatory effects therefore it may contribute to suppress systemic low-grade inflammation (Mattusch et al., 2000; Stewart et al., 2007; Goldhammer, et al., 2005). Overall, both endurance and resistance training decrease C-Reactive Protein (CRP) (Martins et al., 2010). In two studies, LIPOXmax training has been shown to decrease CRP (Ben Ounis et al., 2010; Brun et al, 2011b). In these studies, inflammatory parameters were also measured and changes in CRP were negatively related to those of lipid oxidation during exercise, suggesting that the improvement in the ability to oxidize lipids during exercise is associated with an anti-inflammatory effect. Further studies are needed.

5.7 LIPOXmax training maintains fat-free mass

All the aforementioned studies show that LIPOXmax training maintains fat-free mass, and in some of them an increase is found. This is a constant finding, while protocols using higher intensities in patients give less consistent result on fat-free mass (Brandou et al., 2005; Brun et al., 2010a). Obviously, it is well demonstrated that correctly performed resistance training is an efficient way to improve fat free mass (Schoenfeld et al., 2010), but low intensity exercise has also been demonstrated to protect lean mass and to prevent protein breakdown. A 45-min walk on a treadmill at 40% VO_2 peak induced short-term increases in muscle and plasma protein synthesis in both younger and older men (Sheffield-Moore et al., 2004).

In a study on dieting postmenopausal women with a total energy expenditure of 700 kcal/wk, ie, 8 kcal.kg body weight^{-1}wk^{-1} with LI being at 45-50% if heart rate reserve (HRR) and HI at 70-75% (vigourous-intensity) of HRR (Nicklas et al., 2009) found that with a similar amount of total weight loss, lean mass is preserved with either moderate- or vigorous-intensity aerobic exercise performed during caloric restriction and concluded that FFM is equally preserved with LI and HI. Both resistance (RE) and endurance (EE) exercise are able to stimulate mixed skeletal muscle protein synthesis, but the phenotypes induced by RE (myofibrillar protein accretion) and EE (mitochondrial expression) training are different and this is probably due to differential stimulation of myofibrillar and mitochondrial protein synthesis (Koulmann et al, 2006; Wilkinson et al., 2008; Harber et al., 2009). A mechanism that may play a role in this protective effect of LI is glycogen sparing. It has been shown that CHO availability influences the rates of skeletal muscle and whole body protein synthesis, degradation and net balance during prolonged exercise in humans (Howarth et al., 2010). On the whole, although more investigation is required, LIPOXmax training is an efficient way to maintain or even to improve fat-free mass by increasing the mass of metabolically active muscle. At the beginning of training protocols in very sedentary patients, it may be used for this purpose. For example, studies in undernutrition situations such as anorexia nervosa are in progress.

5.8 Comparison between high intensity (HI) and low intensity (LI) training

It is clear that during LI even more if it is targeted at the LIPOXmax quite important quantities of lipids are oxidized. By contrast, HI oxidizes mostly or exclusively CHO. HI is sometimes followed by a slight rise in oxidation of lipids, but this quantity of lipids oxidized postexercise remains low (Chenevière et al., 2009a; Warren et al., 2009) even more when HI is not continuous (interval training [INT]). Therefore, LI and HI or INT are not equivalent tools and have distinct properties.

This is clearly evidenced in a recent study comparing INT and LIPOX training in T2D (Brun et al., 2010a). 63 type-2 diabetics were compared over a period of 3 months without nutritional intervention: 39 were trained at the LIPOXmax determined with exercise calorimetry, 12 were submitted to a square wave endurance exercise-test (SWEET) protocol of training, and 12 untrained patients served as controls. After 3 months, both training procedures increased VO_{2max} (SWEET training +42% vs LIPOXmax training +14%) and this effect was stronger with SWEET than with LIPOXmax. SWEET training reduced resting systolic blood pressure (-12mmHg) and total cholesterol (-0.29 mmol/l), while LIPOXmax training did not. Both procedures decreased weight and BMI. As expected, the LIPOXmax training improved the ability to oxidize lipids (maximum lipid oxidation rate +53 mg/min) shifted to a higher power intensity (+21 watts), decreased fat mass (-1 kg), increased fat-free

Author	Journal	number	population	protocol	Duration (month)	Weight (Kg)	Waist circumference (cm)	Change in Fat Mass (Kg)	Change in total cholesterol (mmol/l)
Ben Ounis et al., 2008	Diabetes & metabolism	8	Obese adolescent	Training	2	-1,9	-1,8	-1,7	-0,21
Ben Ounis et al., 2008	Diabetes & metabolism	8	Obese adolescent	Training +diet	2	-11,5	-12,3	-11,2	-0,51
Brandou et al., 2003	Diabetes & metabolism	14	Obese adolescent	Training	2	-3,72	-3,73		0,04
Brandou et al., 2005	Diabetes & metabolism	7	Obese adolescent	Training +diet	3	-5,2		-5,07	
Dumortier et al. 2003	Diabetes & metabolism	28	Metabolic syndrome	Training	2	-2,6	-3,53	-1,4	
Fedou et al., 2008	Science et Sport	10	AIDS	Training	12	-0,92		-0,01	-0,28
Ben Ounis et al., 2009a	Science et Sport	18	Obese adolescent	Training	2	-2	-2,9	-2	
Ben Ounis et al., 2009a	Science et Sport	18	Obese adolescent	Training +diet	2	-6	-6,9	-7	
Dumortier et al., 2002	Clinical Hemorheology	21		Training	2				0
Bordenave et al., 2008	Diabetes & metabolism	11	T2D	Training	2			-3,13	
Ben Ounis et al., 2009b	Annales d'endocrinologie	9	Obese adolescent	Training	2	-1,2		-1,4	
Ben Ounis et al., 2009b	Annales d'endocrinologie	9	Obese adolescent	Training +diet	2	-9,5		-5,9	
Jean et al., 2006	Annales d'endocrinologie	28	T2D	Training	3	-1,3	-3,94	-0,66	-0,01
Romain et al., 2009	Science et Sport	17	Neuroleptic treated	Training	3	-2,9			
Venables & Jeukendrup, 2008	Med Sci Sports Exerc	8	Obese	training	2*4 wk	-0,2		-0,1	
Mogensen et al., 2009	diabetes, obesity and metabolism	12	T2D	training	2,5	0	-2,8	-1,5	
		7	Obese adolescent Obese	training Training	2	-1,7			
Elloumi et al., 2009	Acta Paediatrica	7	adolescent	+diet	2	-12,3	-10,5	-12,1	
Brun et al., 2010a	Diabetologia	39	T2D	Training	3	-2,23			

Table 5. Studies of training at the LIPOXmax/FATmax

mass (+1 kg), decreased waist circumference (-3.8 cm) and hip circumference (-2.2 cm) while SWEET training did not significantly modify any of those parameters. Over this short period, the effects of training on HbA1c were significant in the LIPOXmax group (-0.15%) but not in the SWEET group.

Roffey (Roffey, 2008) compared, in a randomized experiment, supervised cycling training at a constant-load FATmax intensity with high intensity interval training (HIIT) with intervals at 85% VO2max, both protocols being matched for total mechanical work volume (11250 kCal). Although both procedures reduced fat mass, the effect was twice more important in FATmax trained subjects than HIIT. A decrease in waist circumference and total cholesterol was evidenced with FATmax but not HIIT. Both procedures decreased systolic blood pressure and increased VO2max.

Put together, these studies show that interval training improves aerobic working capacity, blood pressure and lipid profile, while low intensity endurance training (LIPOXmax training) improves the ability to oxidize lipids during exercise, increases fat free mass, decreases fat mass and decreases HbA1c. The benefits of these two procedures are thus quite different and both are probably interesting to associate in the management of 2 type 2 diabetes.

The psychological tolerability of LIPOXmax training, and more generally low intensity endurance training, compared to high intensity training is poorly known. There is no specific study about the psychological tolerance of LIPOXmax training but some information exists about the effects of prescribing moderate vs higher levels of intensity and frequency on adherence to exercise prescriptions (Perri et al., 2002). In 376 sedentary adults randomly assigned to walk 30 min per day at a frequency of either 3-4 or 5-7 days per week, at an intensity of either 45-55% or 65-75% of maximum heart rate reserve, analyses of percentage of prescribed exercise completed showed greater adherence in the moderate intensity condition. The authors concluded that prescribing a lower frequency increased the accumulation of exercise without a decline in adherence, whereas prescribing a higher intensity decreased adherence and resulted in the completion of less exercise.

Interestingly, Roffey (Roffey, 2008) in his randomized work comparing FATmax training and HIIT, observed a number of clinically significant improvements in health-related quality of life in the FATmax but not the HIIT group.

5.9 Which exercise for diabetes?

Both endurance as well as resistance-type training have been shown to improve whole body insulin sensitivity and/or glucose tolerance and are of therapeutic use in diabetic and insulin-resistant subjects (Praet et al., 2007). Prolonged endurance-type exercise training has been shown to improve insulin sensitivity in both young, elderly and/or insulin-resistant subjects, due to the concomitant induction of weight loss, the upregulation of skeletal muscle glucose transporters GLUT4 expression, improved nitric oxide-mediated skeletal muscle blood flow, reduced hormonal stimulation of hepatic glucose production, and the normalization of blood lipid profiles.

Long-term resistance-type exercise interventions have also been reported to improve glucose tolerance and/or whole body insulin sensitivity. Other than the consecutive effects of each successive bout of exercise, resistance-type exercise training has been associated with a substantial gain in skeletal muscle mass, assumed improve whole body glucose-disposal capacity on the basis on the undemonstrated belief that the higher fat free mass, the higher insulin sensitivity.

While a recent meta-analysis concluded that the effects of both procedures on glucose homeostasis were similar, achieving a reduction in HbA1c by 0.6 to 0.8 (Snowling & Hopkins, 2006; Praet & Van Loon, 2009), a more recent one, after rigourous selection of papers for their methodology, concluded that endurance exercise alone improves Hba1c, blood pressure, and triglycerides, while RT has no demonstrable effects (Chudyk & Petrella, 2011). This issue remains thus controversial, and clearly the best demonstrated method remains endurance training.

When applying endurance-type exercise, energy expenditure should be equivalent to 1.7-2.1 MJ (400-500 kcal) per exercise bout on 3 but preferably 4-5 days/wk, since many of the benefits of exercise are temporary. More vigorous exercise in uncomplicated insulin-resistant states will further improve glycemic control and enhance cardiorespiratory fitness and microvascular function.

Endurance-type exercise combined with resistance (ie, intermittent intensity-type exercise) forms a lower cardiovascular challenge and improves functional performance capacity to a similar extent. Therefore, the combination of endurance- and resistance-type exercise is generally recommended, since its increases the diversity and, as such, the adherence to the exercise intervention program. This is in agreement with the above-reported study in which we compared INT and LIPOX training in T2D (Brun et al., 2010a) and which evidenced that SWEET training improves aerobic working capacity, blood pressure and lipid profile, while low intensity endurance training (LIPOXmax training) improves the ability to oxidize lipids at exercise, increases fat free mass, decreases fat mass and decreases HbA1c. This study shows that benefits of two procedures are rather different and both are probably interesting to associate in the management of type 2 diabetes. A study comparing LIPOX training to more traditional protocols is currently in progress.

Another important advance in this issue comes from a meta-analysis in diabetes (Umpierre et al, 2011) which shows that structured exercise is much more efficient for improving HbA1c than exercise advice alone, and that more than 150 minutes of endurance per week is twice more efficient than exercise performed less than 150 minutes per week.

6. Conclusions

LIPOXmax/Fatmax is a parameter that can be measured with validated protocols. It appears to be a reproducible measurement, although modifiable by several physiological conditions (training, previous exercise or meal). Its measurement closely predicts the amount of lipids that will be oxidized over a 45-60 min of low to medium intensity training performed at the corresponding intensity. It might be a marker of metabolic fitness, and reflects mitochondrial respiration. LIPOXmax is related to catecholamine status and the growth-hormone IGF-1 axis. Its changes are related to alterations in muscular levels of citrate synthase, and to the mitochondrial ability to oxidize lipids during exercise, reducing blood pressure and HbA1c in type 2 diabetes and decreasing circulating cholesterol. Whether the specific targeting on lipid oxidation during exercise has beneficial effects superior to those obtained by a similar energy deficit obtained by other protocols of exercise is suggested by recent studies but remains a current matter of research.

Little is known about the usefulness of these parameters in sports, but classification of athletes according to their metabolic profile during exercise may help to understand their ability to perform endurance sports or short term all of out exercise, and to detect overtraining-related alterations in metabolic adaptation to exercise.

7. References

Achten, J., Gleeson, M., & Jeukendrup, A.E. (2002). Determination of the exercise intensity that elicits maximal fat oxidation. *Med Sci Sports Exerc*, Vol. 34, pp. 92-97.

Achten, J., & Jeukendrup, A.E. (2003) Maximal fat oxidation during exercise in trained men. Int J Sports Med, 24, 603-608.

Achten, J., Venables, M.C., & Jeukendrup, A.E. (2003). Fat oxidation rates are higher during running compared with cycling over a wide range of intensities. *Metab Clin Exp*, Vol. 52, pp. 747-752.

Achten, J., & Jeukendrup, A.E. (2004). Optimizing fat oxidation through exercise and diet. *Nutrition*, Vol. 20, pp. 716-727.

Ahlborg, G., Felig, P., Hagenfeldt, L., Hendler, R., & Wahren, J. (1974). Substrate turnover during prolonged exercise in man. Splanchnic and leg metabolism of glucose, free fatty acids, and amino acids. *J Clin Invest*, Vol. 53, pp. 1080-1090.

Aloulou I. (2002). Le coût glucidique du watt sur ergocycle : une constante biologique? Carbohydrate cost of the watt on ergocycle: a reproducible biological parameter? *Sci Sport*, Vol. 17, pp. 315-317.

Aloulou, I.; Manetta, J; Dumortier, M.; Brandou, F.; Varlet-Marie, E.; Fédou, C.; Mercier, J.; and Brun, J.F. (2003). Effets en miroir de l'entraînement et du surentraînement sur la fonction somatotrope et la balance glucidolipidique à l'exercice *Sci Sport*, Vol. 18, pp. 305-307.

Angevaren, M., Aufdemkampe, G., Verhaar, H.J.J., Aleman, A., & Vanhees, L. (2008). Physical activity and enhanced fitness to improve cognitive function in older people without known cognitive impairment. *Cochrane Database Syst Rev*, CD005381.

Aucouturier, J., Rance, M., Meyer, M., Isacco, L., Thivel, D., & Fellmann, N. (2009). Determination of the maximal fat oxidation point in obese children and adolescents: validity of methods to assess maximal aerobic power. *Eur J Appl Physiol*, Vol. 105, pp. 325-331.

Blanc, S., Normand, S., Pachiaudi, C., Fortrat, J.O., Laville, M., & Gharib, C. (2000). Fuel homeostasis during physical inactivity induced by bed rest. *J Clin Endocrinol Metab*, Vol. 85, pp. 2223-2233.

Barwell, N.D., Malkova, D., Leggate, M., & Gill J.M.R. (2009). Individual responsiveness to exercise-induced fat loss is associated with change in resting substrate utilization. *Metab Clin Exp*, Vol. 58, pp. 1320-1328.

Ben Ounis, O., Elloumi, M., Ben Chiekh, I., Zbidi, A., Amri, M., & Lac, G. (2008). Effects of two-month physical-endurance and diet-restriction programmes on lipid profiles and insulin resistance in obese adolescent boys. *Diabetes Metab*, Vol. 34, pp. 595–600.

Ben Ounis, O., Elloumi, M., Amri, M., Trabelsi, Y., Lac, G., & Tabka, Z. (2009a). Impact of training and hypocaloric diet on fat oxidation and body composition in obese adolescents. *Sci Sports*, Vol. 24, pp. 178-185.

Ben Ounis, O., Elloumi M., Lac, G., Makni, E., Van Praagh, E., & Zouhal, H. (2009b). Two-month effects of individualized exercise training with or without caloric restriction on plasma adipocytokine levels in obese female adolescents. *Ann Endocrinol*, Vol. 70, pp. 235-241.

Ben Ounis, O., Elloumi, M., Zouhal, H., Makni, E., Denguezli, M., & Amri, M. (2010). Effect of individualized exercise training combined with diet restriction on inflammatory markers and IGF-1/IGFBP-3 in obese children. *Ann Nutr Metab*, Vol. 56, pp. 260-266.

Bensimhon, D.R., Kraus, W.E., & Donahue, M.P. (2006). Obesity and physical activity: a review. Am Heart J, 151, 598-603.

Bergman, B.C., & Brooks G.A. (1999) Respiratory gas-exchange ratios during graded exercise in fed and fasted trained and untrained men. *J Appl Physiol*, Vol. 86, pp. 479-487.

Blaak, E.E. & Saris, W.H.M. (2002). Substrate oxidation, obesity and exercise training. *Best Pract Res Clin Endocrinol Metab*, Vol. 16, pp. 667-678.

Blaak, E.E. (2004). Basic disturbances in skeletal muscle fatty acid metabolism in obesity and type 2 diabetes mellitus. *Proc Nutr Soc*, Vol. 63, pp. 323-330.

Bordenave, S., Flavier, S., Fedou, C., Brun, J., Mercier, J. (2007). Exercise calorimetry in sedentary patients: procedures based on short 3 min steps underestimate carbohydrate oxidation and overestimate lipid oxidation. *Diabetes Metab*, Vol. 33, pp. 379-384.

Bordenave, S., Metz, L., Flavier, S., Lambert, K., Ghanassia, E., & Dupuy. A. (2008). Training-induced improvement in lipid oxidation in type 2 diabetes mellitus is related to alterations in muscle mitochondrial activity. Effect of endurance training in type 2 diabetes. *Diabetes Metab*, Vol. 34, pp. 162-168.

Bouchard, C., Tremblay, A., Nadeau, A., Dussault, J., Després, J.P., & Theriault, G. (1990). Long-term exercise training with constant energy intake. 1: Effect on body composition and selected metabolic variables. *Int J Obes*, Vol. 14, pp. 57-73.

Brandou, F., Dumortier, M., Garandeau, P., Mercier, J., & Brun, J.F. (2003). Effects of a two-month rehabilitation program on substrate utilization during exercise in obese adolescents. *Diabetes Metab*, Vol. 29, pp. 20-27.

Brandou, F., Savy-Pacaux, A.M., Marie, J., Bauloz, M., Maret-Fleuret, I., & Borrocoso, S. (2005). Impact of high- and low-intensity targeted exercise training on the type of substrate utilization in obese boys submitted to a hypocaloric diet. *Diabetes Metab*, Vol. 31, pp. 327-335.

Brandou, F., Aloulou, I., Razimbaud, A., Fédou, C., Mercier, J., & Brun, J.F. (2006a). Lower ability to oxidize lipids in adult patients with growth hormone (GH) deficiency: reversal under GH treatment. *Clin Endocrinol* (Oxf), Vol.65, pp. 423-428.

Brandou, F., Savy-Pacaux, A.M., Marie, J., Brun, J.F., & Mercier, J. (2006b). Comparison of the type of substrate oxidation during exercise between pre and post pubertal markedly obese boys. *Int J Sports Med*, Vol. 27, pp. 407-414.

Brooks, G.A., & Mercier, J. (1994). Balance of carbohydrate and lipid utilization during exercise: the "crossover" concept. J Appl Physiol, Vol. 76, pp. 2253-2261.

Brun, J.F., Perez-Martin, A., Fedou, C., & Mercier, J. (2000). Paramètres quantifiant la balance des substrats à l'exercice chez la femme: font-ils double emploi, sont-ils prédictibles par l'anthropométrie? *Ann Endocrinol* (Paris), Vol. 61, pp. 387.

Brun, J.F., Fedou, C., Chaze, D., Perez-Martin, A., Lumbroso, S., & Sultan, C. (1999). Relations entre les proportions respectives de lipides et de glucides oxydés à différents niveaux d'exercice et l'axe GH-IGF-I- IGFBPs chez des sportifs entraînés. *Ann Endocrinol*, Vol. 60.

Brun, J., Jean, E., Ghanassia, E., Flavier, S., & Mercier, J. (2007). Metabolic training: new paradigms of exercise training for metabolic diseases with exercise calorimetry targeting individuals. *Ann Readapt Med Phys*, 50, 528-534.

Brun, J., Fedou, C., Grubka, E., Karafiat, M., Varlet-Marie E., & Mercier J. (2008). Moindre utilisation des lipides à l'exercice chez le diabétique de type 1. *Sci Sports*, Vol. 23, pp. 198-200.

Brun, J., Boegner, C., Raynaud, E., Mercier, J. (2009a). Contrairement à une idée reçue, les femmes n'oxydent pas plus de lipides à l'effort que les hommes, mais leur Lipoxmax survient à une puissance plus élevée. *Sci Sports*, Vol. 24, pp. 45-48.

Brun, J.F., Halbeher, C., Fédou, C., & Mercier, J. (2009b). Le LIPOXmax (niveau d'oxydation maximal des lipides à l'exercice) peut-il être déterminé sans effectuer de calorimétrie d'effort ? *Diabetes Metab*, Vol. 35, A86-A86.

Brun, J., Maurie, J., Jean, E., Romain, A., & Mercier J. (2010a). Comparison of Square-Wave Endurance Exercise Test (SWEET) training with endurance training targeted at the level of maximal lipid oxidation in type 2 diabetics. *Diabetologia*, Vol. 53.

Brun J.F., Varlet-Marie E., Connes P., & Aloulou I. (2010a). Hemorheological alterations related to training and overtraining. *Biorheology*, Vol. 47, pp. 95-115.

Brun, J.F., Romain, A.J., & Mercier, J. (2011a). Maximal lipid oxidation during exercise (Lipoxmax): From physiological measurements to clinical applications. Facts and uncertainties. *Science & Sports*, Vol. 26 No. 2, pp. 57-71.

Brun, J.F., Fedou, C., Bordenave, S., Metz, L., Lambert, K., & Dupuy A. (2011b). L'amélioration de l'oxydation des lipides induite par l'entrainement ciblé au LIPOXmax chez des diabétiques de type 2 s'accompagne d'une diminution de la protéine C-réactive (CRP). *Ann Endocrinol*, Vol. 71, p 416 (abstract P272)

Brun, J.F., Halbeher, C., Fédou, C., & Mercier, J. (2011c). J.-F. Brun, C. Halbeher, C. Fédou, J. MercierWhat are the limits of normality of the LIPOXmax? Can it be predict without exercise calorimetry? *Science & Sports*, Vol. 26 pp. 166-169

Burgomaster, K.A., Howarth, K.R., Phillips, S.M., Rakobowchuk, M., Macdonald, M.J., & McGee, S.L. (2008). Similar metabolic adaptations during exercise after low volume sprint interval and traditional endurance training in humans. *J Physiol* (Lond), Vol. 586, pp. 151-160.

Byrne, N.M., Meerkin, J.D., Laukkanen, R., Ross, R., Fogelholm, M., & Hills A.P. (2006). Weight loss strategies for obese adults: personalized weight management program *vs.* standard care. *Obesity* (Silver Spring). Vol.14, pp. 1777-1788.

P Caudwell, P Hopkins, M King, N A. Stubbs, R J. and Blundell, J E. (2009) Exercise alone is not enough : weight loss also needs a healthy (Mediterranean) diet? Public Health Nutrition, 12(9A). pp. 1663-1666.

Chambliss, H.O. (2005) Exercise duration and intensity in a weight-loss program. Clin J Sport Med, Vol. 15, pp. 113-115.

Chenevière, X., Borrani, F., Ebenegger, V., Gojanovic, B., & Malatesta, D. (2009a). Effect of a 1-hour single bout of moderate-intensity exercise on fat oxidation kinetics. *Metab Clin Exp*, Vol. 58, pp.1778-1786.

Chenevière, X., Malatesta, D., Peters, E.M., & Borrani, F. (2009b). A mathematical model to describe fat oxidation kinetics during graded exercise. *Med Sci Sports Exerc*, Vol. 41, pp. 1615-1625.

Chenevière, X, Borrani, F, Sangsue, D, Gojanovic, B, Malatesta, D. (2011). Gender differences in whole-body fat oxidation kinetics during exercise. *Appl Physiol Nutr Metab*, Vol. 36 No. 1, pp. 88-95.

Christensen, E.H. & Hansen, O. (1939). Arbeitsfähigkeit und Ernährung. Scand Arch Physiol, Vol. 81, pp. 60-171.

Christmass, M.A., Dawson, B., Passeretto, P., Arthur, P.G. (1999). A comparison of skeletal muscle oxygenation and fuel use in sustained continuous and intermittent exercice. *Eur J Appl Physiol*, Vol. 80, pp. 423-435.

Chudyk, A. & Petrella, R.J (2011). Effects of exercise on cardiovascular risk factors in type 2 diabetes: a meta-analysis. *Diabetes Care* Vol. 34 pp. 1228-37.

Corpeleijn, E., Mensink, M., Kooi, M.E., Roekaerts, P.M.H.J., Saris, W.H.M., & Blaak, E.E. (2008). Impaired skeletal muscle substrate oxidation in glucose-intolerant men improves after weight loss. *Obesity* (Silver Spring), Vol. 16, pp. 1025-1032.

Corpeleijn, E., Saris, W.H.M., & Blaak, E.E. (2009). Metabolic flexibility in the development of insulin resistance and type 2 diabetes: effects of lifestyle. *Obes Rev*, Vol. 10, pp. 178-193.

Coyle, E.F., Jeukendrup, A.E., Oseto, M.C., Hodgkinson, B.J., & Zderic, T.W. (2001). Low-fat diet alters intramuscular substrates and reduces lipolysis and fat oxidation during exercise. Am J Physiol Endocrinol Metab, Vol. 280, E391.

Coyle, E.F., Jeukendrup, A.E., Wagenmakers, A.J., & Saris, W.H. (1997). Fatty acid oxidation is directly regulated by carbohydrate metabolism during exercise. *Am J Physiol*, Vol. 273, E268-75.

De Glisezinski, I., Larrouy, D., Bajzova, M., Koppo, K., Polak, J., & Berlan, M. (2009). Adrenaline but not noradrenaline is a determinant of exercise-induced lipid mobilization in human subcutaneous adipose tissue. *J Physiol* (Lond), Vol. 587, pp. 3393-3404.

Del Coso, J.; Hamouti,N.; Ortega, J.F., Mora-Rodriguez, R. (2010) Aerobic fitness determines whole-body fat oxidation rate during exercise in the heat. *Appl Physiol Nutr Metab.* Vol; 35, pp 741-8.

Dériaz, O., Dumont, M., Bergeron, N., Després, J.P., Brochu, M., & Prud'homme, D. (2001). Skeletal muscle low attenuation area and maximal fat oxidation rate during submaximal exercise in male obese individuals. *Int J Obes Relat Metab Disord*, Vol. 25, pp. 1579-1584.

Desplan, M., Avignon, A., Mestejanot, C., Outters, M., Sardinoux, M., & Fedou, C. (2010). Impaired ability to oxidize lipids at exercise in severe vs. mild to moderate sleep apnea/hypopnea obstructive sleep syndrome (OSAS). *Fund Clin Pharmacol*, Vol. 24, pp. 66.

Donnelly, J.E., Blair, S.N., Jakicic, J.M., Manore, M.M., Rankin, J.W., & Smith, B.K. (2009). American College of Sports Medicine Position Stand. Appropriate physical activity intervention strategies for weight loss and prevention of weight regain for adults. *Med Sci Sports Exerc*, Vol. 41, pp. 459-471.

Duclos, M., Duché, P., Guezennec, C., Richard, R., Rivière, D., & Vidalin, H. (2010). Position de consensus : activité physique et obésité chez l'enfant et chez l'adulte. *Sci Sports*, Vol. 25, pp. 207-225.

Dumortier, M., Pérez-Martin, A., Pierrisnard, E., Mercier, J., & Brun, J.F. (2002). Regular exercise (3x45 min/wk) decreases plasma viscosity in sedentary obese, insulin resistant patients parallel to an improvement in fitness and a shift in substrate oxidation balance. *Clin Hemorheol Microcirc*, Vol. 26, pp. 219-229.

Dumortier, M., Brandou, F., Perez-Martin, A., Fedou, C., Mercier, J., & Brun, J.F. (2003). Low intensity endurance exercise targeted for lipid oxidation improves body composition and insulin sensitivity in patients with the metabolic syndrome. *Diabetes Metab*, Vol. 29, pp. 509-518.

Dyck, D.J. (2009). Adipokines as regulators of muscle metabolism and insulin sensitivity. *Appl Physiol Nutr Metab*, Vol. 34, pp. 396-402.

Elloumi, M., Ben Ounis, O., Makni, E., Van Praagh, E., Tabka, Z., & Lac, G. (2009). Effect of individualized weight-loss programmes on adiponectin, leptin and resistin levels in obese adolescent boys. *Acta Paediatr*, Vol. 98, pp. 1487-1493.

Fabre, C., Chamari, K., Mucci, P., Massé-Biron, J., & Préfaut, C. (2002). Improvement of cognitive function by mental and/or individualized aerobic training in healthy elderly subjects. *Int J Sports Med*, Vol. 23, pp. 415-421.

Febbraio, M.A., Snow R.J., Hargreaves M., Stathis C.G., Martin I.K., Carey M.F. (1994) Muscle metabolism during exercise and heat stress in trained men: effect of acclimation. *J Appl Physiol*. Vol. 76, pp. 589-97.

Fedou, C., Fabre, J., Baillat, V., Reynes J., Brun, J.F., & Mercier, J. (2008). Balance des substrats à l'exercice chez des patients infectés par le VIH 1 et présentant un syndrome lipodystrophique: Effet d'un réentraînement ciblé par la calorimétrie d'effort. *Sci Sports*, Vol. 23, pp. 189-192.

Folch, N., Péronnet, F., Massicotte, D., Duclos, M., Lavoie, C., & Hillaire-Marcel, C. (2001). Metabolic response to small and large 13C-labelled pasta meals following rest or exercise in man. *Br J Nutr*, Vol. 85, pp 671-680.

Friedlander, A.L., Casazza, G.A., Horning, M.A., Buddinger, T.F., & Brooks, G.A. (1998a). Effects of exercise intensity and training on lipid metabolism in young women. *Am J Physiol Endocrinol Metab*, Vol. 275, E853-863.

Friedlander, A.L., Casazza, G.A, Horning, M.A., Huie, M.J., Piacentini, M.F., Trimmer, J.K. (1998b). Training-induced alterations of carbohydrate metabolism in women: women respond differently from men. *J Appl Physiol*, Vol. 85, pp. 1175-1186.

Friedlander, A.L., Jacobs, K.A., Fattor, J.A., Horning, M.A., Hagobian T.A., & Bauer T.A. (2007). Contributions of working muscle to whole body lipid metabolism are altered by exercise intensity and training. *Am J Physiol Endocrinol Metab*, Vol. 292, E107-116.

Fritz, T., Krämer, D.K.,. Karlsson, H.K.R, Galuska, D., Engfeldt, P., & Zierath, J.R. (2006). Low-intensity exercise increases skeletal muscle protein expression of PPARdelta and UCP3 in type 2 diabetic patients. *Diabetes Metab Res Rev*, Vol. 22, pp. 492-498.

Gautier, J., Berne, C., Grimm, J., Lobel, B., Coliche, V., & Mollet, E. (1998). Activité physique et diabète. *Diabetes Metab*, Vol. 24, pp. 281-290.

Gautier, J. (2004) Physical activity as a therapeutic tool in type 2 diabetes: the rationale. Ann Endocrinol, Vol. 65, pp. 44-51.

Ghanassia, E., Brun, J.F., Fedou, C., Raynaud, E., & Mercier, J. (2006). Substrate oxidation during exercise: type 2 diabetes is associated with a decrease in lipid oxidation and an earlier shift towards carbohydrate utilization. *Diabetes* Metab, Vol. 32, pp. 604-610.

Gmada, N., Marzouki , H., Haboubi, M. , Tabka, Z., Shephard, R.J., Bouhlel, E. (2011). The cross-over point and maximal fat oxidation in sedentary healthy subjects: methodological issues. *Diabetes Metab* (in press)

Goldhammer, E., Tanchilevitch, A., Maor, I., Beniamini, Y., Rosenschein, U., & Sagiv, M. (2005). Exercise training modulates cytokines activity in coronary heart disease patients. *Int J Cardiol*, Vol. 100, pp. 93-99.

González-Haro, C., Galilea, P.A., González-de-Suso, J.M., Drobnic, F., & Escanero, J.F. (2007). Maximal lipidic power in high competitive level triathletes and cyclists. *Br J Sports Med*, Vol. 41, pp. 23 -28.

Guha, N., Sönksen, P.H., & Holt, R.I. (2009). IGF-I abuse in sport: Current knowledge and future prospects for detection. *Growth Horm IGF Res*, Vol. 19, pp. 408-411.

Guidelines for the rehabilitation of chronic obstructive pulmonary disease. French Language Society of Pneumology, (2005). *Rev Mal Respir*, Vol. 22, 7S8-7S14.

Harber, M.P., Konopka, A.R., Douglass, M.D., Minchev, K., Kaminsky, L.A., & Trappe, T.A. (2009). Aerobic exercise training improves whole muscle and single myofiber size and function in older women. *Am J Physiol Regul Integr Comp Physiol*, Vol. 297, R1452-1459.

Hoene, M., & Weigert, C. (2008). The role of interleukin-6 in insulin resistance, body fat distribution and energy balance. *Obes Rev*, Vol. 9, pp. 20-29.

Hopkins, M., Jeukendrup, A., King, N.A., & Blundell, J.E. (2011). The Relationship between Substrate Metabolism, Exercise and Appetite Control: Does Glycogen Availability Influence the Motivation to Eat, Energy Intake or Food Choice? *Sports Med*, Vol. 41 No. 6, pp. 507-521.

Howarth, K.R., Phillips, S.M., MacDonald, M.J., Richards, D., Moreau, N.A., & Gibala, M.J. (2010). Effect of glycogen availability on human skeletal muscle protein turnover during exercise and recovery. *J Appl Physiol*, Vol. 109, pp. 431-438.

Jakicic, J.M., & Otto, A.D. (2005). Physical activity considerations for the treatment and prevention of obesity. *Am J Clin Nutr*, Vol. 82, 226S-229S.

Jakicic, J.M. & Otto, A.D. (2006) Treatment and prevention of obesity: what is the role of exercise? *Nutr Rev*, 64, S57-61.

Janssen, I., Heymsfield, S.B., Baumgartner, R.N., Ross, R. (2000). Estimation of skeletal muscle mass by bioelectrical impedance analysis. *J Appl Physiol*, Vol. 89, pp. 465-471.

Jean, E., Grubka, E., Karafiat, M., Flavier, S., Fédou, C., & Mercier, J. (2006). Effets d'un entraînement en endurance ciblé par la calorimétrie à l'effort chez des diabétiques de type 2. *Ann Endocrinol*, Vol. 67, pp. 462.

Jean, E., Flavier, S., Mercier, & J., Brun, J.F. (2007). Exercise calorimetry with 6 min steps closely predicts the lipid oxidation flow rate of a 45 min steady state targeted training session at the level of maximal lipid oxidation (LIPOXmax). *Fund Clin Pharmacol*, Vol. 21, pp. 95.

Jeukendrup, A.E., Saris, W.H., & Wagenmakers, A.J. (1998). Fat metabolism during exercise: a review. Part I: fatty acid mobilization and muscle metabolism. *Int J Sports Med*, Vol. 19 No. 4, pp. 231-44.

Jeukendrup, A.E. (2003). Modulation of carbohydrate and fat utilization by diet, exercise and environment. *Biochem Soc Trans*, Vol. 31, pp. 1270-1273.

Jeukendrup, A.E., Wallis, G.A. (2005). Measurement of substrate oxidation during exercise by means of gas exchange measurements. *Int J Sports Med*, Vol. 26, S28-37.

Kelley, D.E., Goodpaster, B., Wing, R.R., & Simoneau, J.A. (1999). Skeletal muscle fatty acid metabolism in association with insulin resistance, obesity, and weight loss, *Am. J Physiol*, Vol. 277, E1130-1141.

Kelley, G.A., Kelley, K.S., Franklin, B. (2006). Aerobic exercise and lipids and lipoproteins in patients with cardiovascular disease: a meta-analysis of randomized controlled trials. *J Cardiopulm Rehabil*, Vol. 26, pp. 131-139.

Kiens, B., & Richter, E.A. (1998). Utilization of skeletal muscle triacylglycerol during postexercise recovery in humans. *Am J Physiol*, Vol. 275, E332-337.

Kim, S.H., Lee, S.J., Kang, E.S., Kang, S., Hur, K.Y., & Lee, H.J. (2006). Effects of lifestyle modification on metabolic parameters and carotid intima-media thickness in patients with type 2 diabetes mellitus. *Metab Clin Exp*, Vol. 55, pp. 1053-1059.

King N.A., Burley V.J., Blundell J.E. (1994) Exercise-induced suppression of appetite: effects on food intake and implications for energy balance. *Eur. J. Clin. Nutr.* Vol 48, pp. 715–725

King, N.A., Caudwell, P.P., Hopkins , M, Stubbs, J.R., Naslund, E., & Blundell, J.E. (2009) Dual-process action of exercise on appetite control : increase in orexigenic drive but improvement in meal-induced satiety. *American Journal of Clinical Nutrition*, Vol 90, pp. 921-927.

King, N.A., Hopkins, M., Caudwell, P., Stubbs, R.J., & Blundell J.E. (2008). Individual variability following 12 weeks of supervised exercise: identification and characterization of compensation for exercise-induced weight loss. *Int J Obes* (Lond), Vol. 32, pp. 177-184.

Kirwan, J.P., Costill, D.L., Mitchell, J.B., Houmard, J.A., Flynn, M.G., & Fink, W.J. (1988). Carbohydrate balance in competitive runners during successive days of intense training. *J Appl Physiol*, 65, 2601-2606.

Koulmann, & N., Bigard, A. (2006). Interaction between signalling pathways involved in skeletal muscle responses to endurance exercise. *Pflugers Arch*, Vol. 452, pp. 125-139.

Krogh, A., & Linhardt, J. (1920). The relative value of fat and carbohydrate as sources of muscular energy. *Bioch J*, Vol. 14, pp. 290-363.

Krogh, J., Nordentoft, M., Sterne, J.A.C., Lawlor, D.A. (2010). The effect of exercise in clinically depressed adults: systematic review and meta-analysis of randomized controlled trials. *J Clin Psychiatry*.

Lavault, P., Deaux, S., Romain, A.J., Fedou, C., Mercier, J., & Brun, J.F. (2011). Intérêt de la quantification de la masse musculaire pour interpréter la calorimétrie d'effort. *Sci Sports*. Vol. 26, pp. 88-91

Lazzer, S., Lafortuna, C., Busti, C., Galli, R., Tinozzi, T., & Agosti, F. (2010). Fat oxidation rate during and after a low- or high-intensity exercise in severely obese Caucasian adolescents. *Eur J Appl Physiol*, Vol. 108, pp. 383-391.

Lazzer, S., Lafortuna, C., Busti, C., Galli, R., Agosti, F.; & Sartorio, A. (2011) Effects of low- and high-intensity exercise training on body composition and substrate metabolism in obese adolescents. *J Endocrinol Invest*. Vol. 34, pp 45-52.

Lefebvre, P., Bringer, J., Renard, E., Boulet, F., Clouet, S., & Jaffiol, C. (1997). Influences of weight, body fat patterning and nutrition on the management of PCOS. *Hum Reprod*, Vol. 12, pp. 72-81.

Lindström, J., Ilanne-Parikka, P., Peltonen, M., Aunola, S., Eriksson, J.G., & Hemiö, K. (2006). Sustained reduction in the incidence of type 2 diabetes by lifestyle intervention: follow-up of the Finnish Diabetes Prevention Study. *Lancet*, Vol. 368, pp. 1673-1679.

MacLean, P.S.; Higgins, J.A.; Wyatt H.R.; Melanson, E.L.; Johnson, G.C.; Jackman, M.R.; Giles, E.D.; Brown, I.E; Hill, J.O. (2009) Regular exercise attenuates the metabolic drive to regain weight after long-term weight loss. *Am J Physiol Regul Integr Comp Physiol*. Vol. 297, pp.R793-802.

MacLean, P.S.; Bergouignan, A.; Cornier, M.A.; Jackman, M.R. (2011) Biology's Response to Dieting: the Impetus for Weight Regain. *Am J Physiol Regul Integr Comp Physiol*. 2011 (in press)

MacRae, H.S., Noakes, T.D., & Dennis, S.C. (1995). Role of decreased carbohydrate oxidation on slower rises in ventilation with increasing exercise intensity after training. *Eur J Appl Physiol Occup Physiol*, Vol. 71, pp. 523-529.

Malatesta, D., Werlen, C., Bulfaro, S., Chenevière, X., & Borrani, F. (2009). Effect of high-intensity interval exercise on lipid oxidation during postexercise recovery. *Med Sci Sports Exerc*, Vol. 41, pp. 364-374.

Malin, S.K., Stephens, B.R., Sharoff, C.G., Hagobian, T.A., Chipkin, S.R., & Braun, B. (2010). Metformin's effect on exercise and postexercise substrate oxidation. *Int J Sport Nutr Exerc Metab*, Vol. 20, pp. 63-71.

Manetta, J., Brun, J.F., Maimoun, L., Galy, O., Coste, O., Raibaut, J.L., & Mercier, J. (2002a). Carbohydrate dependence during hard-intensity exercise in trained cyclists in the competitive season: importance of training status. *Int J Sports Med*, Vol. 23, pp. 516-523.

Manetta, J., Perez-Martin, A., Brun, J.F., Callis, A., Prefaut, C., & Mercier, J. (2002b). Fuel oxidation during exercise in middle-aged men: effect of training and glucose disposal. *Med Sci Sports Exerc*, Vol. 34, pp. 423-429.

Manetta, J., Brun, J.F., Prefaut, C., & Mercier, J. (2005). Substrate oxidation during exercise at moderate and hard intensity in middle-aged and young athletes versus sedentary men. *Metabolism*, Vol. 54 No. 11, pp. 1411-1419.

Martins, R.A., Neves, A.P., Coelho-Silva, M.J., Veríssimo, M.T., & Teixeira, A.M. (2010). The effect of aerobic versus strength-based training on high-sensitivity C-reactive protein in older adults. *Eur J Appl Physiol*, Vol. 110, pp. 161-169.

Marwick, T.H., Hordern, M.D., Miller, T., Chyun, D.A., Bertoni, A.G., & Blumenthal, R.S. (2009). Exercise Training for Type 2 Diabetes Mellitus: Impact on Cardiovascular Risk: A Scientific Statement From the American Heart Association. *Circulation*, Vol. 119, pp. 3244-3262.

Mattusch, F., Dufaux, B, Heine, O., Mertens, I., & Rost, R. (2000). Reduction of the plasma concentration of C-reactive protein following nine months of endurance training. *Int J Sports Med*, Vol. 21, pp. 21-24.

Melanson, E.L., Sharp, T.A., Seagle, H.M., Horton, T.J., Donahoo, W.T., & Grunwald, G.K. (2002). Effect of exercise intensity on 24-h energy expenditure and nutrient oxidation. *J Appl Physiol*, Vol. 92, pp. 1045-1052.

Melanson K.J., Westerterp-Plantenga M.S., Campfield L.A., Saris W.H. (1999). Appetite and blood glucose profiles in humans after glycogen-depleting exercise. *J Appl Physiol*. Vol 87, pp 947-54.

Mensink, M., Blaak, E.E., van Baak, M.A., Wagenmakers, A.J., & Saris, W.H. (2001). Plasma free Fatty Acid uptake and oxidation are already diminished in subjects at high risk for developing type 2 diabetes. *Diabetes*, 50, 2548-2554.

Meyer, T., Folz, C., Rosenberger, F., & Kindermann, W. (2009). The reliability of fat. Scand J Med Sci Sports, Vol. 19, pp. 213-221

Meyer, T., Gässler, N., & Kindermann, W. (2007). Determination of "Fatmax"with 1 h cycling protocols of constant load. *Appl Physiol Nutr Metab*, Vol. 32, pp. 249-256.

Michallet, A., Bricout, V., Wuyam, B., Guinot, M., Favre-Juvin, A., & Lévy, P. (2006). Aspects méthodologiques de la mesure du PCGL et du Lipoxmax. *Rev Mal Respir*, Vol. 23, pp. 396.

Michallet, A., Tonini, J., Regnier, J., Guinot, M., Favre-Juvin, A., & Bricout, V. (2008). Methodological aspects of crossover and maximum fat-oxidation rate point determination. *Diabetes Metab*, Vol. 34, pp. 514-523.

Mogensen, M., Vind, B.F., Højlund, K., Beck-Nielsen, H., & Sahlin, K. (2009). Maximal lipid oxidation in patients with type 2 diabetes is normal and shows an adequate increase in response to aerobic training. *Diabetes Obes Metab*, Vol. 11, pp. 874-883.

Møller, N., Jørgensen, J.O., Alberti, K.G., Flyvbjerg, A., & Schmitz, O. (1990a). Short-term effects of growth hormone on fuel oxidation and regional substrate metabolism in normal man. J Clin Endocrinol Metab, 70, 1179-1186.

Møller, N., Jørgensen, J.O., Schmitz, O., Møller, J., Christiansen, J., & Alberti, K.G. (1990b). Effects of a growth hormone pulse on total and forearm substrate fluxes in humans. *Am J Physiol*, Vol. 258, E86-91.

Nicklas, B.J., Wang, X., You, T., Lyles, M.F., Demons, J., & Easter, L. (2009). Effect of exercise intensity on abdominal fat loss during calorie restriction in overweight and obese postmenopausal women: a randomized, controlled trial. *Am J Clin Nutr*, Vol. 89, pp. 1043-1052.

Nordby, P., Saltin, B., & Helge, J.W. (2006). Whole-body fat oxidation determined by graded exercise and indirect calorimetry: a role for muscle oxidative capacity? *Scand J Med Sci Sports*, Vol. 16, pp. 209-214.

Perez-Martin, A., Raynaud, E., Aïssa Benhaddad, A., Fedou, C., Brun, J.F., & Mercier, J. (2000). Utilisation des substrats énergétiques à l'effort chez les sujets obèses et les diabétiques de type 2. *Diabetes & Metabolism*, Vol. 26, XXXVII.

Perez-Martin, A., Dumortier, M., Raynaud, E., Brun, J.F., Fédou, C., & Bringer, J. (2001). Balance of substrate oxidation during submaximal exercise in lean and obese people. *Diabetes Metab*, Vol. 27, pp. 466-474.

Perez-Martin, A., & Mercier, J. (2001). Stress tests and exercise training program for diabetics - Initial metabolic evaluation. *Ann Endocrinol*, Vol. 62, pp. 291-293.

Perri, M.G., Anton, S.D., Durning, P.E., Ketterson, T.U., Sydeman, S.J., & Berlant, N.E. (2002). Adherence to exercise prescriptions: effects of prescribing moderate versus higher levels of intensity and frequency. *Health Psychol*, Vol. 21, pp. 452-458.

Pescatello, L.S., Franklin, B.A., Fagard, R., Farquhar, W.B., Kelley, G.A., Ray, C.A. (2004). American College of Sports Medicine position stand. Exercise and hypertension. *Med Sci Sports Exerc*, Vol. 36, pp. 533-553.

Pescatello, L.S. (2005). Exercise and hypertension: recent advances in exercise prescription. *Curr Hypertens Rep*, Vol. 7, pp. 281-286.

Poehlman, E.T., Gardner, A.W., Arciero, P.J., Goran, M.I., & Calles-Escandon, J. (1994). Effects of endurance training on total fat oxidation in elderly persons. *J Appl Physiol*, Vol. 76, pp. 2281-2287.

Praet S.F.E., van Loon L.J.C. (2007). Optimizing the therapeutic benefits of exercise in Type 2 diabetes. *J Appl Physiol*, Vol. 103, pp. 1113-1120.

Praet S.F.E., van Loon L.J.C. (2009). Exercise therapy in type 2 diabetes. Acta Diabetol, Vol. 46, pp. 263-278.

Richter, W.O., Kerscher, P., & Schwandt, P. (1983). Beta-endorphin stimulates in vivo lipolysis in the rabbit. *Life Sci*, Vol. 33 Suppl 1, pp. 743-746.

Richter, W.O., Naudé, R.J., Oelofsen, W., & Schwandt, P. (1987). In vitro lipolytic activity of beta-endorphin and its partial sequences. *Endocrinology*, Vol. 120, pp. 1472-1476.

Riddell, M.C., Jamnik, V.K., Iscoe, K.E., Timmons, B.W., & Gledhill, N. (2008). Fat oxidation rate and the exercise intensity that elicits maximal fat oxidation decreases with pubertal status in young male subjects. *J Appl Physiol*, Vol. 105, pp. 742-748.

Rochester, C.L. (2003). Exercise training in chronic obstructive pulmonary disease. *J Rehabil Res Dev*, Vol. 40, pp. 59-80.

Roffey, D.M. (2008) Exercise intensity, exercise training and energy metabolism in overweight and obese males. PhD thesis, Queensland University of Technology.

Romain, A., Attal, J., Hermès, A., Capdevielle, D., Raimondi, R., & Boulenger J. (2009). Effets d'un réentraînement en endurance au LIPOXmax chez des patients psychiatriques traités par psychotropes. *Sci Sports*, Vol. 24, pp. 265-268.

Romain, A., Fedou, C., Mercier, J., & Brun, J. (2010). Exercise targeted at the level of maximal lipid oxidation in overweight and obesity: a meta-analysis. *Obes Rev*, Vol. 11, pp. 229.

Romijn, J.A., Coyle, E.F., Hibbert, J., & Wolfe, R.R. (1992). Comparison of indirect calorimetry and a new breath 13C/12C ratio method during strenuous exercise. *Am J Physiol*, Vol. 263, E64-71.

Romijn, J.A., Coyle, E.F., Sidossis, L.S., Gastaldelli, A., Horowitz, J.F., & Endert, E. (1993). Regulation of endogenous fat and carbohydrate metabolism in relation to exercise intensity and duration. *Am J Physiol*, Vol. 265, E380-391.

Ross, R., Dagnone, D., Jones, P.J., Smith, H., Paddags, A., & Hudson, R. (2000). Reduction in obesity and related comorbid conditions after diet-induced weight loss or exercise-induced weight loss in men. A randomized, controlled trial. *Ann Intern Med*, Vol. 133, pp. 92-103.

Sahlin, K., Sallstedt, E., Bishop, D., & Tonkonogi, M. (2008). Turning down lipid oxidation during heavy exercise-what is the mechanism? *J Physiol Pharmacol*, Vol. 59 Suppl 7, pp. 19-30.

Sardinoux, M., Brun, J.F., Lefebvre, P., Bringer, J., Fabre, G., & Salsano, V. (2009). Influence of bariatric surgery on exercice maximal lipid oxydation point in grade 3 obese patients. Fund Clin Pharmacol, Vol. 23, pp. 57.

Schoenfeld, B.J. (2010). The mechanisms of muscle hypertrophy and their application to resistance training. *J Strength Cond Res*, Vol. 24, pp. 2857-2872.

Schrauwen, P., van Aggel-Leijssen, D.P.C., Hul, G, Wagenmakers, A.J.M., Vidal, H., & Saris, W.H.M. (2002). The effect of a 3-month low-intensity endurance training program on fat oxidation and acetyl-CoA carboxylase-2 expression. *Diabetes*, Vol. 51, pp. 2220-2226.

Sheffield-Moore, M., Yeckel, C.W., Volpi, E., Wolf, S.E., Morio, B., & Chinkes, D.L. (2004). Postexercise protein metabolism in older and younger men following moderate-intensity aerobic exercise, *Am J Physiol Endocrinol Metab*, Vol. 287, E513-522.

Slentz, C.A., Duscha, B.D., Johnson, J.L., Ketchum, K., Aiken, L.B., & Samsa, G.P. (2004). Effects of the amount of exercise on body weight, body composition, and measures of central obesity: STRRIDE--a randomized controlled study. *Arch Intern Med*, Vol. 164, pp. 31-39.

Snowling, N.J. & Hopkins, W.G. (2006). Effects of different modes of exercise training on glucose control and risk factors for complications in type 2 diabetic patients: a meta-analysis. *Diabetes Care*, Vol. 29, pp. 2518-2527.

Snyder, K.A., Donnelly, J.E., Jabobsen, D.J., Hertner, G., & Jakicic, J.M. (1997). The effects of long-term, moderate intensity, intermittent exercise on aerobic capacity, body composition, blood lipids, insulin and glucose in overweight females. *Int J Obes Relat Metab Disord*, Vol. 21, pp. 1180-1189.

Starritt, E.C., Howlett, R.A., Heigenhauser, G.J., & Spriet, L.L. (2000). Sensitivity of CPT I to malonyl-CoA in trained and untrained human skeletal muscle. *Am J Physiol, Endocrinol Metab*, Vol. 278, E462-468.

Stewart, L.K., Flynn, M.G., Campbell, W.W., Craig, B.A., Robinson, J.P., & Timmerman, K.L. (2007). The influence of exercise training on inflammatory cytokines and C-reactive protein. *Med Sci Sports Exerc*, Vol. 39, pp. 1714-1719.

Stisen, A.B., Stougaard, O., Langfort, J., Helge, J.W., Sahlin, K., & Madsen, K. (2006). Maximal fat oxidation rates in endurance trained and untrained women. *Eur J Appl Physiol*, Vol. 98 No. 5, pp. 497-506.

Strasser, B., Spreitzer, A., & Haber, P. (2007). Fat loss depends on energy deficit only, independently of the method for weight loss. *Ann Nutr Metab*, Vol. 51, pp. 428-432.

Talanian, J.L., Galloway, S.D.R., Heigenhauser, G.J.F., Bonen, A., & Spriet, L.L. (2007). Two weeks of high-intensity aerobic interval training increases the capacity for fat oxidation during exercise in women. *J Appl Physiol*, Vol. 102, pp. 1439-1447.

Thompson, D.L., Townsend, K.M., Boughey, R., Patterson, K., & Bassett, D.R. (1998). Substrate use during and following moderate- and low-intensity exercise: implications for weight control. *Eur J Appl Physiol Occup Physiol*, Vol. 78, pp. 43-49.

Thomson, J.A., Green, H.J., & Houston, M.E. (1979). Muscle glycogen depletion patterns in fast twitch fibre subgroups of man during submaximal and supramaximal exercise. *Pflugers Arch*, Vol. 379, pp. 105-108.

Tolfrey, K., Jeukendrup, A.E., & Batterham, A.M. (2010). Group- and individual-level coincidence of the 'Fatmax' and lactate accumulation in adolescents. *Eur J Appl Physiol*, Vol. 109 No. 6, pp. 1145-53.

Trenell, M.I., Hollingsworth, K.G., Lim, E.L., & Taylor R. (2008). Increased daily walking improves lipid oxidation without changes in mitochondrial function in type 2 diabetes. *Diabetes Care*, Vol. 31, pp. 1644-1649.

Umpierre, D.; Ribeiro, P.; Kramer, C.; Leitao, C.; Zucatti, A.; Azevedo, M.; Gross, J.; Ribeiro, J.; Schaan, B. (2011) Physical Activity Advice Only or Structured Exercise Training and Association With HbA1c Levels in Type 2 Diabetes. A Systematic Review and Meta-analysis. *JAMA*, Vol. 305, pp. 1790-1799.

Vallet, G., Ahmaidi, S., Serres, I., Fabre, C., Bourgouin, D., & Desplan, J. (1997). Comparison of two training programmes in chronic airway limitation patients: Standardized versus individualized protocols. *Eur Resp J*, Vol. 10, pp. 114-122.

Van Aggel-Leijssen, D.P., Saris, W.H., Wagenmakers, A.J., Hul, G.B., & van Baak, M.A. (2001). The effect of low-intensity exercise training on fat metabolism of obese women. *Obes Res*, Vol. 9, pp. 86-96.

Varlet-Marie, E., Brun, J.F., Fedou, C., & Mercier, J. (2006). Balance of substrates used for oxidation at exercise in ahletes: lipodependent vs glucodependent sports. *Fund Clin Pharmacol*, Vol. 20, pp. 220.

Venables, M.C., Achten, J., & Jeukendrup, A.E. (2005). Determinants of fat oxidation during exercise in healthy men and women: a cross-sectional study. *J Appl Physiol*, Vol. 98, pp. 160-167.

Venables, M.C., & Jeukendrup, A.E. (2008). Endurance Training and Obesity. Med Sci Sports Exerc, Vol. 40, pp. 495-502.

Venables, M.C., & Jeukendrup, A.E. (2009). Physical inactivity and obesity: links with insulin resistance and type 2 diabetes mellitus. *Diabetes Metab Res Rev*, Vol. 25, S18-23.

Vijayakumar, A., Novosyadlyy, R., Wu, Y., Yakar, S., & LeRoith, D. (2010). Biological effects of growth hormone on carbohydrate and lipid metabolism. *Growth Horm IGF Res*, Vol. 20, pp. 1-7.

Warren, A., Howden, E.J., Williams, A.D., Fell, J.W., & Johnson, N.A. (2009). Postexercise fat oxidation: effect of exercise duration, intensity, and modality. *Int J Sport Nutr Exerc Metab*, Vol. 19, pp. 607-623.

Watt, M.J., Steinberg, G.R., Heigenhauser, G.J.F., Spriet, L.L., & Dyck, D.J. (2003). Hormone-sensitive lipase activity and triacylglycerol hydrolysis are decreased in rat soleus muscle by cyclopiazonic acid. *Am J Physiol Endocrinol Metab*, Vol. 285, E412-419.

Westerterp-Plantenga M. S., Verwegen C. R. T., Ijedema M. J. W., Wijkmans N. E. G., Saris W. H. M.(1997) Acute effects of exercise or sauna on appetite in obese and non-obese men. *Physiol. Behav.* Vol 62, 1345–1354.

Wilkinson, S.B., Phillips, S.M., Atherton, P.J., Patel, R., Yarasheski, K.E., & Tarnopolsky, M.A. (2008). Differential effects of resistance and endurance exercise in the fed state on signalling molecule phosphorylation and protein synthesis in human muscle. *J Physiol* (Lond), Vol. 586, pp. 3701-3717.

Wu, T., Gao, X., Chen, M., & van Dam, R.M. (2009). Long-term effectiveness of diet-plus-exercise interventions vs. diet-only interventions for weight loss: a meta-analysis. *Obes Rev*, Vol. 10, pp. 313-323.

Zakrzewski, J.K., & Tolfrey, K. (2011a). Exercise protocols to estimate Fatmax and maximal fat oxidation in children. *Pediatr Exerc Sci*, Vol. 23 No. 1, pp. 122-135.

Zakrzewski, J.K., & Tolfrey, K. (2011b). Comparison of fat oxidation over a range of intensities during treadmill and cycling exercise in children. *Eur J Appl Physiol*, Vol. 21.

Zuntz, N. (1901). Über die Bedeutung der verschiedenen Nährstoffe als Erzeuger der Muskelkraft. *Pflugers Arch*, Vol. 83, pp. 557-571.

2

Physical Activity Measures in Children – Which Method to Use?

Juliette Hussey
F.T.C.D. Discipline of Physiotherapy, School of Medicine,
Trinity Centre for Health Sciences, St James's Hospital, Dublin
Ireland

1. Introduction

There is increasing evidence supporting the health benefits of physical activity in children both in the immediate term in terms of body composition and in the longer term in the prevention of risk factors for cardiovascular disease, type-2 diabetes osteoporosis and certain cancers (Lee at al, 2000; Mohan et al, 2005; Blair et al, 1999; Pan et al, 1997; Tuomilehto et al, 2001; Colditz et al, 2005; Samad et al, 2005).

Physical activity is defined as body movement produced by skeletal muscles which results in energy expenditure (Caspersen et al, 1985). It can be difficult to measure physical activity as it is a variable with many dimensions including type, frequency, duration and intensity. The context and location where activity takes place may also be of interest. As a behaviour physical activity is unstable, as habitual levels of activity vary during the day, throughout the week and at different times of the year. Children have less regular patterns of activity than adults and therefore a picture of overall activity may be more difficult to capture. Spontaneous un-planned activity is typical of children, particularly younger children, and may be due to opportunities that present within their environment such as play facilities and other children. Even in older children who do engage in regular planned sporting activities, there may be a degree of unplanned activity.

The "gold standard" method of measuring energy expenditure as a result of physical activity is by the use of doubly labelled water (DLW). The technique uses stable isotopes of hydrogen and oxygen i.e. deuterium (^{2}H) and oxygen (^{18}O) ingested as water. Oxygen uptake and therefore energy expenditure are then calculated from the rate at which these isotopes are eliminated from the body. The difference between these is the amount of CO_2 produced. DLW is not a technique that is generally suitable for use in field studies due to the resources required. Even if cost were not a consideration the information gained pertains to total energy expenditure over a time period e.g. a number of days/ weeks and does not permit the examination of acute patterns of physical activity such as time spent in specific activities or intensity of specific exercise sessions.

The methods that can be used in field and most clinical studies are generally divided into the following; subjective methods such as observation and questionnaires and objective methods such as heart rate monitoring and motion sensors. The advantages and limitations of these methods will be outlined below. Before discussing these methods a synopsis of energy expenditure in children will be presented.

2. Energy expenditure in children

The largest factor that determines total daily energy expenditure (TDEE) is the basal or resting metabolic rate. It refers to the energy expended during normal cellular and organ functioning during post-absorptive resting conditions and accounts for roughly 60-75% TDEE. The second factor is the thermic effect of feeding and it accounts for approximately 10% of TDEE. The third component is the energy expended during physical activity. This can occur as a result of volitional mechanical work, such as exercise and daily activities, and non-volitional activity, such as fidgeting, spontaneous muscle contractions, and maintaining posture. It is the most modifiable component of TDEE and accounts for 20-30% of TDEE. As the output of physical activity energy expenditure (PAEE) is the most modifiable component of total daily EE, it may elicit the greatest response to intervention and subsequently, produce a beneficial impact on health related issues.

A sum of the estimation of energy expended in activity can be calculated from the data provided in questionnaires. The concept of measuring energy expenditure as a multiple of an individual's basal metabolic rate is used and examples of many activities are presented in the form of tables and published in compendiums. The compendia express EE in METs which are multiples of the resting metabolic rate (RMR).

The concept of denoting energy expenditure as a multiple of an individual's basal metabolic rate (BMR) has been referred to as 1 MET. In 1955 Passmore and Durnin published a review of measurements of human energy expenditure of various activities made by indirect calorimetry. This enabled the calculation of an individual's daily energy expenditure by the total of the metabolic cost of each activity by its duration. Initial work in this area was performed using a human calorimeter where the heat produced by a subject's metabolism was directly related to the temperature change in a contained environment, but more recent studies have used indirect calorimetry where expired air is continuously sampled.

In adults the resting metabolic rate (RMR) is taken as 3.5 mL O_2/kg/min. However despite the widespread acceptance of the 1 MET = 3.5 mL O_2/kg/min studies that have made such measures in specific cohorts have found different mean values. Byrne et al (2005) found that average resting VO_2 was 2.56 +/- 0.4 ml/O_2/kg and in this case if the 1 MET of 3.5 was used the resting metabolic rate would have been overestimated by 35%.

The RMR is higher in children and teenagers due to a number of factors including growth and puberty. RMR has been found to be higher than the generic adult value for each age group of children and Tanner stage of pubertal development and significantly higher in younger children (Harrell et al, 2005). Boys have been found to have a higher RMR than girls (Goran et al, 1997). Variation in energy expenditure in typical activity in adolescent girls of approximately 20-25% has been found (Pfeiffer et al, 2006). While a number of studies have found higher RMR in overweight children, the differences are negated when corrected for Fat Mass/Fat Free Mass (Treuth et al, 1998; Molnar & Schutz, 1997; Dietz et al, 1994).

The actual energy cost of adult type activities may also be higher due to the smaller muscle mass in children. Generally it is believed that the adult MET values should be multiplied by the child's RMR for an estimation of EE. Clearly in light of the increasing prevalence of childhood obesity there is a need for further work into the actual energy expenditure due to physical activity in children.

3. Observation methods

Observation methods of determining physical activity are generally used only in documenting workplace activity or in young children who are confined to a physical area e.g. a school playground. Observers are trained to note behavioural information about the types of activities, the time spent in each activity and the frequency of such. Short time periods may not be reflective of habitual physical activity but observing for longer periods can be tedious and may lead to inaccuracies in reporting information. Recording can also be done by video recording providing a permanent record. In order to obtain a complete picture of physical activity of children a number of time periods such as during school break times, lunch times and physical education classes may be required.

Information on the physical surroundings which may influence physical activity levels can be obtained in observational studies, and thus these studies can provide added data which may partly explain the reasons for particular findings e.g. environmental factors such as few public play areas which may explain low levels of activity (Johns & Ha, 1999). While accurate information on the intensity of activity cannot be captured by observation methods they may be useful where classification of activity is all that is required (Chen et al, 2002). Observation methods also allow data to be collected on inactivity as the length of intervals between activities can be determined. With the advent of lightweight activity monitors there may be less need for observation studies in children.

4. Questionnaires

Questionnaires and interviews are frequently the method of collecting data on physical activity in studies involving large numbers of subjects where simple, inexpensive methods are required. Questionnaires measuring activity in adults usually include questions on occupational, transport and leisure time activity. As data is collected after its occurrence the procedure does not influence performance. The validity of questionnaires measuring physical activity is difficult to establish due to the lack of a gold standard criterion against which to compare them and the problems with long term recall of activities and the likelihood of overestimation of time and intensity of activity.

The use of questionnaires in children requires specific considerations. Below the age of 10-12 years children can only give limited information about their activity patterns. Parents, teachers or other adults may give details of the child's physical activity but this information may be estimated especially for outside activities. Regular planned activity is relatively easy to remember in the short term but so much of childrens' activity is spontaneous, unplanned and of a stop start nature and therefore activity may be difficult to recall. Children can also have difficulties estimating the duration of activities and time frames may need to be provided for the child in terms of *"on the way to school, break time, way home from school, before dinner"* etc. Questions about participation in Physical Education (P.E.), method of transport to and from school and extra-curricular activities may be included to gain information on childrens' overall activity levels. Providing a list of activities can aid recall.

The Modifiable Activity Questionnaire for Adolescents (MAQA) assesses physical activity over the previous year (Aaron et al, 1993). It includes questions on the number of times in the previous 14 days the subject engaged in at least 20 minutes of hard and of light exercise. Hours per days spent watching television, videos, playing computer games each day and the number of competitive activities the adolescent participates in is assessed, as is the energy expended in regular physical activity each week.

5. Heart rate monitoring

Heart rate (HR) monitoring is an objective method of measuring physical activity. HR monitoring can provide details on the time, intensity and frequency of specific activities based on the heart rate response to such activity. It is an indirect measure which is based on the linear relationship between heart rate and oxygen uptake, so the relative stress placed on the cardiopulmonary system due to physical activity is assessed. Advances in technology have made it possible to detect and store impulses over a number of weeks prior to being downloaded to a PC. While athletes commonly use heart rate recorders to determine and monitor exercise training zones these instruments can also be used in research and in clinical practice. Heart rates above a percentage of maximum can be identified and the data can be classified into time spent in specific zones for the time measured. Inactivity can be classified from heart rates close to baseline. However if heart rate is elevated for a period of time during inactivity (e.g. due to caffeine), on data analysis it can appear that this was related to activity. Heart rate can also be influenced by emotional stress, ambient temperature, humidity, and drugs and there may be some day to day variation. In addition resting heart rate and heart rate for any given workload is influenced by exercise tolerance. Fitter subjects have higher stroke volumes and hence lower the heart rates for any given workload.

The definition of resting heart rate and its' method of determination has an impact on the apparent level of activity (Logan et al, 2000). The interpretation of physical activity level depends on the threshold used and different thresholds will lead to different overall results. In terms of providing the most accurate results individual fitness testing would need to be performed prior to using heart rate monitoring so that data obtained can be correctly interpreted. Without individual data on exercise tolerance and/or the specifics of the activities being measured, lower heart rate data could be due to less activity in someone unfit or more intense activity for an individual who had a higher fitness level. In those who are less fit the return of heart rate to baseline after activity is slower than for those more fit but in the absence of this information it could appear that a less fit person is active for longer.

In summary heart rate monitoring is a useful method of measuring overall activity in children but interpretation of how active the child is depends on the fitness of the child and the definition of resting heart rate used. In addition heart rate may be influenced by other factors not related to physical activity.

6. Motion sensors

In recent years there has been a move away from other methods as described above to the use of instruments to detect body movement. The selection of motion sensors is ever increasing and ranges from simple pedometers to electronic accelerometers which reflect not only the occurrence of body movement but its intensity and in some instances its location. Pedometers record acceleration and deceleration of the waist in the vertical direction but do not record the intensity of movement. For large studies, where total activity is of interest, the pedometer may be useful and particularly in adults where Sequeia et al (1995) have demonstrated that the pedometer could differentiate between various levels of occupational activity (sitting, standing and moderate effort occupational categories). No differentiation could be made between heavy and moderate work, where heavy work involved much static work such as lifting but in assessing overall activity in large numbers this may not be that important. In adults and children much of the activity accumulated during the day is by walking which can be captured by pedometers.

These monitors have become more available and less expensive. Their use in epidemiological studies is helping to add significantly to our understanding of activity and health status as has been demonstrated by Craig et al (2010) in CANPLAY (Canadian Physical Activity Levels Among Youth) where pedometer data on almost 20,000 children was measured. Validity, reliability and accuracy need to be determined for all pedometers used in research. The Walk4Life 2505 has been found to be within 5.3% of actual time across all speeds and was thus recommended for the quantification of physical activity in children (Beets et al, 2005). However in those with intellectual disability Pitetti et al (2009) found an underestimation of approximately 11% in registered steps and an overestimation of 8.7% in time spent in activity when the Walk4Life was compared to video-recorded activity. Outputs from different pedometers may not be comparable. In addition as stride lengths will vary considerably with different age groups of children data from similar instruments may not be comparable across age groups when distance is the variable of interest. While pedometers may be used in large scale studies due to relatively low cost it is only total ambulatory activity over the measured time period that can be captured. Data on intensity, duration or frequency of activity bouts within that period cannot be obtained.

The assessment of physical activity by accelerometry is based on the measurement of body movement or the dynamic component of activity and accelerometers may be uni-axial, bi-axial or tri-axial. Uni-axial accelerometers such as the Caltrac or the Computer Science Application (CSA) incorporate a single, vertical axis piezoelectric bender element which is displaced with movement, and this generates a signal which is proportional to the force of the movement that produced it (Puyau et al. 2002). A study examining the validity of the CSA in children walking and running on a treadmill found the activity counts were strongly correlated with energy expenditure by indirect calorimetry (Trost et al, 1998). In addition to walking and running other activities typical in children such as Nintendo, arts and crafts, aerobic warm up, and Tae Bo were measured by CSA and the Mini-Mitter Actiwatch (MM) (Puyau et al, 2002) and data was compared to by room respiration calorimetry, and heart rate measured by telemetry. Correlations of r=0.78 ± 0.06 and r=0.80±0.05 were found for the MM and r=0.66± 0.08 and r=0.73± 0.07 for the CSA for the right and left hips respectively.

While uni-axial accelerometers can only measure movement in one plane most movements in the saggital and horizontal planes are accompanied by movement in the vertical plane and some would argue that a uni-dimensional (vertical axis) activity monitor may be just as valid as a three dimensional monitor. However as many activities in young children (such as crawling and climbing) may be captured better by tri-axial accelerometers. The Tritrac R3D is a three dimensional motion sensor which measures the acceleration in three planes and integrates values to a vector magnitude. Vector magnitude is calculated as the square root of the sum squared of activity counts in each vector.

Data from the Tritrac accelerometer has been compared to the energy expenditure measured by indirect calorimetry for treadmill walking and running in 60 young adults who walked and ran on a treadmill at speeds of 3.2, 6.4 and 9.7 km.h[-1] (Nichols et al, 1999). The mean differences between energy expenditure measured by indirect calorimetry and that measured by the Tritrac ranged from 0.0082 kcal.kg[-1].min[-1] at 3.2 km.h[-1] to 0.0320kcal.kg[1].min[1] at 9.7 km.h[1] with the Tritrac consistently overestimating EE during horizontal treadmill walking. Overall it was found that the Tritrac accurately distinguished between the various intensities of walking and running on level ground, was highly reliable from day to day and was sensitive to changes in speed of movement but not to incline.

The RT3 (Stayhealthy Inc, Monrovia, CA) has followed on from the Tritrac and although smaller it has a similar output to its predecessor. The validity of the RT3 in the assessment of physical activities which included walking on a treadmill, kicking a ball, playing hopscotch and sitting quietly was examined in 10 boys and 10 adult males (Rowlands et al, 2004). The RT3 vector magnitude correlated significantly with oxygen consumption in boys and in men. When compared to oxygen uptake excellent correlations with the RT3 have been found in 7-12 year olds (Hussey et al, 2009) and 12-14 year olds r-0,96, p< 001 (Sun et al, 2008). The measurements of inactivity, low activity, and moderate activity are very accurate with the RT3. The limits of agreement for vigorous activity are wider but this may not be highly important in measuring overall physical activity where short time periods are spent in vigorous activity each day and the classification of vigorous activity is needed but the absolute measure may not be required. Up to three weeks data can be acquired when the vector magnitude is sampled every minute. Data can be downloaded to a PC and saved in an excel files so data can be presented as required. The data can be manipulated in a number of ways depending on the needs of the project in question.

In our experience one of the most useful methods in the manipulation of the data has been to calculate the mean number of minutes per day spent in different classifications of activity e.g. inactivity, light activity, moderate activity, and vigorous activity. Alternatively the energy expended in activity may be used. However the intensity thresholds used need to be standardised if data is to be compared across groups. Where intensity is defined into categories on specific cut off points there will still be a wide variation in energy expended in subjects depending on where most of the activity within a wide range occurs. Two subjects may be classified as having spent the same amount of time in moderate/vigorous activity in a day yet one may have been at the lower range and the other at the higher and yet the data analysed will be the same. Thresholds for sedentary behaviour also need to be agreed as slight changes will have considerable impact on time spent sedentary per day as most of the day is spent either sedentary or in light activity. Reilly et al (2008) have demonstrated how using the cut off points provided by different researchers on the same data set can lead to significant differences in the time spent either sedentary or in moderate to vigorous activity. There is a real need for consensus on how data is analysed so data can be compared across studies. This needs to be done in children as well as adults and in children age may need to be a factor considered.

In the past decade there has been a substantial increase in the use of portable accelerometers and examples include the BioTrainer Pro and the SenseWear Armband. The former is a biaxial accelerometer that can sample data between 15 seconds and 5 minute intervals and can store up to 112 days of data. The SenseWear Armband is also a biaxial accelerometer with a heart rate receiver and thermocoupler which can measure heat production. The monitor is a wireless armband and is worn on the upper arm in contact with the skin surface. These newer monitors along with the CSA, the Tritrac R3D and the RT3 (King et al, 2004) were evaluated against indirect calorimetry for treadmill walking and running. No significant difference was found between the mean energy expenditure of the activity monitors at all speeds. The SenseWear Armband, Tritrac and RT3 had significant increases in mean EE as the speeds increased.

Another recent accelerometer is the IDEEA which provides an advantage over other acclerometers as it employs a more sophisticated motion-capture system using two dimensional accelerometers which are placed on the thighs, feet and sternum in conjunction with pattern recognition software which allows movement patterns to be detected (Zhang et al, 2004). A particular attraction of the IDEEA is the data on the type of activity performed e.g. walking, running. The IDEEA is a portable device and consists of 5 sensors that are attached to the body and a small data collection device (or microcomputer). The basic working principle of the IDEEA is that the sensors are attached to the body in specific areas. One sensor is attached to the sternum (preferably just below the sternal angle that is supposedly perpendicular to the vertical axis of the upper body, its correct alignment is crucial for distinguishing between sitting, reclining and lying down), two sensors are placed on the anterior sides of the upper legs, halfway between the hip and the knee, and the other two sensors are placed on the inferior side of the feet. The IDEEA system monitors the body and limb motions constantly through these sensors and the different combinations of signals from the sensors represent different physical activities, which are coded for as different numbers. The monitor collects 32 samples/second while continuously distinguishing among different postures and gaits to identify the type of physical activity.

The ability of the IDEEA to correctly identify the type of activity and to quantify PA intensity allows for calculations of EE in free-living conditions. The IDEEA device has in-built equations that determine the EE in kcal.min^{-1} or kJ.min^{-1}. Recent work in our laboratory was performed with the objective of examining the validity of the IDEEA in the estimation of energy expenditure during rest, walking and running in 28 young adults against the criterion method of physiological energy expenditure by indirect calorimetry (Oxycon mobile VIASYS). Good correlations in rest and walking were detected (r=0.73, p<0.0001 at rest to r=0.49, p< 001 at 6 km/h). The IDEEA was able to differentiate between inactivity, light, moderate and vigorous activities and can provide a valid estimate of energy expenditure in rest and walking (Mc Creddin & Hussey, 2009). A particular beneficial feature of the IDEEA is identification of type of activity, gait analysis during walking and running and identifying most postures.

The multisensory monitors the IDEEA and the Sense Wear Pro Armband have also been evaluated in children along with the ActiReg. While it was found that all three needed further development, the IDEEA had the highest ability in assesses energy cost (Arvidsson et al, 2009). The Actireg contains two pairs of sensors worn over the sternum and right thigh. These sensors can determine body position and motion. Along with the data processor the body positions and motion captured are given an "Activity factor" based on a multiple of basal metabolic rate. All three monitors were comparable for resting and sitting but none accurately measured stationary cycling, jumping on a trampoline or playing basketball. The IDEEA was the only one to accurately measure stair walking. In walking and running activities the IDEEA showed a close estimate of EE where the Sense Wear accurately measured slow to normal walking but underestimated higher speeds. In health related research accurate measures of inactivity and light activity may be more important than differentiating between more vigorous activity.

Global positioning systems are potentially valuable in the assessment of physical activity. The technology permits the identification of location and such data is important in our understanding of physical activity behaviours in children. A Global Position System receiver position is calculated by measuring its distance from a number of GPS satellites. Once switched on the GPS device constantly receives signals from satellites and can calculate the distance from each. In addition to providing a profile of the child's activity patterns the GPS data can be combined with a GIS (Geographical Information Systems) database to provide information on where activity occurs and how the built environment/ transport options may influence activity behaviours (Maddison & Ni Mhurchu, 2009). GPS systems may be combined with accelerometry or other methods to provide richer data. Ideally these should be incorporated into one monitor. A small pilot study that examined how well the combination of GPS and accelerometer data predicted activity modes. Using three variables 91% of observations were correctly classified by the combined methods (Troped et al, 2008) A feasibility study in combining heart rate and GPS data was performed on 39 children during a confined time period (Duncan et al, 2009) and the system was found it to be a promising method for measuring play related energy expenditure. In this instance location, distance, speed and HR data were captured every second using the F500 model.

A limitation to the use of GPS is that it can only be used out doors and even then high buildings and trees may effect the use. The location of the GPS system may effect sitting postures as typically it has been situated on the back in harness/backpack. Increased battery life for devices such as the Garmin is required in order to establish activity patterns in children where at least four days of monitoring is recommended (Trost et al, 2000).

In summary: accelerometers are designed to measure physical movement without impeding activity in free- living situations and can measure periods of inactivity as well as quantity and intensity of movement. The ability of newer accelerometers to store data over a number of weeks permits measurement of habitual activity. Motion sensors are for the most part small unobtrusive devices that have the capacity to store movement data for prolonged time periods. The development of wireless communication to the data collection device could reduce the inconvenience associated with wearing the multiple sensors.

7. Conclusion

Increased time spent inactive has been cited as one reason for the epidemic of childhood obesity and therefore it is important to be able to obtain valid measures. This review has concentrated on methods of measuring physical activity in both clinical and laboratory settings. Observational studies are time consuming, labour intensive and involve many observers who may require intense training. Their cost may be prohibitive in epidemiological or large scale studies where the use of questionnaires may be more appropriate. While assessing physical activity through the use of questionnaires has some limitations, it is the only feasible approach for epidemiologic investigations. Heart rate monitoring can distinguish between different intensities of activity in children and therefore can be used to determine light, moderate and vigorous activity. However as higher degrees of fitness are associated with lower resting heart rates, fitness may need to be individually assessed before measurement. This would be very difficult in large cohort studies. Accelerometers can measure habitual physical activity and inactivity, are easy to wear and do not interfere or influence movement. An additional benefit of accelerometry is the ability to measure intensity of activity. The ultimate choice of activity measure will depend on the question to be studied, the size of the cohort and the resources available.

8. References

Aaron D.J.; Kriska, A.M. ; Dearwater, S.R.; Anderson, R.L.; Olsen, T.L.; Cauley, J.A., et al (1993). The epidemiology of leisure physical activity in an adolescent population.

Medicine and Science in Sports and Exercise, Vol. 25, No. 7 (July 1993), pp. 847-53, ISSN 0195-9131

Arvidsson, D.; Slinde, F.; Larrson, S. & Hulthien, L.(2009). Energy cost in children assessed by multisensor activity monitors. *Medicine and Science in Sports and Exercise*, Vol. 41, No. 3 (March 2009), pp. 603-611, ISSN 0195-9131

Beets, M.W.; Patton, M.M. & Edwards, S.(2005). The accuracy of pedometer steps and time during walking in children. *Medicine and Science in Sports and Exercise*, Vol. 37, No.3 (March 2005), pp. 513-20 ISSN 0195-9131

Blair, S.N.& Brodney, S. (1999). Effects of physical inactivity and obesity on morbidity and mortality: current evidence and research issues. *Medicine and Science in Sports and Exercise*, Vol. 31, No 11 Suppl), pp. S646-62, ISSN 0195-9131

Byrne, N.M.; Hills, A.P.; Hunter, G.R.; Weissier R.L.& Schutz, Y.(2005). Metabolic equivalent: one size does not fit all. *Journal of Applied Physiology* ,Vol. 99, No.3 (September 2005), pp. 1112-9, ISSN 8750-7587

Caspersen, C.J.; Powell, K.E. & Christenson, G.M. (1985). Physical activity, exercise, and physical fitness: definitions and distinctions for health-related research. *Public Health Reports*, Vol. 100, No.2, (March-April 1985), pp.126-31, ISSN 0033-3549

Chen, X. ; Sekine, M. ; Hamanishi, S. ; Wang, H. ; Hayashikawa, Y. ; Yamagami, T. et al.(2002). The validity of nursery teachers' report on the physical activity of young children. *Journal of Epidemiology*, Vol. 12, No. 5 (September 2002), pp. 367-74, ISSN 0141-7681

Colditz, G.A.; Sellers, T.A. & Trapido, E. (2006). Epidemiology-identifying the causes and preventability of cancer? *Nature Reviews Cancer*, Vol. 6, No. 1 (January 2006), pp. 75-83, ISSN 1474-1768

Craig, C.L.; Cameron, C.; Griggiths, J.M.& Tudor-Locke, C.(2010). Descriptive epidemiology of youth pedometer-determined physical activity: CANPLAY. *Medicine and Science in Sports and Exercise* ,Vol. 42, No. 9, (September 2010), pp. 1639-43, ISSN 0195-9131

Dietz, W.H.; Bandolini, .LG.; Morelli, J.A.; Peers, K.F.&, Ching P.L.(1994). Effect of sedentary activities on resting metabolic rate. *American Journal of Clinical Nutrition*, Vol. 59, No. 3 (March 1994), pp. 556-9, ISSN 0002-9165

Duncan, J.S.; Badland, H.M.& Schofield, G. (2009). Combining GPS with heart rate monitoring to measure physical activity in children: A feasibility study. *Journal of Science and Medicine in Sport*, Vol. 12, No. 5, (September 2009), pp. 583-585, ISSN 0813-6289,

Goran, M.I.; Hunter, G.; Nagy, T.R.& Johnson, R.(1997). Physical activity related energy expenditure and fat mass in young children. *International Journal of Obesity* , Vol 21, No.3 , (March 1997), pp. 171-8, ISSN 0307-0565

Harrell, J.S.; McMurray, R.G.; Baggett, C.D.; Pennell, M.L.; Pearce, P.F. & Bangdiwala, S.I .(2005). Energy costs of physical activities in children and adolescents. *Medicine and Science in Sports and Exercise*, Vol. 3, No.2 (February 2005), pp. 329-336, ISSN 0195-9131

Hussey, J.; Bennett, K.; Dwyer, J.O.; Langford, S.; Bell, C. & Gormley J .(2009). Validation of the RT3 in the measurement of physical activity in children. *Journal of Science and Medicine in Sport*, Vol. 12, No. 1 (January 2009), pp.130-133, ISSN 0813-6289

Johns, D.P.& Ha, A.S. (1999). Home and recess physical activity of Hong Kong children. *Research Quarterly Exercise and Sport*, Vol. 70, No.3 (September 1999), pp. 319-23, ISSN 0270-1367

King, G.A.; Torres, N.; Potter, C.; Brooks, T.J. & Coleman, K.J.(2004). Comparison of activity monitors to estimate energy cost of treadmill exercise. *Medicine and Science in Sports and Exercise*, Vol. 36, No. 7, (July 2004), pp. 1244-51, ISSN 0195-9131

Lee, IM. & Paffenbarger, R.S.(2000). Associations of light, moderate, and vigorous intensity physical activity. The Harvard Alumni Health Study. *American Journal of Epidemiology*, Vol. 151, No. 3, (February 2000), pp. 293-9, ISSN 0002-9262

Logan, N.; Reilly, .J.J; Grant, S. & Paton, J.Y. (2000). Resting heart rate definition and its effect on apparent levels of physical activity in young children. *Medicine and Science in Sports and Exercise*, Vol. 32. No. 1, (January 2000), pp. 162-6, 0195-9131

Maddison, R. & Ni Mhurchu, C.(2009). Global positioning system: a new opportunity in physical activity measurement. *International Journal of Behavioural Nutrition and Physical Activity*, Vol. 73. No. 6, (November 2009), pp. 73, ISSN 1479-5868

Mc Creddin, S, Hussey J. The validity of the IDEEA in the measurement of energy expenditure during treadmill walking and running. *International Journal of Pediatric Obesity*, Vol. 4, No. (X 2009), pp. ISSN 1747-7166

Mohan, V.; Gokulakrishnan, K.; Deepa, R.; Snthirani, C.S, & Datta, M. (2005). Association of physical inactivity with components of the metabolic syndrome and coronary artery disease- the Chennai Urban Population Study (CUPS no. 15). *Diabetes Medicine*, Vol. 22, No. 9 (September 2005), pp. 1206-11, ISSN 0742-3071

Molnar, D. & Schutz, Y.(1997). The effect of oesity, age, puberty and gender on resting metabolic rate in children and adolescents. *European Journal of Pediatrics*, Vol. 156, No. 5, (May 1997), pp. 376-81, ISSN 1122-7672

Nichols, J.F.; Morgan, C.G.; Sarkin, J.A.; Sallis, J,F. & Calfas, K.J. (1999). Validity, reliability, and calibratrion of the Tritrac accelerometer as a measure of physical activity. *Medicine and Science in Sports and Exercise*, Vol. 31, No. 6, (June 1999), pp. 908-12, ISSN 0195-9131

Pan, X.R.; Li, G.W.; Hu, Y.H.; Wang, J.X.; Yang, W.Y.; An, Z.X. & Hu, Z.X. et al.(1997). Effects of diet and exercise in preventing NIDDM in people with impaired glucose tolerance. The Da Qing IGT and Diabetes Study. *Diabetes Care*, Vol. 20, No. 4, (April 1997), pp. 537-44, ISSN 0149-5992

Passmore, R. & Durin, J. V. G. A. (1955). Human Energy Expenditure. *Physiology Reviews*, Vol. 35, No. 4, (October 1955), pp. 801-840, ISSN 8750-7587

Pfeiffer, K.A.; Schmitz, K.H.; Mc Murray, R.G.; Treuth, M.S.; Murray, D.M. & Pate, R.(2006). Physical activities in adolescent girls: variability in energy expenditure. *American Journal of Preventive Medicine*, Vol, 31, No. 4, (October 2006), pp. 328-31, ISSN 0749-3797

Pitetti, K.H.; Beets, M.W. & Combs, C. (2009). Physical activity levels of children with intellectual disabilities during school. *Medicine and Science in Sports and Exercise,* Vol. 41, No. 8, (August 2009), pp. 1580-1586, ISSN 0915-9131

Puyau, M.R.; Adolph, A.L.; Vohra, F.A. & Butte, N.F. (2002). Validation and calibration of physical activity monitors in children. *Obesity Research,* Vol. 10, No. 3, (March 2002), pp. 150-57, ISSN 1071-7323

Reilly, J.J.; Penpraze, V.; Hislop, J.; Davies, G.; Grant, S. & Paton, J.Y. (2008). Objective measurement of physical activity and sedentary behaviour: review with new data. *Archives of Diseases in Childhood,* Vol. 93, No. 7, (July 2008), pp. 614-619, ISSN 1743-0585

Rowlands, A.V.; Thomas, P.W.M.; Eston, R.G. & Topping O.R. (2004). Validation of the RT3 triaxial accelerometer for the assessment of physical activity. *Medicine and Science in Sports and Exercise, Vol. 36, No. 3, (March 2004), pp.* 518-524, ISSN 0195-9131

Samad, A.K.; Taylor, R.S.; Marshall, T. & Chapman, M.A.(2005). A meta-analysis of physical activity with reduced risk of colorectal cancer. *Colorectal Disease,* Vol. 7, No. 3, (May 2005), pp. 204-13, ISSN 1463-1318

Sequeia, M.M.; Rickenbach, M.; Wietlisbach, V.; Tullen, B. & Schutz, Y.(1995). Physical activity assessment using a pedometer and its comparison with a questionnaire in a large population survey. *American Journal of Epidemiology,* Vol. 42, No. 9 (November 1995), pp. 989-99, ISSN 0002-9262

Sun, D.X.; Schmidt, G.& Teo-Koh, S.M. (2008). Validation of the RT3 accelerometer for measuring physical activity of children in simulated free-living conditions. *Pediatric Exercise Science,* Vol. 20, No. 2, (May 2008), pp. 181-97, ISSN 0899-8493

Tuomilehto, J.; Lindstrom, J.; Eriksson, J.G.; Valle, T.T.; Hamalainen, H.; Ilanne-Parikka, P. et al. (Finnish Diabetes Prevention Study Group). (2001). Prevention of type 2 diabetes mellitus by changes in lifestyle among subjects with impaired glucose tolerance. *New England Journal of Medicine,* Vol. 344, No. 18, (May 2001), pp. 1343-50, ISSN 0028-4793

Treuth, M.S.; Figueroa- Colon, R.; Hunter, G.R.; Weinsier, R.L.; Butte, N.F. & Goran, M.I.(1998). Energy expenditure and physical fitness in overweight vs non-overweight prepubertal girls. *International Journal of Obesity and Related Metabolic Disorders,* Vol. 22, No. 5, (May 1998), pp. 440-7, ISSN 0307-0565

Troped, P.J.; Oliveira, M.S.; Mathews, C.E.; Cromley, E.K.; Melly, S.J. & Craig, B.A. (2008). Prediction of activity mode with global positioning system and accelerometer data. *Medicine and Science in Sports and Exercise,* Vol. 40, No. 5, (May 2008), pp. 972-8, ISSN 0195-9131

Trost, S.G.; Pate, R.R.; Freedson, P.S.; Sallis, J.F.; & Taylor, W.C. (2000). Using objective physical activity measures with youth: how many days of monitoring are needed? *Medicine and Science in Sports and Exercise,* Vol. 32, No.2, (February 2000), pp. 426-431, ISSN 0195-9131

Trost, S.G.; Ward, D.S.; Moorehead, S.M.; Watson, P.D.; Riner, W. & Burke, J.R .(1998). Validity of the computer science and applications (CSA) activity monitor in children. *Medicine and Science in Sports and Exercise,* Vol. 30, No. 4, (April 1998), pp. 629-633, ISSN 0195-9131

Zhang, K.; Pi- Sunyer, F.X. & Booger, C.N. (2004). Improving energy expenditure estimation
    for physical activities. *Medicine and Science in Sports and Exercise,* Vol. 36, No. 5, (
    May 2004), pp. 883-9, ISSN 0195-9131

3

Glutamine and Glutamate Reference Intervals as a Clinical Tool to Detect Training Intolerance During Training and Overtraining

Rodrigo Hohl[1], Lázaro Alessandro Soares Nunes[1],
Rafael Alkmin Reis[1], René Brenzikofer[1], Rodrigo Perroni Ferraresso[1],
Foued Salmen Spindola[2] and Denise Vaz Macedo[1]
[1]Laboratory of Exercise Biochemistry (LABEX), Biology Institute,
University State of Campinas (UNICAMP),
[2]Laboratory of Biochemistry and Molecular Biology (LABIBI),
Federal University of Uberlândia (UFU)
Brazil

1. Introduction

1.1 Training and overtraining

A training process consists of a sum of repeated exercise sessions with gradual overloads that are performed in a systematised and programmed way. The workload can be manipulated through variables such as weight load resistance, speed, duration, pauses between stimuli, muscular action, movement speed, amplitude, weekly frequency, number of sessions per day, number of exercises per session and the combination of different exercises in the same session.

Exercise triggers the synthesis of several enzymes and structural proteins that adapt tissues, organs and systems to changes in cellular homeostasis, in a task-oriented way and depending on the exercise stimulus. This set of chronic physiological and metabolic changes, currently termed supercompensation, allows for a more efficient and sustainable physiological environment during voluntary physical activity. Supercompensation supplies energy economy for habitual physical activities or enhances the energy supply during exercises of high metabolic demands. Recently, our group demonstrated, using proteomic analyses of rat muscle, that only one stimulus of exhaustive, incremental exercise (approximately 30 min) is enough to produce an acute, generalised, metabolic response in the muscular fibre (Gandra et al., 2010). This probably occurs to minimise the stress that will occur in a subsequent exercise session and, in the long term, the cumulative effects of exercise on gene expression lead to specific muscle phenotypic alterations, which is a major aspect of performance enhancement.

However, supercompensation is only achieved when the ratio between overload and recovery time is individually balanced. Damaged tissue structures resulting from the exercise stimulus are repaired during recovery, when rest and food intake are crucial for the energy supply that is required for the synthesis of new proteins and cellular components.

On the other hand, an excess of rest and a lack of exercise load may cause a loss of phenotypic adaptation, or performance stagnation. Therefore, athletes routinely use a continuous process of intense training to achieve maximal competitive performance (Bompa & Haff, 2009; Meeusen et al. 2006). The training load can be manipulated through substantial increases in duration, frequency, intensity or multiple variables simultaneously, along with a reduction of the regenerative period. However, a persistent imbalance between exercise load and recovery time can also lead to a state of chronic fatigue associated with previously acquired performance decrement, generally called overtraining (OT).

Throughout the years, different nomenclatures have been used to describe this loss of performance in previously well-adapted individuals, such as overtraining, overtraining syndrome (OTS), overreaching, non-functional overreaching (NFOR), staleness and chronic fatigue. Independent of the terminology, decreased performance seems to be the only critical feature of OT in human beings (Halson & Jeukendrup, 2004; Meeusen et al., 2006). Furthermore, OT may cause financial loss and emotional distress to trainers and athletes.

The European College of Sport Science proposed a change in terminology for OT (Meeusen et al., 2006). They defined OT as a continuous process of intense training that can generate different outcomes, depending on performance states. Upkeep, or a possible increase in performance after a brief recovery period (days to weeks), was named functional overreaching (FOR); meanwhile, a prolonged decay in performance, reversed only by a long regenerative period (weeks to months) was named non-functional overreaching (NFOR). Finally, the extreme state of the OT process was named OTS, where recovery may take years or may never happen.

The NFOR and OTS states can be associated with one or more symptoms, including accentuated catabolic state; physiological, immunological and biochemical alterations; increased incidence of injury; and mood alterations (Halson & Jeukendrup, 2004). Still, there is no set of conclusive characteristics that define the NFOR and OTS states. Diagnosis is only possible when a decrease in performance cannot be explained by other factors, such as high levels of muscle microtrauma (which is characterised by increased blood concentrations of muscle injury markers such as creatine kinase and lactate dehydrogenase), contusions, diseases, infections, allergies and abnormal cardiac symptoms (Meeusen et al., 2006). Elite athletes are susceptible to OT outcomes because they are constantly submitted to OT to maintain high physical performance during the training season. However, amateur sportsmen who do not respect the time for recovery between stimuli are also susceptible to undesirable OT outcomes.

There are many theories regarding the biological basis of the training–OT *continuum*, but the underlying mechanisms remain to be validated experimentally. Experimental difficulties that have impeded progress in this field include variability of research studies, the contradiction of applying a training program that aims to reduce functional physiological capacity and the lack of volunteer athletes willing to risk losing a season of training and competitions (Halson & Jeukendrup, 2004). These obstacles limit data collection to anecdotes from athletes who have been diagnosed as overtrained (Halson & Jeukendrup, 2004) due to the intensification of the training process (i.e., OT), which is routinely utilised by athletes who hope to improve their performance. Thus, physiological and psychological limits dictate a need for research that addresses the avoidance of the undesirable outcomes of OT, maximises recovery and successfully negotiates the fine line between high and excessive training loads (Kellmann, 2010).

1.2 Overtraining animal model

Experiments in humans must meet ethical requirements to protect the physical and emotional well-being of the volunteer subjects. Those subjects must also be aware of all possible benefits and disadvantages of the experimental protocol. Therefore, one must consider the risks of possible damage to the athlete's professional and social life when he or she is subjected to an OT induction protocol. Therefore, the study of OT in animal models is endorsed by The American Physiological Society (APS, 2006), which states that '...experimental protocols that use animal subjects are therefore developed when it would not be appropriate to use human subjects for studies of exercise's impact.'

Currently, animal models are used in all biological research areas. Claude Bernard (1865) advanced the principle of studying animal models and showed how findings in animal models could be translated to human physiology. A model is an imitation object that must have similar characteristics to the imitated object and the capacity to be manipulated without the limitations of the imitated object. Therefore, an OT animal model should display a set of similar alterations that would be expected in humans. In this vein, our group standardised an 11-week treadmill endurance training model using Wistar rats, where a gradual reduction in the recovery time between exercise sessions was introduced during the last three weeks (Hohl et al., 2009). Six incremental performance tests to exhaustion were performed during the training protocol, which is described in Table 1.

Experimental Weeks	Performance tests	Training Speed (m/min)	Training Time (min)	Number of Daily sessions	Recovery between training sessions (h)
	1	(–)	(–)	(–)	(–)
1st	no tests	15	20	1	24
2nd	no tests	20	30	1	24
3th	no tests	22.5	45	1	24
4th	2	25	60	1	24
5th to 7th	no tests	25	60	1	24
8th	3	25	60	1	24
9th	4	25	60	2	4
10th	5	25	60	3	3
11th	6	25	60	4	2

Table 1. Overtraining animal model protocol

This OT animal model was characterised by an adaptive training period (1st to 8th week) followed by a period of increased daily training sessions (9th, 10th and 11th weeks). This OT model is also unique because it allows for the comparison of two distinct groups of animals separated by performance *a posteriori*. One group show continuous performance improvement after 60 hours of complete rest, characterising the FOR state; and the other group show improvement followed by a sharp drop in performance that persists for two weeks, characterising the NFOR state (Fig. 1).

Analysis of performance during training was the parameter used both for selection criteria and to define the experimental FOR and NFOR groups. Thus, similar changes observed in the training groups (i.e., FOR and NFOR) as compared to a control group likely reflect the common response to OT, whereas differences that are unique to the NFOR group reflect the intolerance of some rats to OT. This generates a performance drop that is related to the effects of OT on the intrinsic characteristics of each animal. As observed in Fig. 1, although

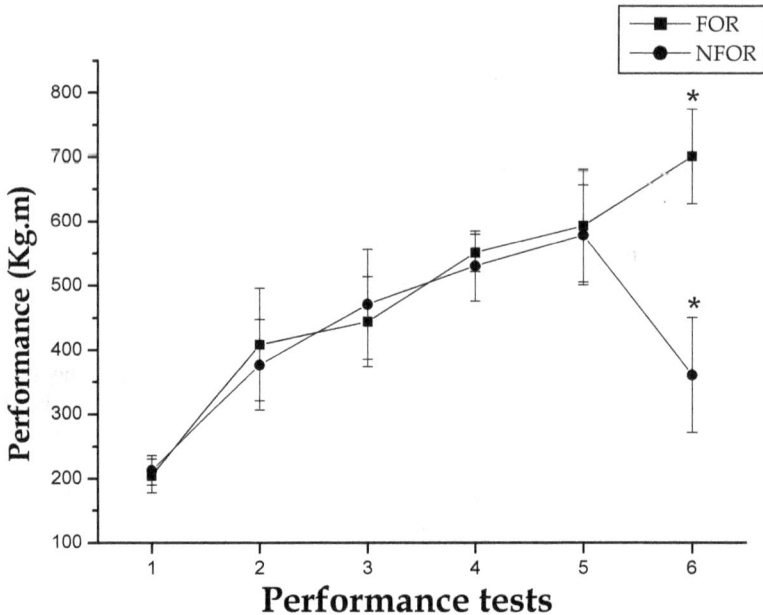

Fig. 1. Performance (mean ± sd) of the FOR (n = 11) and NFOR (n = 8) groups in the six performance tests performed during the 11-week training described in Table 1. * Significant difference between test 6 and test 5 in the paired *t* test analysis of FOR and NFOR groups (p < 0.01 for FOR and p < 0.001 for NFOR).

OT is necessary to maximise the increase in performance, it is also detrimental to the adaptive process for some animals. Lehmann et al. (1993) reported that inter-individual variability in recovery potential, exercise capacity and stress training tolerance explains the different vulnerabilities of athletes to OT under identical training stimuli. Therefore, OT is a process that deserves careful and individualised control of appropriate training loads and recovery times.

The animal model proposed by Hohl et al. (2009) has been a useful tool in seeking tissue and blood biomarkers for use in studying undesirable OT outcomes (i.e., NFOR/OTS) that are associated with an animal's tolerance or intolerance to the same OT protocol. This method can be used to compare the effects of OT in FOR and NFOR group of rats.

1.3 Glutamine and glutamate as potential biomarkers for training intolerance

Some blood biomarkers have been proposed to be associated with OT in humans (Petibois et al., 2002), but there is currently no consensus for all OT cases. One possible biomarker that could be used is the ratio of the concentration of glutamine to glutamate (Gm/Ga) in the blood. A decreased Gm/Ga ratio, due to a decrease in the glutamine blood concentration (Parry-Billings et al., 1992) and/or an increase in glutamate concentration (Coutts et al., 2007; Smith & Norris, 2000) after exercise, has been observed in overtrained humans (Coutts et al., 2007; Halson et al., 2003; Smith & Norris, 2000).

Keast et al. (1995) reported mean plasma glutamine decay from 630 µM to 328 µM in five highly trained male subjects who underwent intensive interval training sessions twice daily for ten days. The authors concluded that 'reduced plasma glutamine concentrations may provide a good indication of severe exercise stress'. Smith and Norris (2000) reported a mean (± standard deviation (sd)) glutamine concentration of 522 ± 53 μM, glutamate concentration of 128 ± 19 μM and Gm/Ga ratio of 4.15 ± 0.57 'as the extreme values for athletes who have not met conditions of overtraining and are thus managing the training load imposed', and they also proposed that 'overreaching which can also lead to overtraining may occur when the Gm/Ga ratio is 3.58'. Additionally, Halson et al. (2003) reported a mean (± sd) glutamine concentration decrease from 631± 21 μM to 475 ± 40 μM, glutamate increase from 158 ± 18 μM to 235 ± 18 μM and Gm/Ga ratio decrease from 4.38 ± 0.49 μM to 2.13 ± 0.26 μM in 'overreached athletes' after two weeks of intense training loads. The terminologies and statements of 'severe exercise stress', 'who have not met conditions of overtraining' and 'overreaching' suggest that blood glutamine and/or glutamate levels change before the dangerous and undesirable outcomes of OT, here termed NFOR or OTS. We have also found the same pattern of plasma glutamine and glutamate responses in rats subjected to OT (Hohl et al., 2009). Hohl et al. (2009) showed a significantly higher glutamate blood concentration in the NFOR group compared to the FOR group. Moreover, blood glutamine level in the NFOR group suggested a trend to a lower plasma concentration than the FOR group. Therefore, the Gm/Ga ratio in the NFOR group was significantly lower than in the FOR group (3.1 ± 0.2 and 4.5 ± 0.9, respectively), confirming previous studies with humans. Together, these data suggest that changes in glutamine and glutamate levels may be early indicators of some critical aspects of metabolism related to the individual training intolerance.

1.4 Glutamine and glutamate changes due to metabolic maladaptation

Changes in glutamine and glutamate concentrations may not be the direct cause of OT outcomes (Keast et al., 1995), but those changes may be linked to many different aspects of metabolism, which may contribute, in different magnitudes, to the undesirable OT outcomes during the training program. Significant plasma glutamine and glutamate changes could be an indication of undesirable maladaptation in progress, in other words, that the training program is becoming more harmful than helpful to the subject.

In response to deleterious challenges, such as burn damage or surgery, plasma glutamine decreases, despite increased mobilisation from muscle (Lobley et al., 2001). This is probably due to increased metabolic usage by the immune system and the liver, due to immunological challenge. Of note, the skeletal muscle is the main glutamine exporter to the blood stream (Krebs, 1980), and glutamine is mainly metabolised by immune cells such as lymphocytes, macrophages and neutrophils, which all depend on glutaminolysis for cell proliferation (Krebs, 1980).

Smith (2000) proposed that OTS is a response to excessive muscle stress, which may induce a local acute inflammatory response that may evolve into chronic inflammation and can lead to systemic inflammation. Circulating monocytes are activated in response to muscle trauma, which may increase the demand for glutamine. In addition, the increases in pro-inflammatory cytokines IL-6 and Tumor necrosis factor (TNF-α) stimulate glutamine and alanine uptake in human hepatocytes (Fischer and Hasselgren, 1991). Increased glutamine uptake by the liver from blood also favours the synthesis of large quantities of inflammatory-related, acute-phase proteins, such as C-reactive protein and haptoglobin (Marks et al., 1996). Serum proteomic analyses have shown increases in other acute-phase proteins in NFOR when compared to FOR rats (Lazarim et al., 2010), which may be linked to the decreased blood glutamine observed by Hohl et al. (2009).

Another complementary hypothesis to be considered for blood glutamine reduction is that a decrease in oxidative capacity is caused by muscle mitochondrial damage. The muscle glutamine synthetase (GS) requires α-oxoglutarate as co-substrate for glutamate synthesis that is actually used as GS substrate for glutamine synthesis with ATP and NH_3^+. It was speculated that mitochondrial injuries could limit the availability of α-oxoglutarate formed by the Krebs cycle, thereby diminishing glutamine production inside the muscle (Rowbottom et al., 1995).

This hypothesis is supported by the uncommon reduction in citrate synthase (CS) activity that we found in the NFOR group from the OT animal model protocol (Hohl et al., 2009). The unexpected chronic performance drop associated with lower oxidative capacity in the NFOR group could be related to the increased generation of reactive oxygen species (ROS, e.g., superoxide anion $[O_2^{\bullet-}]$, hydrogen peroxide $[H_2O_2]$ and hydroxyl radical $[OH^{\cdot}]$). Ji et al. (1988) have shown that increased ROS production in muscles of rats during prolonged and exhaustive exercise causes an alteration in the intra-mitochondrial redox state. This occurs by the oxidation of thiol groups (-SH) of mitochondrial enzymes (e.g., CS, malate dehydrogenase and aminotransferase alanine), linking this alteration to the reductions in the activities of these enzymes for 48 hours after exercise. We observed oxidative stress in the NFOR rat group red gastrocnemius, along with decreased CS and mitochondrial Complex IV activities, 60 hours after the last training session (at 11th week in Table 1) (Hohl et al., 2010).

The increase in blood glutamate is less understood than the decrease in glutamine during OT. A possible explanation for the increase in blood glutamate in the NFOR/OTS states is that excessive skeletal muscle microtrauma causes a reduction in the electrochemical gradient in the muscle by increasing intracellular Na^+ (Hack et al., 1996).Glutamate is carried in the cell by Na^+-dependent transporters; therefore, increased intracellular Na^+ will result in decreased glutamate carried into the cell (McGivan & Pastor-Anglada, 1994). This problem was verified in hypercatabolism (cachexia) (Hack et al., 1996), which entails a great loss of body cell mass. In addition, excess tissue trauma may be associated with reduced food intake, causing gluconeogenesis to be up-regulated in order to maintain blood glucose level (Smith, 2000). Because alanine and glutamine are the main precursors for gluconeogenesis, glutamine will decrease in this case (Wagenmakers, 1998). Muscle microtrauma and up-regulation of liver gluconeogenesis could link the blood glutamate increase and glutamine decrease in a feedback loop.

Although measuring blood glutamine and glutamate may be useful to monitor the effects of exercise programs, they can only be used to individualise medical/nutritional programs or exercise training interventions if the blood values are increased or decreased in relation to a well-defined reference population. So far, there have been no reports describing the reference intervals for blood glutamine and glutamate that can be applied in the exercise/sport sciences.

1.5 Reference interval as a clinical tool

The results of laboratory tests are often used in the clinic to diagnose, monitor or prevent many different pathological states. The most commonly used interpretation task is to compare individual blood parameter values with reference intervals that have been obtained from a defined population. Reference intervals refer to the range of values for a laboratory test that are observed in a specific population, typically described by upper and lower reference limits.

The International Federation of Clinical Chemistry (IFCC) Expert Panel on Theory of Reference Values in 1986 established the terminology, analytical procedures and statistical analyses of reference intervals (Solberg, 1987a). A *reference individual* is an individual selected for comparison using defined criteria (Solberg, 1987a). For sport science studies, it is important to consider that physical training promotes significant alterations in blood cells, enzyme activities, and protein and metabolite concentrations (Lazarim et al., 2009; Nunes et al., 2010; Sawka 2000). The training characteristics, or sport modalities, can promote different adaptive responses that can be reflected in each analyte. For example, endurance athletes have lower haematocrit, haemoglobin and red blood cell count compared to individuals who perform strength training (Schumacher et al., 2002). In addition, biochemical and haematological biomarkers may be influenced by age, body mass, genotype, ethnicity, sex, diet, circadian rhythm (Ritchie & Palomaki, 2004) and biological variation (Nunes et al., 2010). Thus, the selection of a reference individual should include the training characteristics or sport modality.

The *reference population* consists of all possible *reference individuals* of a *reference sample group*. The IFCC recommend a minimum of 120 subjects to obtain reliable estimates and confidence intervals (Solberg, 1987a). This may be a problem when one decides to estimate reference intervals for team sports, such as soccer, volleyball or individual sports. One alternative is to obtain reference intervals in co-operation with laboratories that use the same methods for screening tests in athletes. Another important issue is the selection criteria for a reference sample group. It is important to consider the training level and adaptive state of each individual. In such a way, a performance test is important to characterise the subjects that will make up an exercised reference sample group. In addition, when the reference sample group is composed of professional athletes, it is important to consider possible variations of blood parameters during the training season and competition periods (Banfi et al., 2011).

The *reference values* are the values obtained in reference individuals for an individual analyte (the constituent that will be analysed) (Solberg, 1987a). The reference values are sensitive to pre-analytical and analytical variation; therefore, sample collection and handling techniques that are adopted should be standardised to minimise the sources of error (Fraser, 2001). Some techniques must be observed to obtain the reference samples: i) taking samples at the same time of day, considering possible circadian variations of the analyte; ii) ensuring that the reference individuals have been subjected to the same conditions (i.e., fasting for at least 10 hours and no consumption of alcohol or medication for at least 2 days before testing, particularly anti-inflammatory drugs); iii) the individual's training load or fitness level should be standardised; iv) taking blood samples with a standard phlebotomy technique (e.g., placing the samples into the same type of collection tubes and preferably having the subjects in a sitting position); and v) no training or exercise for at least 48 hours before the collection to avoid the acute haemodilution effects that can occur on the blood samples (Sawka, 2000). Also, the sample transport and handling should be carefully monitored to avoid haemolysis and to keep the analytes stable.

Analysis of reference samples sometimes requires many methodological steps. Therefore, applying the same equipment, reagents and calibrators is critical to ensure that the results are accurate. The analytical variation can be estimated by calculating the analytical coefficient of variation, obtained from the mean and standard deviation of the quality control analysis. The internal quality control should analyse a sample that simulates the reference values samples (e.g., serum, plasma, whole blood, urine or saliva).

After the reference sample assay, a histogram should be generated to inspect the distribution of the data (Fig. 2). We found that glutamine and glutamate show a Gaussian (Fig. 2A) and non-Gaussian distribution (Fig. 2B), respectively. In the visual histogram analysis, it is also possible to detect aberrant values (*outliers*) and to identify possible data errors. A number of statistical tests should also be performed to detect *outliers*. The IFCC do not recommend any particular method, but the Dixon test is commonly used, and it is relatively 'insensitive to moderate deviation from the Gaussian distribution' (Solberg, 1987b). However, this method often fails when several outliers are present. The *Horn's* algorithm (Horn et al., 2001) attempts to solve this problem by employing two stages. In the first stage, the data are transformed in a Gaussian distribution, and in the second stage, the extreme values are detected based on 50% of the transformed sample (Horn et al., 2001). The aberrant values, which are identified as *outliers*, should be removed following rational criteria: the pre-analytical process should be re-evaluated, the analytical process should be checked or samples re-assayed to discharge possible mistakes (Solberg, 1987b).

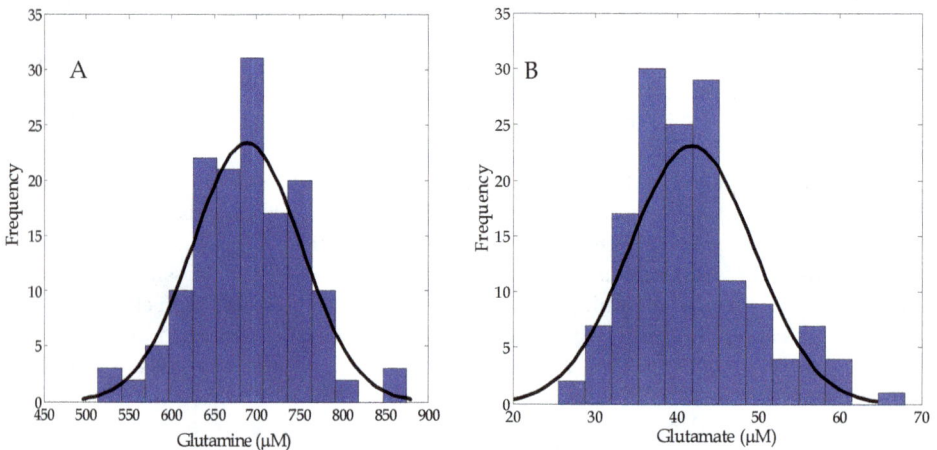

Fig. 2. Histograms representing the reference distributions of glutamine (A) and glutamate (B) in a physically active population (n = 146). The black line represents a normal fit.

Several types of reference intervals have been proposed in the literature: inter-percentile interval, tolerance interval and prediction interval. Most frequently, the reference intervals are estimated to be the lower and upper percentiles in the central 95% of the results (Solberg 1987b). This procedure is recommended because the reference intervals are easily estimated by parametric and non-parametric procedures. Other percentiles (e.g., 90%) can be adopted to narrow the intervals.

The percentiles may be estimated by parametric (Gaussian distribution) or by non-parametric methods (non-Gaussian distribution). There are several non-parametric methods for estimating reference intervals. The rank-based method is simple to apply manually or by using a computer, and it is also recommended by the IFCC and well described by Reed et al. (1971). As parametric estimates are more precise, we can transform the non-Gaussian distribution into a Gaussian distribution by applying statistical techniques (e.g., logarithms or square roots of the values) (Solberg, 1987b). To calculate reference intervals by parametric methods, we first need to test a Gaussian distribution by applying a goodness-of-fit test, such as an Anderson-Darling or Kolmogorov-Smirnov test (Solberg, 1986). The calculation will use the mean - 1.96 x sd to estimate the 2.5th percentile and mean + 1.96 x sd for the 97.5th percentile of the reference intervals (Horn & Pesce, 2003). The RefVal program, developed by Solberg (2004), is a computer program that performs many statistical routines described above, including procedures and algorithms in accordance with the IFCC recommendations. It has a simple data input routine and intuitive interface.

One difficulty in assessing the effects of training on blood parameters is the lack of appropriate reference intervals obtained from a reference population that practices regular and systematised physical activity and following the IFCC rules. The aim of this study was to obtain glutamine, glutamate and Gm/Ga reference intervals, according to IFCC rules, using automated equipment that does not require extensive laboratory skills. The reference population consisted of a cohort of young men who had increased performance in a 3000-m time trial test after four months of periodic training, when compared with their performances at the beginning of training. Secondly, we present a suggestion for a practical method to follow training effects that combines routine performance analyses with glutamine level, glutamate level and Gm/Ga ratio.

2. Material and methods

2.1 Subjects
Male volunteers (n=526), with an average age of 18 ± 1 years, participated in this study. All volunteers were students in the first stage of physical and educational preparation for a career in the army. The participants responded to a questionnaire about their use of medication and their complaints of pain and injuries caused by training. Those who were using medications or were injured were not included in the study. Volunteer subjects were duly informed about the research and signed a free informed consent form. They participated for nine months (February to October) in a regular and strictly controlled exercise program, which consisted predominantly of aerobic activities (high volume and low intensity) for three hours daily. They trained five days per week, with two days of rest. This work was approved by the Human Research Ethics Committee of the Campinas State University (CAAE: 0200.0.146.000-08).

2.2 Performance test and subject selection for a reference population
All subjects performed four freely paced 3000-m time trial tests during the training period. The tests were performed in February, April, May and October, respectively, with all subjects performing them within the same one-week period. The time trial test is a feasible way to test the endurance capacity of the subjects, considering the large sample size. Each subject ran 3000 m with a numbered wristband. At the end of the 3000-m trial, the subjects placed their wristbands on a pole. A total of five poles were placed at the end line, and one evaluator stopped a memory stopwatch every time a wristband was placed on the pole. Later, the sequences on the wristbands were matched with the stopwatch times.

The students were highly motivated for the time trial test. The 3000-m time trial was graded by members of the army school, and students failed the year if they did not perform the 3000 m in at least 14′ 59″ in the last test (October). A maximum grade (10) was obtained when the cadet performed below 11′ 30″, and the grade dropped 0.5 per every additional 10″.

Software was developed to facilitate the visualisation, identification and selection of subjects from this large sample. It is based on the use of scatter plots and allows the user, in an interactive way, to observe trends and patterns of the group's results, providing the position of the individual within the group and showing the current results of the subjects compared to previous results (Reis et al., 2011).

The example shown in Fig. 3 illustrates the comparison between the time achieved for a 3000-m time trial performed in February and May. This type of comparison allowed for visualisation of the progress of the students during the training period between tests. By clicking on 'Identity Line', a straight line is drawn with a slope equal to 1 and an intercept equal to 0, which divides the graph diagonally. This line represents the set of identical results in both tests. The points below the identity line represent the students who responded well to the physical training program, as they performed the 3000-m time trial with a lower time in May than in February. There were also a few students positioned above the identity line who, for some reason, performed the test more slowly in May than in February.

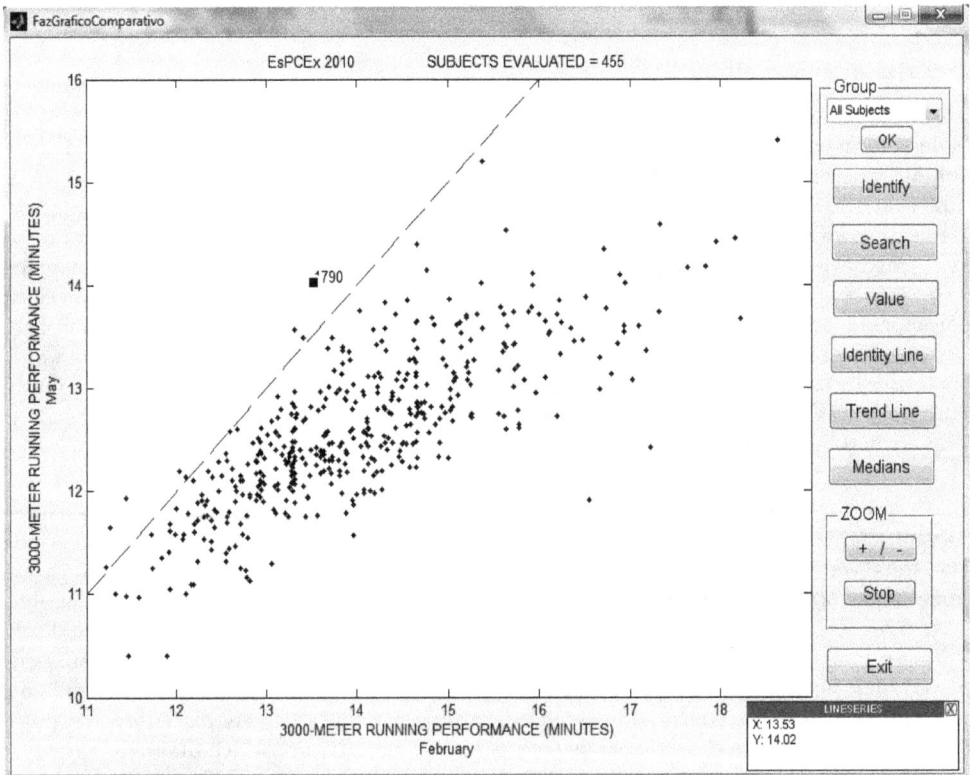

Fig. 3. Comparison between 3000-m time trials performed in February (x-axis) and May (y-axis). The dashed line represents the identity line. The text box indicates the exact value obtained by subject 1790 on both dates.

Figure 4 shows a zoom of a specific region of the graph and the selected students chosen to compose the reference population (points circled in gray). Thus, the glutamine and glutamate reference intervals presented here represent a population of young, physically active, healthy men who responded to 4 months of training.

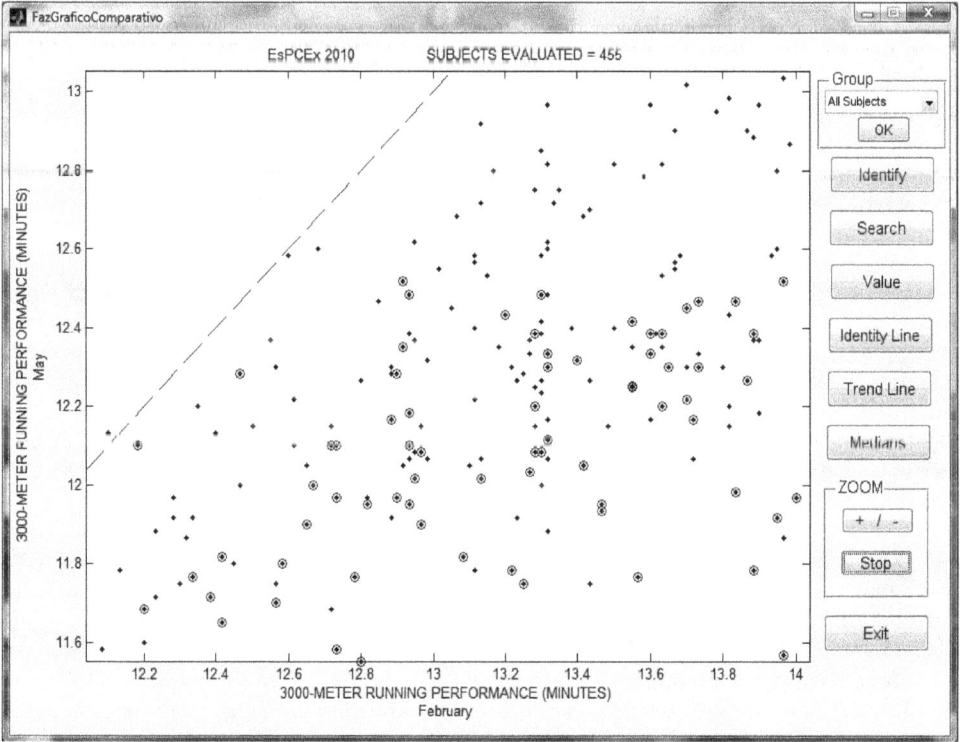

Fig. 4. Zoom applied on Fig.3. Comparison between 3000-m time trials performed in February (x-axis) and May (y-axis). The points circled in grey represent the individuals selected to establish the reference values for glutamine and glutamate. The dashed line represents the identity line.

The performances of the students in the 3000-m time trial tests between May and October were used to choose candidates to test the use of plasma glutamine level, glutamate level and Gm/Ga ratio as biomarkers of tolerance or intolerance to the same training protocol. Twenty-five subjects who were above the identity line were randomly selected as the non-responders to training (NRT), and an additional 25 subjects who fell below the identity line were randomly selected as responders to training (RT).

2.3 Collection of blood samples

All blood samples were collected after two days of rest to avoid the effects of hemodynamic variations and acute haemodilution that are induced by exercise. Blood samples were collected under standardised conditions. Eight millilitres of venous blood was collected in heparin tubes with a Vacuette® (Greiner Bio-one) gel separator to obtain plasma for glutamine and glutamate assays. Blood samples were collected in the morning after 12 hours of fasting with subjects in a seated position, transported at 4°C to the laboratory within 30 min, centrifuged under refrigeration (4°C) at 1,800 x g for 10 minutes, and then immediately separated and protected from light. Plasma samples were finally stored at -80°C and analysed within 2 months.

2.4 Assays for glutamine and glutamate measurements

Glutamine and glutamate analyses were conducted with a dual-channel YSI 2700® Select Biochemistry automated analyser (Yellow Springs Instrument Co., Ohio, USA), according to the manufacturer's recommendations. This analyser uses a platinum electrode to measure the current generated by two enzyme-impregnated membranes. When a sample is injected into the sample chamber, the glutamine diffuses to the glutamine membrane, which contains glutaminase and glutamate oxidase. The glutamine is deaminated to glutamate and ammonia by glutaminase. In the presence of glutamate oxidase, glutamate is oxidised to hydrogen peroxide, α-ketoglutarate, and ammonia. The hydrogen peroxide is detected amperometrically at the platinum electrode surface. The current flow at the electrode is directly proportional to the hydrogen peroxide concentration and thus to the glutamate concentration. The glutamate in the sample is also oxidised at the glutamate and glutamine membranes by glutamate oxidase, producing hydrogen peroxide, α-ketoglutarate, and ammonia. Glutamine concentration is calculated as the concentration measured by the glutamine electrode minus that detected by the glutamate electrode.

We used 1 mM glutamine and 0.500 mM glutamate standards to calibrate the machine after every four measurements (sample size 65 µl). The standard solutions (5 mM) were provided by the manufacturer (Yellow Springs Instrument Co., Ohio, USA) and were diluted in Milli-Q water (Millipore Corporation, MA, USA).

The 146 samples used for the reference interval were analysed within two days, and the linearity of the enzyme membranes was evaluated every day before sample analysis. The 50 samples (RT, n = 25; NRT, n = 25) were analysed within the same day with other enzyme membranes and standard kits, after evaluation of membrane linearity. All plasma samples were measured in duplicate, and the mean of the duplicate runs was used in subsequent calculations. The linearity for glutamine and glutamate was calculated with diluted standards in three concentrations: 0.300 mM, 0.500 mM and 0.900 mM for glutamine and 0.05 mM, 0.100 mM and 0.200 mM for glutamate. In all linearity analyses, the correlation coefficient and the slope (r) were approximately 1.

We used one plasma pool to evaluate the within-day coefficient of variation (CVw) and four different plasma pools to evaluate the between-day coefficient of variation (CVb). The CVw of glutamine and glutamate were 0.60% and 1.20%, respectively (n = 20 using one plasma pool). The mean CVb, within three consecutive days, of glutamine and glutamate were 2.0% and 3.8%, respectively.

The accuracy of the YSI 2700D, when analysing the amino acids in non-deproteinated plasma, was evaluated by adding four different standard concentrations into four vials of the same plasma sample. Glutamine and glutamate standard concentrations that were diluted in plasma were thus calculated by subtracting the real glutamine and glutamate concentrations previously measured in plasma. We added 0.600 mM, 0.700 mM, 0.800 mM and 0.900 mM of glutamine standard into four different vials of one plasma sample, and the standard concentrations detected were 0.620 mM, 0.692 mM, 0.812 mM and 0.892 mM, respectively. The same procedure was done for glutamate: the added standard concentrations were 0.020 mM, 0.030 mM, 0.040 mM and 0.050 mM, and the standard concentrations detected were 0.021 mM, 0.030 mM, 0.039 mM and 0.053 mM, respectively.

2.5 Statistical analysis

Initially, all data from the 3000-m time trial tests were organised using Microsoft Excel and were checked for consistency between the recorded values and their identities with the evaluated subjects. After this initial organisation, all data were imported into Matlab® 7.0, which is the platform on which the software that was designed for this study was developed. Despite having been developed in this environment, the software was compiled and can run on any computer using Microsoft Windows and does not require the installation of Matlab® 7.0. The software, Origin 6.0, was used to perform statistical analyses and to generate graphs. An unpaired t test was used to compare RT and NRT glutamine and glutamate measurements; $p < 0.05$ was considered significant. The *Horn's* algorithm was applied to detect and remove outliers (Horn et al., 2001). The RefVal program (Solberg 2004), including practical approaches and formulas recommended by the IFCC, was used to calculate the 97.5th and 2.5th percentiles of the subjects and their respective 0.90 confidence intervals. This was achieved by using parametric estimates of the glutamine levels, glutamate levels and Gm/Ga ratios that were obtained from plasma samples of the 146 volunteers after four months of daily, periodic physical activity.

3. Results

Table 2 shows the reference intervals (upper and lower limits) and the confidence intervals for healthy, physically active young men.

Analysis	Reference Interval	0.90 Confidence Interval		Subjects (n)	Outliers	Subjects Ref. Interval (n)
	2.5th - 97.5th	2.5th	97.5th			
Glutamine (µM)	566 - 798	546 - 586	782 - 813	146	514, 867, 875	143
Glutamate (µM)	31 - 59	30 - 32	55 - 62	146	26, 28, 68	143
Gm/Ga	12 - 23	12 - 12	22 - 24	146	10, 10, 26	143

Table 2. Reference intervals for glutamine level, glutamate level and Gm/Ga ratio for healthy, physically active young men.

Figure 5 presents the performance analyses of the test subjects for the 3000-m time trial, over the span of one training year. At the end of the training year (May x October, Fig. 4C) almost all subjects performed below 14' 59'' (cut off) and the 3000-m times were more homogenous than at the beginning of the year (February x April, Fig. 4A). However, the regression line in Fig. 4C approaches the line of identity due to the increase in the amount of time it took some the test subjects (n = 222) to complete the 3000-m trial in October compared to May.

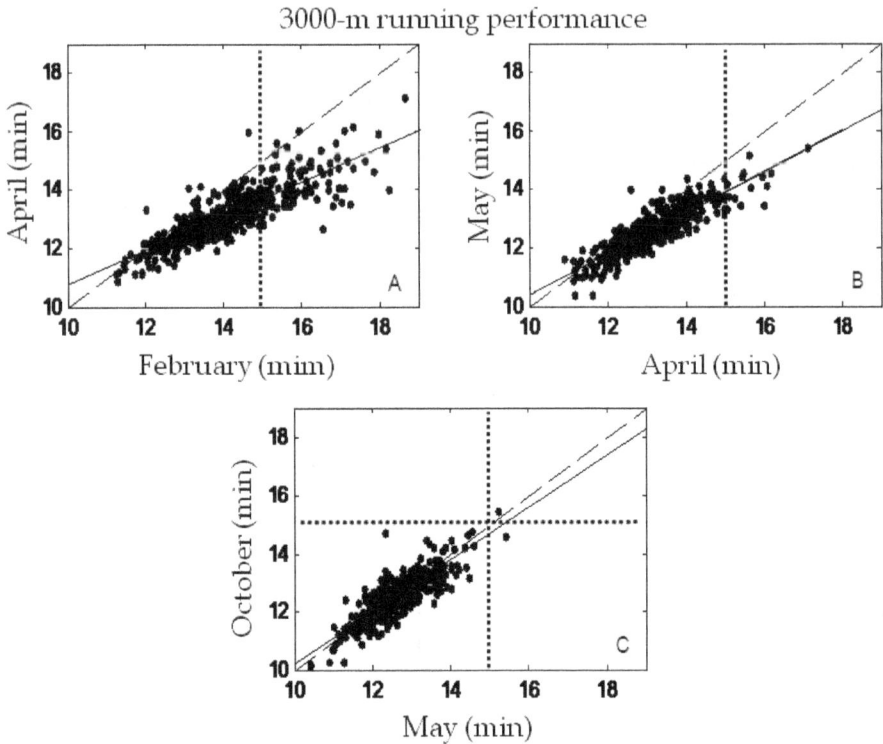

Fig. 5. Comparisons of 3000-m time trial tests over the training year. In these charts, the identity lines are dashed and the regression lines are solid. The identity line is the reference for time changes between the two tests. Subjects who fell below the identity line showed lower 3000-m times from one test to the next, so the performance was improved. The regression line shows the trend between the two 3000-m time trial tests over the year. Dotted lines show the Army School's cutting time in 14'59''.

Table 3 shows the comparisons of glutamine, glutamate and Gm/Ga between the RT and NRT groups. We observed a tendency of lower glutamine, significantly higher glutamate and significantly lower Gm/Ga ratio in the NRT group compared to the RT group.

	RT	NRT
Glutamine (µM)	669 ± 49	645 ± 63
Glutamate (µM)	41 ± 5	46 ± 6 *
Gm/Ga	16 ± 2	14 ± 2 *

Table 3. Glutamine, glutamate and Gm/Ga ratio in the RT group vs. the NRT group. RT: Responders to training (n = 25). NRT: Non-responders to training (n = 25). * Unpaired t test: significant difference between groups (glutamate, $p = 0.002$ and Gm/Ga, $p = 0.0003$).

Figure 6 presents the blood glutamine and glutamate levels of responders and non-responders to training in relation to the 97.5th and 2.5th percentile reference interval. Only four NRT subjects had Gm/Ga ratios below the reference interval, and one of them also presented a glutamine concentration below the reference interval (subject "X").

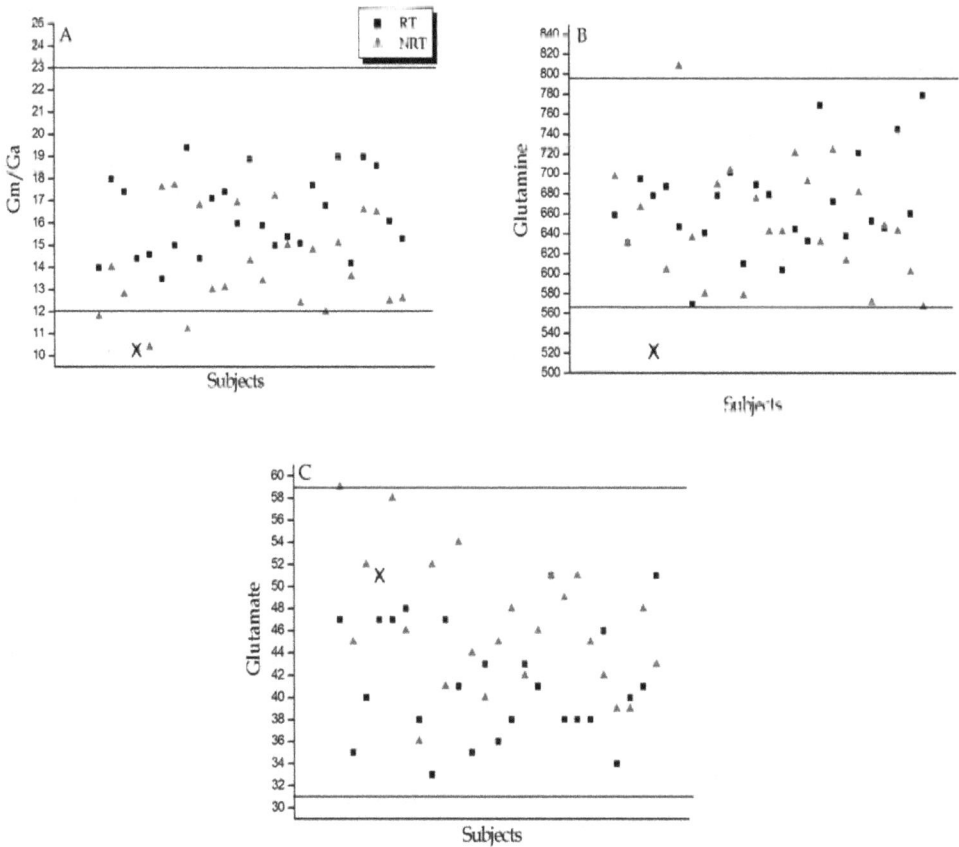

Fig. 6. Gm/Ga (A), glutamine (B) and glutamate (C) plasma levels (μM) of responders and non-responders to training (NRT; n = 25). Solid lines are the reference intervals. X identifies one subject with low Gm/Ga ratio and glutamine.

4. Discussion

This is the first study to establish reference intervals for glutamine, glutamate and Gm/Ga ratio in the plasma of test subjects, according to the IFCC recommendations. The reference intervals presented here are not comparable to other studies regarding the subject selection criteria or number (n= 143), sample preparation, sample storage or the equipment used for glutamine and glutamate measurements (i.e., YSI 2700).

4.1 Methodological aspects and confounding factors in measuring plasma glutamine and glutamate

To date, three different methods have been used to measure glutamine and glutamate concentrations: high-performance liquid chromatography (HPLC), the enzymatic method and a glutamine-dependent *Escherichia coli* bioassay (Hiscock & Pedersen, 2002). According to Hiscock and Pedersen (2002), the major difference amongst the three is in the concentrations of glutamine that is detected. When measured by the bioassay, the glutamine concentration is 40% higher than by HPLC. In addition, plasma glutamate measured by the enzymatic assay seems to be more than 200% higher than HPLC. The reason for disagreement amongst these methods is speculative. However, the discrepancies may be verified by noting the plasma glutamate values between 100 and 200 µM measured by the enzymatic assay (Halson et al., 2003; Keast et al., 1995; Smith & Norris, 2000) with values between 28 and 55 µM measured by HPLC (Abdulrazzaq & Ibrahim, 2001; de Jonge & Breuer, 1995; Van Eijk et al., 1994).

HPLC has been widely used in methodological studies that evaluate the stability of amino acids in non-deproteinated, deproteinated and neutralised samples at several storage temperatures (Abdulrazzaq & Ibrahim, 2001; de Jonge & Breuer, 1995; Van Eijk et al., 1994). Although HPLC is considered a reliable method for amino acid measurements, it also requires highly skilled laboratory personnel to guarantee reliability. According to the manufacturer (Yellow Springs Instrument Co., Ohio, USA), the YSI 2700 electrode method is highly correlated with HPLC glutamine measurements (slope 0.94 and $r^2=0.99$), with the advantage of being much more user-friendly than the HPLC method. The reliability tests performed in this study also showed outstanding accuracy in measuring glutamine and glutamate standards in plasma, good linearity and small within-day and between-day variability.

Blood plasma storage and deproteination add systematic errors that can influence inter-laboratorial comparisons of data (de Jonge & Breuer, 1996). Blood acid deproteination is frequently used to stop enzymatic activity; however, glutamine is particularly influenced by sample acid deproteination because a low storage pH accelerates the spontaneous degradation of glutamine in pyroglutamate (Khan et al., 1991). Nevertheless, the systematic error caused by deproteination is negligible when samples are stored below -70°C (Van Eijk et al., 1994). Glutamine and glutamate are stable for at least 6 months in non-deproteinated samples that are stored below -70°C (Van Eijk et al., 1994) but are not stable when stored at -20°C for more than 4 weeks (Abdulrazzaq & Ibrahim, 2001; de Jonge & Breuer, 1996). Therefore, based on those previous studies, non-deproteinated plasma stored at -80°C was used in this study.

Plasma glutamine and glutamate seem to not be affected by sex or age. Van Eijk et al. (1994) used deproteinated plasma and HPLC as their measurement technique. They showed mean glutamine levels between 663 and 693 µM and mean glutamate levels between 49 and 55 µM in healthy males 20–69 years old, with no significant differences in those amino acids between males and females. Planche et al. (2002) showed no differences in plasma glutamine and or glutamate between healthy children (12–71 months) and healthy adults (age not specified) using the YSI 2700. They observed a mean value (range min–max) of 532 (485–577) µM for glutamine and 32 (28–43) µM for glutamate. Both Planche et al. (2002) and Van Eijk et al. (1994) used only 8–12 subjects, which are insufficient numbers to consider those glutamine and glutamate values as references, according to the IFCC, who recommend a

minimum of 120 subjects (Solberg, 2004). However, those glutamine and glutamate values
are slightly lower than the upper limits of the reference intervals found in this study (Table
2), probably due to the regular physical training effect. Particularly, glutamine may increase
due to endurance training. Rowbottom et al. (1997) identified a positive correlation between
the level of plasma glutamine and improved endurance performance. In addition, Kargotich
et al. (2006) showed increased plasma Gm, VO$_2$max and time to exhaustion after 6 weeks of
endurance training (3 to 6 × 90-minute sessions per week at 70% VO$_2$ max) in active, not
well trained subjects.

Plasma glutamine level is also influenced by acute exercise. The effect of acute exercise on
plasma glutamine seems to depend on the intensity and duration of the exercise (Hiscock &
Pedersen, 2002). For instance, intermittent, high-intensity bouts of activity decrease plasma
glutamine (Walsh et al., 1998), but a single, short, high-intensity bout increases (Babij et al.,
1983) or maintains glutamine (Sewell et al., 1994). Other studies have shown that blood
glutamine decreases for 2–4 hours after acute exercise lasting more than 2 hours (Castell et
al., 1997; Rohde et al., 1996). Therefore, to use the glutamine and glutamate reference
intervals as a training monitoring tool, it is advised not to withdraw blood samples right
after acute exercise of any type. Otherwise, the effect of acute exercise may overcome the
chronic training effect on glutamine metabolism.

As well as being influenced by exercise, blood glutamine level may also change due
carbohydrate (CHO) intake. Wagenmakers et al. (1991) showed that both plasma glutamine
and glutamate decrease after glycogen depletion, compared to CHO loading during
exercise. This change is probably due to increased deamination of amino acids. Blanchand et
al. (2001) showed that resting mean plasma glutamine of test subjects was significantly
higher after 14 days of rich CHO intake (70% of total energy; mean plasma glutamine of 857
µM) than in subjects with poor CHO intake (45% of total energy; mean plasma glutamine of
610 µM). In practice, athletes and coaches should carefully plan the CHO intake of the
athlete because it can also negatively affect performance (Maughan et al., 1997). If
performance decreases and glutamine falls below the reference interval, but CHO intake is
sufficient for maintenance of liver and muscular glycogen levels during the training
program, then intolerance to training may have occurred.

For the reasons expressed so far, the reference intervals for glutamine and glutamate
presented here should be used whether the measurement conditions (i.e., storage,
preparation and assay technique) are reproduced faithfully. Sufficient CHO energy intake
for the maintenance of glycogen stores is recommended in order to avoid
glutamine/glutamate changes associated with performance decay related to poor nutrition.
Overnight fasting and 8 to 12 hours of recovery from a previous training session should be
considered before blood sample withdrawal. Finally, it is advised, for endurance training
monitoring, to use glutamine, glutamate and Gm/Ga reference intervals that have been
established from endurance-trained subjects, as presented here.

4.2 Training monitoring using self-paced time trials and glutamine and glutamate reference intervals

To test the glutamine and glutamate reference intervals, 25 subjects were randomly selected
as responders to training, due to their decreased times in the self-paced 3000-m time trial in
October compared to May (subjects below identity line, Fig. 5C). The self-paced time trial is

influenced by an anticipatory component, which, in turn, is influenced by physiological inputs prior to exercise that are related to the fitness level, expected exercise distance/duration and previous experience of the test subject (Tucker, 2009). The army students were experienced in the 3000-m time trial because they had previously performed many trials throughout the year in addition to the four officially valid ones for the army school records. In addition, they were task-motivated, due to the internal competition amongst themselves and also to the army school grading. However, many students showed poorer performance in October compared to May (subjects above identity line, Fig. 5C), and therefore, an additional 25 subjects were randomly selected from this group to test the reference intervals. No additional symptoms, such as mood alterations or increased incidence of injuries, which would also be characteristic of NFOR/OTS, were observed (Meeusen et al., 2006); therefore, those subjects were considered non-responders to training.

The same exercise-training stimulus may be either efficient or insufficient in improving performance and physiological adaptation when applied to many different subjects. An insufficient training stimulus may cause unexpected stagnation or a mild decrease in performance in self-paced time trials of subjects who are not responding (i.e., adapting) to training. The pacing strategy also depends on external factors such as the environment, race situation and the influence of other competitors (Tucker, 2009). Therefore, decreased performance may not be caused only by physiological maladaptation, but may also be a result of stagnation and test variability. In this sense, the army training program does not aim for high performance levels, as in professional athletes; the goal, in this case, is to homogenise the fitness level of young cadets on their first step in an army career. To reduce the differences amongst the 3000-m time trials, all students were subjected to a similar training program and load.

Figures 5A to 5C show that the army training program was effective in improving the 3000-m time trial for those subjects with higher initial 3000-m times (above ~15 min). However, the training program was less effective in decreasing the 3000-m time trial for subjects who performed below 14 minutes. The scattered points behaviour suggest that the army endurance training program was an insufficient stimulus for students already performing the 3000-m time trial below ~14 min early in the season (Figs. 5A and B).

However, the self-pacing time trial is also the result of a complex, physiological, integrative model of exercise. It has been stated that 'pacing is controlled by the brain, which regulates exercise intensity and alters the adopted pacing strategy to ensure that potentially catastrophic derangements to homeostasis do not occur' (Noakes et al., 2005). This definition holds that during self-paced exercise, when one is able to select an exercise work rate, performance is regulated by a central governor (i.e., brain) to prevent changes in physiological systems that may be harmful during exercise (Noakes et al., 2005; Tucker, 2009). We hypothesize that glutamine and glutamate are related to many of the chronic and acute metabolic aspects related to exercise (topic 1.4 in this chapter) which could interfere with the central governor regulation. In this sense, glutamine and glutamate reference intervals may be used as additional tools for deciding between heavier training loads to avoid detraining/stagnation, or extended recovery to avoid maladaptation. In practice, when the performance decreases and the glutamine, glutamate or Gm/Ga ratio falls within the reference interval limits, then an adjustment in the training load should be considered.

On the other hand, when the performance decreases and the biomarker levels fall outside the reference interval limits, then extended recovery should be considered.

4.3 Practical use of glutamine, glutamate and Gm/Ga ratio reference intervals

Any blood biomarker that is measured during training monitoring would be useful when the detectable changes in blood happen before NFOR/OTS outcomes. In this sense, previous studies that have measured glutamine and glutamate before and after a period of intense training loads seem to agree that changes in these amino acids occur before the extreme OT outcomes, independent of the terminologies used to define them (Halson et al., 2003; Keast et al., 1995; Smith & Norris, 2000; Souza et al., 2005). Nevertheless, intense exercise is related to the context of biological individuality and fitness level.

The occurrence of mean lower glutamine, a significantly lower Gm/Ga ratio and higher glutamate in the NRT group compared to the RT group may indicate slight differences in glutamine and glutamate metabolism (Table 2). However, mean glutamine, glutamate and Gm/Ga ratio of the NRT group were all within the population reference interval. Therefore, glutamine and glutamate mean values may be indicative of higher training stress or lower endurance capacity within a group but are meaningless regarding individual intervention.

When the reference intervals were used, only four subjects from the NRT group showed Gm/Ga ratios below the reference interval, and one of them also showed low glutamine (Fig. 6). Of note, all 25 subjects in the RT group showed glutamine and glutamate levels, and Gm/Ga ratios within the reference intervals (Fig. 6).

These results suggest that only those four subjects, and particularly the subject with low glutamine concentration (X-mark in Fig. 6), should continue the training program with close daily or weekly monitoring of their mood profiles. The remaining 21 NRT subjects probably were not responsive to the training program in the last four months; therefore, the 3000-m time trial test probably reflects stagnation and the inherent variation of the test.

5. Conclusion

For most trainers and sportsmen, the main sign that an athlete has developed NFOR/OTS is sustained poor performance and fatigue. Poor performance and fatigue, however, can also be due to many other factors, such as inadequate training sessions and poor nutrition, respectively, as well as to extraneous factors such as loss of confidence, pressure outside of the sport, and sleep disturbances. The reference intervals of glutamine, glutamate and Gm/Ga ratio presented here may therefore be useful tools to monitor adaptation to training and to thereby identify those athletes who show early signs of OT before prolonged fatigue. In addition, glutamine and glutamate blood concentrations may identify those athletes who are intolerant to a training program versus those who are not responsive to the training program because of insufficient workload.

6. Acknowledgements

The authors thank Ana Maria Marçal Porto and Ismair Teodoro Reis for technical support. This study was financially supported by the Sao Paulo State Research Support Foundation (FAPESP) and Campinas State University Foundation (FUNCAMP). Rodrigo Hohl

(09/51125-2) and Rodrigo Luiz Perroni Ferraresso (07/57512-2), receiveid scholarship from FAPESP.

7. References

APS (The American Physiological Society). (2006) Resource Book for the Design of Animal Exercise Protocols. 21/06/2011. Available from: http://www.the-aps.org/.

Abdulrazzaq, YM. & Ibrahim, A. (2001). Determination of amino acids by ion-exchange chromatography on filter paper spotted blood samples stored at different temperatures and for different periods: comparison with capillary and venous blood. *Clinical Biochemistry*, Vol. 34, No.5 (Jul), pp. 399–406.

Babij, P., Matthews, SM., & Rennie, MJ. (1983). Changes in blood ammonia, lactate and amino acids in relation to workload during bicycle ergometer exercise in man. *Eur J Appl Physiol*, Vol. 50, No. 3, pp. 405– 411.

Bernard C. (1865) An introduction to the study of experimental medicine. In: *Images from the history of medicine division*. 21/06/2011. Available from: National Library of Medicine. http://www.ihm.nlm.nih.gov.

Banfi, G., Lundby, G., Robach, P., & Lippi, G. (2011). Seasonal variations of haematological parameters in athletes. *Eur J Appl Physiol*. Vol. 111, No. 1 (Jan), pp. 9–16.

Blanchard, MA., Jordan, G., Desbrow, B., Mackinnon, LT., & Jenkins, DG. (2001) The influence of diet and exercise on muscle and plasma glutamine concentrations. *Med. Sci. Sports Exerc.*, Vol. 33, No. 1(Jan), pp. 69-74.

Bompa, TO. & Haff, GG. (2009). The Basis for training (2009) In: *Periodization: theory and methodology of training*, pp. 3-26, 5th ed. : Human Kinetics; United States.

Castell, LM., Poortmans, JR., Leclercq R, Brasseur M, Duchateau J, & Newsholme EA.(1997). Some aspects of the acute phase response after a marathon race, and the effects of glutamine supplementation. *Eur J Appl Physiol*, Vol. 75, No.1, pp. 47–53.

Coutts, AJ., Reaburn, P., Piva, TJ. & Rowsell, GJ. (2007). Monitoring for overreaching in rugby league players. *Eur J Appl Physiol*. Vol. 99, No. 3 (Feb) pp.313–324.

De Jonge, LH. & Breuer, M. (1996). Evaluation of systematic errors due to deproteinization, calibration and storage of plasma for amino to acid assay by ion-exchange chromatography. *Journal of Chromatography*, Vol. 677, No. 1 (Feb),pp. 61-68.

Fischer, J., & Hasselgren, PO. (1991). Cytokines and glucocorticoids in the regulation of the "hepato-skeletal muscle axis"in sepsis. *Am. J. Surg.* Vol. 161, No. 2 (Feb) pp.266-271.

Fraser, CG. (2001). The utility of population-based reference intervals, In: *Biological variation: from principles to practice*, 91-116, ISBN 1-890883-49-2, AACC Press, Washington DC.

Gandra, PG., Valente, RH., Perales, J., Pacheco, AG., & Macedo, DV. (2010). Proteomic analysis of rat skeletal muscle submitted to one bout of incremental exercise. *Scand J Med Sci Sports*, 21: n.d.

Hack, V., Stütz, O., Kinscherf, R., Schykowski, M., Kellerer, M., Holm, E., & Dröge W. (1996). Elevated venous glutamate levels in (pré) catabolic conditions result at least partly from a decreased glutamate transport activity. *J. Mol. Med.* Vol. 74, No. 6 (Jun), pp. 337-343.

Halson, SL. & Jeukendrup, AE. (2004). Does overtraining exist? An analysis of overreaching and overtraining research. *Sports Med*, Vol. 34, pp. 967-981.

Halson, SL., Lancaster, GI., Jeukendrup, AE., & Glesson, M. (2003). Immunological responses to overreaching in cyclists. *Med Sci Sports Exerc.* Vol. 35, No. 5 (May), pp. 854-861.

Hiscock, N., & Pedersen, BK. (2002). Exercise-induced immunodepression–plasma glutamine is not the link. *J Appl Physiol*, Vol.93, No. 3 (Sep), pp.813–822.

Hohl, R., Ferraresso, RLP., Buscariolli, R., Costa, KG., & Macedo, DV. (2010). Muscular Oxidative Stress and Mitochondrial Activity in an Overtraining Animal Model. In: *15th Annual Congress of the European College of Sports Science*, Book Of Abstracts, Antalya, Turkey, June, 2010.

Hohl, R., Ferraresso, RLP., Oliveira, RB., Lucco, R., Brenzikofer, R., & Macedo, D. V. (2009). Development and characterization of an overtraining animal model. *Med. Sci. Sports Exerc*, Vol.41, No. 5 (May) pp. 1155-1163.

Horn, PS., Feng, L., Li, Y., & Pesce, AJ. (2001). Effect of outliers and nonhealthy individuals on reference interval estimation. *Clin Chem*, Vol.47, No 12 (Dec), pp. 2137-2145.

Horn, PS. & Pesce, AJ. (2003). Reference intervals: an update. *Clin Chim Acta*, Vol. 334, No. 1-2 (Aug) pp.5-23.

Ji, LL., Stratman, FW.; & Lardy, HA. (1988). Enzymatic down regulation with exercise in rat skeletal muscle. *Arch. Biochem. Biophys.* Vol. 263, No. 1 (May), pp. 137-149.

Kargotich, S., Keast, D., Goodman, C., Bhagat, CI., Joske, DJ., Dawson, B., & Morton, AR. (2007). Monitoring 6 Weeks of Progressive Endurance Training with Plasma Glutamine. *Int J Sports Med*, Vol. 28, No. 3 (Mar), pp. 211–216. ISSN 0172-4622.

Keast, D., Arstein, D., Harper, W., Fry, R., & Morton A. (1995). Depression of plasma glutamine following exercise stress and its possible influence on the immune system. *Med J*, Vol. 162, No.1 (Jan) pp. 15–18.

Kellmann, M. (2010). Preventing overtraining in athletes in high-intensity sports and stress/recovery monitoring. *Scandinavian Journal of Medicine & Science in Sports*, 20 Suppl Vol. 2 *(Oct)*, pp. 95-102.

Khan, K., Blaak, E., & Elia, M. (1991). Quantifying intermediary metabolites in whole blood after a simple deproteinization step with sulfosahcylic acid. *Clin Chem*, Vol. 37, No. 5 (May), pp. 728-733.

Krebs, H. (1980). Glutamine metabolism in the animal body. In: *Glutamine: metabolism, enzymology and regulation*. Ed. Mora J & Palacios R, pp. 319-29, New York.

Lazarim, FL., Valente, RH., & Macedo, DV. (2010). Serum proteomic analysis of rats submitted to a protocol that induces the continnum training-overtraining. In: *15th Annual Congress of the European College of Sports Science, Book of Abstracts*, Anatlya. Turkey, June, 2010.

Lazarim, FL., Antunes-Neto, JMF., Oliveira da Silva, FC., Nunes, LAS., Cameron, AB., Cameron, LC., Alves, AA., Brenzikofer, R., & Macedo, DV. (2009). The upper values of creatine kinase of professional soccer players during a Brazilian national championship. *J Sci Med Sport.* Vol.12, No. 1 (Jan), pp. 85-90.

Lehmann, M., Foster, C., & Keul, J. (1993). Overtraining in endurance athletes: a brief review. *Med. Sci.Sports Exerc.* Vol. 25, No. 7 (Jul), pp. 854-862.

Lobley, GE., Hoskin, SO, & McNeil CJ.(2001). Glutamine in Animal Science and Production *J. Nutr.* Vol. 131, pp. 2525S-2531S.

Marks, DB., Marks, AD., & Smith CM. (1996). Intertissue relationships in the metabolism of amino acids. *In: Basic Medical Biochemistry* (1st Ed). Willians and Wilkins, pp. 647-666, Baltimore.

Maughan, R J., Greenhaff, PL., Leiper, JB., Ball, D., Lambert, CP., & Glesson, K. (1997). Diet composition, and the performance of high-intensity exercise. *J. Sports Sci,*Vol. 15, No. 3 (Jun) pp. 265-275.

McGivan, JD., Pastor-Anglada, M. (1994). Regulatory and molecular aspects of mammalian amino acid transport. *Biochem. J.* Vol. 229 (Apr), pp. 321-334.

Meeusen, R.; Duclos, M.; Gleeson, M.; Rietjens, G.; Steinacker, J.; & Urhaus. NA. (2006) Prevention, diagnosis and treatment of the overtraining syndrome. *Eur. J. Sports Sc,* Vol.6, No.1 (Mar), pp. 1-14.

Noakes, TD., St Clair Gibson, A., & Lambert, EV. (2005). From catastrophe to complexity: a novel model of integrative central neural regulation of effort and fatigue during exercise in humans: summary and conclusions. *Br J Sports Med*, Vol. 39, No. 2 (Feb), pp. 120-124.

Nunes, LAS., Brenzikofer, R., & Macedo, DV. (2010) Reference change values of blood analytes from physically active subjects. *Eur J Appl Physiol*, Vol. 110, No. 1 (Sep), pp. 191-198.

Parry-Billings, M., Budgett, R., Koutedakis, Y., Blomstrand, E., Brooks, S., Williams, C., Calder, PC., Pilling, S., Baigrie, R., & Newsholme EA. (1992). Plasma amino acid concentrations in the overtraining syndrome: possible effects on the immune system. *Med Sci Sports Exerc.* Vol. 24, No. 12 (Dec), pp. 1353-1358.

Petibois, C., Cazorla, G., Poortmans, JR., & Déléris G. (2002). Biochemical Aspects of Overtraining in Endurance Sports. *Sports Med*, Vol. 32, No. 13, pp. 867-878.

Planche, T., Dzeing, A., Emmerson, AC., Onanga, M., Kremsner, PG., Engel, K., Kombila, M., Ngou-Milama, E., & Krishna S. (2002). Plasma glutamine and glutamate concentrations in Gabonese children with Plasmodium falciparum infection. *Q J Med*, Vol. 95, No.2 (Feb), pp. 89–97.

Reed, AH., Henry, RJ., & Mason, WB. (1971). Influence of Statistical Method Used on the Resulting Estimate of Normal Range. *Clin Chem*, Vol. 17, No 4, pp. 275-284.

Reis, RA., Macedo, DV., & Brenzikofer, R. (2011). New Software For The Identification OfIndividualized Responses To Physical Tests In Large Groups Of Subjects. *Port. J. Sports Sci.Vol.*11, Suppl. 2, pp. 927-930.

Ritchie, RF. & Palomaki, G. (2004). Selecting clinically relevant populations for reference intervals. *Clin Chem Lab Med*. Vol.42, No. 7 (Jul), pp. 702-709.

Rohde, T., MacLean, DA., Hartkopp, A., & Pedersen, BK. (1996). The immune system and serum glutamine during a triathlon. *Eur J Appl Physiol*, Vol. 74, No. 5, pp. 428–434.

Rowbottom D, Keast D, Garcia-Webb P, & Morton A. (1997). Training adaptation and biological changes among well treined male atlets. *Med Sci Sports Exerc*, Vol. 29, No. 9 (Sep), pp. 1233–1239.

Rowbottom, DG., Keast, C., & Goodman, C. (1995). The haematological, biochemical and immonulogical profile of athletes suffering from the overtraining syndrome. *Eur. J. Appl. Physiol.* Vol. 70, pp. 502-509.

Sawka, MN., Convertino, VA., Eichner, R., Schinieder, SM., & Young, AG. (2000). Blood volume: importance and adaptations to exercise training, environmental stresses, and trauma/sickness. *Med Sci Sports Exerc*, V. 32, No.2 (Feb), pp. 332-348.

Schumacher, YO., Schmid, A., Grathwohl, D., Bultermann, D., & Berg, A. (2002). Hematological indices and iron status in athletes of various sports and performances. *Med. Sci. Sports Exerc.* Vol. 34, No. 5 (May), pp.869-875.

Sewell, DA., Gleeson, M., & Blannin, AK. (1994). Hyperammonaemia in relation to high-intensity exercise duration in man. *Eur J Appl Physiol*, Vol. 69, No. 4, pp. 350–354.

Smith LL. (2000). Cytokine hypothesis of overtraining: a physiological adaptation to excessive stress? *Med Sci Sports Exerc.* Vol. 32, No. 2 (Feb), pp. 317-331.

Smith, DJ. & Norris, SR. (2000). Changes in glutamine and glutamate concentrations for tracking training tolerance. *Med. Sci. Sports Exerc.* Vol. 32, No. 3 (Mar), pp. 684-689.

Solberg, HE. (2004). The IFCC recommendations on estimation of reference intervals. The RefVal Program. *Clin Chem Lab Med*, Vol.42, No.7 (Jul), pp. 710-714.

Solberg, HE. (1987a). Approved recommendation (1986) on the theory of reference values. 1. The concept of reference values. *Clin Chim Acta*, Vol.165, pp. 111-118.

Solberg, HE. (1987b). Approved recommendation (1987) on the theory of reference values. 5. Statistical treatment of collected reference values - determination of reference limits. *Clin Chim Acta* Vol.170 (Nov), pp. S13-32.

Solberg, HE. (1986). Statistical treatment of reference values in laboratory medicine: testing the goodness-of-fit of an observed distribution to the Gaussian distribution. *Scand J Clin Lab Invest Suppl*, Vol. 184, pp.125-132.

Souza, HAC., Santos, RVT., Souza, EJC., Rogeri, P., Uchida, MC., Lancha Junior, AH., & Costa Rosa, LFBP. (2005). Plasma glutamine and glutamate in road cyclists during two seasons of training and races. *Rev. bras. Educ. Fís. Esp.*, Vol.19, No.4 (oct/dec), pp.295-306.

Tucker R. (2009). The anticipatory regulation of performance: the physiological basis for pacing strategies and the development of a perception-based model for exercise performance. Br J Sports Med, Vol. 43, No. 6 (Jun), pp. 392-400.

Van Eijk,HMH., Dejong, CHC., Deutz, NEP., & Soeters, PB. (1994) Influence of storage conditions on normal plasma amino-acid concentrations. *Clin Nutrition* Vol. 13, No.6 (Dec) 374-380.

Wagenmakers, AJ., Beckers, EJ., Brouns, F., Kuipers, H., Soeters, PB., Van der Vusse, GJ., & Saris, WH.(1991). Carbohydrate supplementation, glycogen depletion, and amino acid metabolism during exercise. *Am. J. Physiol.* Vol.260, No (6 pt 1) (Jun), pp. E883-E890.

Wagenmakers, JM. (1998). Muscle amino acid metabolism at rest and during exercise: role in human physiology and metabolism. In: Exercise and Sport Sciences Reviews, J.O Hollosky (Ed.), pp. 287-314, Willians and Wilkins, Baltimore.

Walsh, NP., Blannin, AK., Robson, PJ., & Gleeson, M. (1998). Glutamine, exercise and immune function: links and possible mechanisms. *Sports Med, Vol.* 26, No. 3 (Sep), pp. 177–191.

4

Applicability of the Reference Interval and Reference Change Value of Hematological and Biochemical Biomarkers to Sport Science

Lázaro Alessandro Soares Nunes, Fernanda Lorenzi Lazarim,
René Brenzikofer and Denise Vaz Macedo
Laboratory of Exercise Biochemistry (LABEX), Biology Institute,
State University of Campinas (UNICAMP),
Laboratory of Instrumentation for Biomechanics, Physical Education Faculty,
State University of Campinas (UNICAMP), Campinas, SP,
Brazil

1. Introduction

The training principle states that tissue adaptation depends upon overload applications. The cumulative effect of these programmed breaks in homeostasis through variations in the intensity, duration and frequency of the exercise is higher performance. However, it is important to point out that the positive adaptive response, which is reflected by increased performance, depends upon an adequate recovery time between each training session and during training sessions to result in phenotypic alterations (Hohl et al., 2009).

Training sessions and nutrition are highly interrelated. Repeated training sessions typically require a diet that can sustain muscle energy stores to execute the training proposed. The phenotypic alterations that lead to increased performance result from an intense process of protein synthesis that occurs during the recovery period and can last up to 24 h after the exercise session. This process is highly influenced by food ingestion, which offers energy and nutrients that are essential to the process and to the recovery of energy reserves (Hawley et al., 2006). Recent evidence shows that some nutrients can potentiate the protein synthesis pathways that are activated by exercise, influencing the adaptive process and performance (Hawley et al., 2011).

Professional athletes, for example, soccer players, are submitted to an annual training and competition routine with periods of recovery that are not always properly adjusted to the workload. The main problem is that the current championship schedule generally does not allow the teams to take the minimum time required for appropriate physical preparation because the different stages (competitions and physical, technical and tactical training) overlap. As a consequence, the athletes may suffer an imbalance between the effort put forth and the recovery time during the competitive season, which increases the likelihood that the workload will be excessive for some players.

Each overload stress results in different degrees of microtrauma in the muscle, connective tissue, and/or bones and joints, which trigger an inflammatory response promoting repair and muscular regeneration. These microtraumas are therefore called adaptive microtrauma (AMT). An AMT may be regarded as an initial phase along an injury *continuum*. Conceivably, this injury might progress from the initial benign AMT stage to a subclinical injury in the athlete who is training strenuously and frequently (Smith, 2000). The main challenge for the better adjustment of physical training methodologies is therefore to program a sequence of exercise stimuli that has an ideal relationship between the amount of exercise and the time to recovery between sessions and that leads to increased performance with a lower energy cost.

The longitudinal evaluation of some blood analytes may reveal markers of previously altered situations, which could prevent the amplification of the response before the performance is affected. A variety of studies using different types of exercise protocols have already demonstrated that biomarkers, such as creatine kinase (muscular overload), urea (protein turnover), creatinine (muscular mass), uric acid (the major antioxidant in plasma) and hematological parameters, suffer some modulation by exercise (Sawka et al., 2000; Pattwell et al., 2004; Lac & Maso 2004; Finaud et al., 2006; Peake et al., 2007; Lippi et al., 2008; Lazarim et al., 2009). However, there is currently no consensus about the applicability of these biomarkers as markers of training effects that effectively contribute to reaching and maintaining a better performance.

1.1 Biomarkers of training effects
1.1.1 Muscular damage

The muscle tissue may be damaged both directly and indirectly. Direct damage may be due to crush injuries (Brancaccio et al., 2010; Cervellin et al., 2010), but the main force responsible for damage is the mechanical stress that occurs during training sessions (Fielding et al., 1993; Tidball, 2005a). Indirect damage can originate from several sources that reduce membrane permeability (e.g., drugs, toxins, electrolyte alterations, bacterial or viral infections and disorders in carbohydrate metabolism) (Brancaccio et al., 2010).

Muscle damage is related to a disorganization of the myofibrillar structure and a disruption of the Z line, extracellular matrix, basal lamina and sarcolemma, allowing some of the proteins present within the cell to be release into the bloodstream (Sayers & Clarkson, 2003). Among them are creatine kinase (CK), lactate dehydrogenase (LDH), aspartate aminotransferase (AST) and myoglobin. These proteins are blood markers of muscle functional status, and an increase in their serum concentrations or activities may be an index for either muscle damage or muscular adaptation to training (Brancaccio et al., 2008; Lazarim et al., 2009).

The enzyme CK is a globular protein with a molecular mass of 43-45 kDa. It influences the availability of energy to the muscles through the exchange of high-energy phosphate from phosphocreatine (PCr) to ADP (adenosine diphosphate) for fast ATP (adenosine triphosphate) production, as follows:

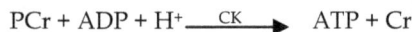

$$PCr + ADP + H^+ \xrightarrow{\text{CK}} ATP + Cr$$

Five isoforms of the enzyme are present in the skeletal muscle, cardiac muscle and brain: three of them are found in the cytoplasm (CK-MM, CK-MB and CK-BB, respectively), and two isoforms are found in the mitochondria. Because of their differential tissue distribution, they provide different information about tissue damage: CK-MM is a marker for muscle damage, CK-MB is a marker for acute myocardial infarction and CK-BB is a marker for brain damage (Brancaccio et al., 2010).

Doubts about the application of CK analysis to the monitoring of the muscular workload in athletes are derived from studies suggesting that this analyte is an unreliable marker for histological muscle lesions (Malm, 2001). Another source of doubt is that the serum CK values measured in individuals exercising to a similar degree showed high variability and a non-Gaussian distribution (Clarkson & Ebbeling, 1988; Lazarim et al., 2009). Studies of subjects performing specific exercises for short, defined periods have shown that the time of CK release into the bloodstream and its clearance from the plasma depends on the training level, type, and intensity as well as the duration of the exercise. Peak serum CK values of approximately twice the baseline levels occur eight hours after strength training (Serrão et al., 2003). After an acute bout of intense plyometric exercise, the serum CK levels reached peak values from 48 through 72 hours of recovery (Chatzinikolaou et al., 2010). Peak serum CK values of approximately sevenfold above the baseline were found 48 h after a soccer game (Fatouros et al., 2010). There are marked differences between the sexes, with lower basal CK values in females than in males. Estrogen levels may be one important factor in maintaining membrane stability post-exercise (Tiidus, 2000). Creatine kinase serum levels can also be influenced by muscle mass and ethnicity (Eliakim et al., 1995).

While these studies make important contributions to the understanding of acute responses, they do not provide enough information for longitudinal, seasonal application in actively competing athletes. An important point to be considered is that serum CK activity can arise in the absence of histological lesions as a consequence of changes in the muscle membrane permeability (Manfredi et al., 1991). Thus, monitoring the changes in serum CK may represent an indirect route for monitoring workload effects and a way to prevent sub-clinical damage due to muscle overload. However, to be a useful tool for individual adjustments in the stimulus/recovery ratio during a competitive season, it is necessary to compare individual blood values with population-based reference intervals. With this knowledge, it is possible to individualize training program interventions to adjust overloads or medical/nutritional programs only when necessary. Prevention thus leads to economy for all.

One difficulty in assessing the effects of training through blood biomarkers is the lack of appropriate reference intervals obtained from a reference population practicing regular and systematized physical activity or sports modality. To solve this problem, we have recently determined the reference interval for the plasma CK activity of blood samples obtained from 128 professional soccer players at different times during the Brazilian Championship (Lazarim et al., 2009). The upper limits of the 97.5th and 90th percentiles for the CK activity were determined according to the International Federation of Clinical Chemistry (IFCC) rules and were 1.338 U/L (CI = 1191−1639 U/L) and 975 U/L (CI = 810−1090 U/L), respectively. These percentile values were markedly higher than the values previously reported in the literature (< 207 U/L) (Rustad et al., 2004). Taking the upper limit of any percentile as the decision limit, the individual plasma CK activity above the upper reference limit may indicate the transition from adaptive microtrauma to a sub-clinical muscular injury, increasing the potential for histological damage.

In this study, we suggest the 90th percentile (975 U/L) as the upper plasma CK limit for the early detection of muscle overload in competing soccer players (Lazarim et al., 2009). We hypothesized that the same muscle membrane alterations that may increase plasma CK activity also affect the release of growth factors by muscle cells (McNeil & Khakee, 1992), explaining why changes in the plasma CK activity could also reflect muscular adaptation when the values are lower than the upper limit values. To test this hypothesis, we evaluated a soccer team monthly throughout the Championship. During the five moments of analyses, we detected only six players with plasma CK values that were higher than 975 U/L. These players were asked to decrease their training for 1 week, after which they presented lower CK values. Only one player with a CK value higher than the decision limit (1800 U/L one day before a game) played on the field, and he was unfortunately injured during the game. The CK activity in all of the other players showed a significant decrease over the course of the Championship, and the values became more homogeneous toward the end.

Later, we showed that the 97.5th percentile for a young population with improved performance after four months of systematic endurance training was similar (< 1309 U/L, CI = 882 – 1464 U/L) to that found in soccer players (Nunes & Macedo, 2008). To us, this finding justified the use of blood samples from this physically active population to establish reference population intervals for analytes that respond to exercise stimulus, such as plasma glutamine and glutamate concentrations, which are discussed in another chapter of this book.

1.1.2 Inflammatory response

The response to AMT is a subsequent inflammation post-exercise, triggering tissue repair and remodeling. The activation of the inflammatory process is both local and systemic and is mediated by different cells and secreted compounds with pro- and anti-inflammatory activities. The objective is to reestablish organ homeostasis after a single bout of exercise or after several exercise sessions. The acute-phase response involves the combined actions of activated leukocytes, cytokines, acute-phase proteins, hormones, and other signaling molecules that control the response to an exercise session and guide the adaptations resulting from training (Gruys et al., 2005).

The leukocytes are the first cells of the immune system to respond to tissue damage (Smith, 2000), and the neutrophils are the first subpopulation to migrate to the damaged site (Tidball, 2005). Neutrophils are produced in the bone marrow and represent 50 to 60% of the total leukocytes in circulation (Toumi & Best, 2003; Tidball, 2005b). Cortisol stimulates their release (Pyne, 1994), and their main function is the removal, by phagocytosis, of undesirable elements that are related to injury. To accomplish this removal, they release proteases to degrade proteins and produce superoxide anions $[O_2^{\bullet-}]$ and subsequently other reactive oxygen species (ROS; hydrogen peroxide $[H_2O_2]$ and hydroxyl radical $[OH^{\bullet}]$) through a respiratory burst that is catalyzed by NADPH oxidase and myeloperoxidase (Pyne, 1994; Tidball, 2005b). This action is the starting point for the subsequent response of repair and tissue growth.

The monocytes are the second subpopulation of leukocytes that migrate to the damaged tissue. In the cells, they undergo differentiation and become macrophages (Tidball, 2005b). Recently, it was proposed that the macrophages that invade the lesion site earlier (between 24-48 h) have different functions than do those that appear later (between 48-96 h). The main function of the first group is the removal of damaged tissue, whereas the later group has a more active function in muscular repair and secrete remodeling molecules, such as insulin-like receptor, cytokines and TGF-α, that act in the recruitment and activation of fibroblasts and collagen secretion, contributing to tissue remodeling (Butterfield et al., 2006). Moreover, macrophages signal the activation, proliferation and differentiation of stem satellite cells, an important pathway for tissue remodeling (Pedersen et al., 1998).

The lymphocytes present a biphasic response to training. There is an increase during and immediately after the effort, especially of the Natural Killer (NK) cells, followed by a decrease that can last for hours (mainly of T and NK cells). The latter effect can lead to a transitory immunosuppressive state that is related to a higher susceptibility for upper respiratory tract infections as an acute effect of exhausting, prolonged exercise (Glesson, 2007; Pedersen et al., 1998). This phenomenon is known as an open window, and it can lead to increased susceptibility for infections post-exercise (Rowbottom & Green, 2000; Glesson, 2007).

The literature related to exercise indicates distinct inflammatory responses to both acute and chronic exercise (Catanho da Silva & Macedo, 2011). In general, acute exercise induces a proinflammatory response that is characterized by transient leukocytosis (neutrophilia, monocytosis, and lymphocytosis), followed by a partial cellular immunosuppressive state. After a single bout of physical activity, there is an increase in the number of circulating leukocytes that is related to the intensity and duration of the exercise (Gleeson, 2007). Other substances related to leukocyte function, including inflammatory cytokines and inflammatory acute phase proteins are also increased. These values are generally normalized to basal concentrations within 3-24 hours (Gleeson, 2006). An increase in the serum concentrations of creatine kinase, C-reactive protein and cell adhesion molecules is also observed, in addition to an increase in the secretion of cortisol and cytokines (Pedersen & Hoffman-Goetz, 2000; Steensberg et al., 2000).

In contrast, chronic exercise (training) seems to result in a local and systemic imbalance in the anti-inflammatory status as compared to the pro-inflammatory status. This imbalance promotes tissue adaptation and protects the organism against the development of chronic inflammatory diseases and against the deleterious effects of overtraining, a condition in which a systemic and chronic proinflammatory and pro-oxidant state seems to prevail (Petersen & Pedersen, 2005; Catanho da Silva & Macedo, 2011). Some studies have shown an attenuation in the production and secretion of acute phase proteins, especially PCR (Kasapis & Thompson, 2005), greater production and secretion of anti-inflammatory proteins (IL-6) (Petersen & Pedersen, 2005) and improved antioxidant status (Petersen & Pedersen, 2005; Ji, 1999). A possible transient alteration in the production of IL-1β and TNF is dependent upon the exercise type, intensity and duration (Petersen & Pedersen, 2005). Adipose tissue also has been investigated in chronic protocols and has shown the same anti-inflammatory pattern (Lira et al., 2009).

In general, there is little evidence available to suggest clinical differences between the immune functions of sedentary and exercised subjects. Some studies have reported a lower frequency of upper respiratory tract infections in persons who are moderately active as compared to those with a sedentary lifestyle (Gleeson, 2007). Cross-sectional studies that have compared leukocyte numbers in sedentary control groups with athletes more than 24 hours after their last training session have generally found few differences (Gleeson, 2006).

We established reference intervals for hemogram in a large population (n = 357) after four months of systematized endurance training. We followed the criteria established by the International Federation of Clinical Chemistry (IFCC). The outliers were detected and removed before the estimation of the reference interval by Horn's algorithm (Horn et al., 2001). The RefVal program (Solberg, 2004), including practical approaches and formulas recommended by the IFCC, was used to calculate the non-parametric 2.5th and 97.5th percentiles, together with their 90% confidence intervals (CI), using a Bootstrap methodology. Table 1 shows the lower limit (2.5th percentile) and upper limit (97.5th percentile) of the reference intervals and their respective 90% confidence intervals for hematological parameters.

Analysis	Reference Interval	90% Confidence Interval		Subjects (n)	Outliers (n)	Total Subjects
	2.5th – 97.5th	2.5th	97.5th			
RBC (10^{12}/L)	4.4 - 5.6	4.3 - 4.5	5.6 - 5.7	357	5	352
Ht (%)	39.5 - 48.0	39.0 - 40.2	47.7 - 48.8	357	3	354
Hgb (g/dL)	13.0 - 16.1	12.8 - 13.2	15.9 - 16.3	357	2	352
MCV (fL)	80.9 - 94.9	80.0 - 82.3	94.3 - 95.4	357	6	351
MCH (pg)	26.1 - 31.6	25.7 - 26.5	31.4 - 31.7	357	9	348
RDW (%)	12.1 - 14.3	12.0 - 12.1	14.1 - 14.4	357	16	341
WBC (10^9/L)	4.5 - 10.1	4.2 - 4.7	9.7 - 10.4	357	12	345
Lym (10^9/L)	1.2 - 3.3	1.2 - 1.3	3.15 - 3.4	357	4	353
Neut (10^9/L)	1.8 - 6.7	1.7 – 2.0	6.5 - 7.0	353	10	343
PLT (10^9/L)	140 – 337	135 – 147	307 – 350	357	4	353

Table 1. Reference intervals, confidence intervals and outliers obtained from a hemogram of physically active individuals.

We found slightly higher values for counts of leukocytes (4.5×10^9 – 10.1 $\times 10^9$/L) and neutrophils (1.8 $\times 10^9$ – 6.7 $\times 10^9$cel/L) in our physically active population as compared to sedentary individuals (3.5×10^9 - 9.8×10^9/L and 1.4 $\times 10^9$ – 6.6×10^9/L, respectively) (Kjeldsberg, 1992). Our reference ranges are narrower than the traditional reference intervals for leukocyte counts, mainly due to the homogeneity of the reference population. The 2.5th and 97.5th percentile of the lymphocyte and platelet counts found were similar to those of healthy, non-exercised population values (Lym = 1.2 – 3.5 x 10^9/L) and (PLT = 145 – 348 x 10^9/L) (Kjeldsberg, 1992; Nordin et al., 2004), indicating no training effects on these parameters.

The erythrogram is a part of the hemogram that evaluates the red blood cell (RBC) number, volume and hemoglobin content. Erythrograms can be useful to diagnose sports anemia, which can impair the athlete's performance (Sottas et al., 2010, Schumacher et al., 2002). Exercise-induced hemolysis has been reported for more than 50 years (Gilligan et al., 1943). This phenomenon is associated with the destruction of red blood cells (RBC), with higher RBC turnovers in runners as compared to non-trained subjects, although it is commonly observed in other modalities (e.g., swimming, weight lifting, rowing) (Telford et al., 2003). A persistent decrease in the hemoglobin concentration, decreases in indices such as the mean corpuscular volume and the hemoglobin corpuscular volume and an increase in red distribution width (RDW) can also indicate iron deficiency (Zoller & Vogel, 2004). Three subjects presented higher RBC values and lower MCV values, characteristics of thalassemia, while four subjects were detected to have microcytosis (MCV < 80.0 fL and RDW>15%) and hypochromia (HCM=26.0 pg), suggestive of an iron deficiency: these subjects were classified as outliers and were excluded from the calculations of the reference intervals.

The data presented in Table 1 show a more narrow reference interval for RBC, hematocrit and hemoglobin in our population as compared to a sedentary subject's values (RBC = 4.4 – 5.9 x 10^{12}/L; hematocrit = 40 – 50% and hemoglobin 13 – 18 g/dL) (Kjeldsberg, 1992). The mean erythrocyte lifespan in athletes and physically active subjects may be shorter than that in non-exercised subjects, mainly due to the exercise-induced hemolysis that is inherent to endurance training (Weight et al., 1991). This lifespan may lead to the narrow values observed in the red blood cell parameters in our study. The accelerated turnover and increased rate of RBC production in endurance trained subjects can lead to a steady state of a population of younger RBCs, which are more efficient at oxygen transportation due partly to higher 2,3-diphosphoglycerate concentrations (Smith, 1995).

1.1.3 Nitrogen compounds

A prolonged, uncontrolled local neutrophil action can damage other cells near the inflammatory site due to increases in ROS production, which compromises the integrity of the muscle cells, contributing to systemic inflammation (Tidball, 2005b). A series of enzymatic and non-enzymatic antioxidants (Ji, 1999) limit the biological activity of ROS. Uric acid is one of the most important non-enzymatic antioxidants in plasma and tissues (Lippi et al., 2008). In addition, the plasma antioxidant system is also composed of other molecules and enzymes, such as ascorbic acid, proteins, vitamin E, bilirubin and peroxidases (Finaud et al., 2006).

Athletes and physically active subjects displayed an enhanced antioxidant capacity (Carlsohn et al., 2008) with increased serum concentrations of uric acid (Finaud et al., 2006). It was suggested that urate quantification could be useful for monitoring athletes in training (Youssef et al., 2008). We have found (Nunes et al., 2010) a slightly higher serum uric acid reference interval in athletes (0.24 – 0.49 mmol/L) than in sedentary subjects (0.23 – 0.47 mmol/L) (Rustad et al., 2004). This difference can be explained by the intensity of the subject's training (Finaud et al., 2006).

Biomarkers, such as serum creatinine and urea, are also used to monitor the effects of training. The urea is an end product of the degradation of nitrogenous compounds from proteins; it is synthesized in the liver and is excreted by kidneys. The main factors influencing the higher urea serum levels found during the training period may be the increased consumption and protein turnover, the reduced water intake and the incomplete replenishment of glycogen after exercise (Hartmann & Mester, 2000). The serum concentrations of urea have been used as a marker of protein catabolism and were found to stimulate gluconeogenesis during higher training loads. It was proposed that monitoring the serum urea concentrations and the CK activity may indicate an acute impairment in exercise tolerance (Urhausen & Kindermann, 2002; Lehmann et al., 1998). The serum urea level seems to respond to exercise training, and the upper limit of the reference interval observed by Nunes & Macedo (2008) (3.0 – 8.51 mmol/L) in physically active subjects at a well-trained stage is higher compared than that of a non-exercised healthy population (3.20 – 8.20 mmol/L) (Rustad et al., 2004).

Serum creatinine concentrations have long been the most widely used and commonly accepted biomarker of renal function in clinical medicine (Perrone et al., 1992). Their concentrations can be modified by age, sex, ethnicity, muscle mass and exercise (Banfi et al., 2009). The serum creatinine concentrations found in professional athletes can vary according to their modality, the training load, their aerobic/anaerobic metabolism, the frequency of their competitions, the lengths of their competition and the annual training period (Banfi et al., 2009). The creatinine reference intervals commonly used for sedentary people are 62.0 – 115.0 μmol/L. In physically active individuals, we observed higher values (77.8 – 132.6 μmol/L) (Nunes & Macedo, 2008), which are typically influenced by the higher muscle mass that is found in exercised populations, as observed by Banfi & Del Fabro (2006).

Our data have shown that the reference intervals were significantly higher in trained subjects than in a non-exercised population, suggesting a training effect on blood analytes, such as the hemogram, which were slightly different from those values reported in the literature for a healthy, non-exercised population (Kjeldsberg, 1992; Nordin et al., 2004). In the biochemical parameters, the main differences found were as follows: urea (3.0 – 8.51 mmol/L), creatinine (77.8 – 132.6 µmol/L), uric acid (0.24 – 0.49 mmol/L), creatine kinase (<1309 U/L), aspartate aminotransferase (<62 U/L) and C-reactive protein (<19.8 mg/L), all of which had higher reference intervals in trained subjects as compared to a non-exercised population (Nunes & Macedo, 2008). Now that the lower and upper reference values for the blood analytes of an exercised population are known, it will be possible to use these biomarkers to differentiate between the adaptation and maladaptation states that are induced by training.

1.2 Biological variation and reference change values

A comparison of individual blood parameter values with the reference intervals obtained from a defined, physically active population has certain limitations, one of which is that the laboratory test results may be influenced by natural fluctuations that are particular to a given analyte: this phenomenon is called biological variation (Fraser, 2004). This biological variation should be assessed in longitudinal studies with serial blood analyses of the same subjects. For example, a determined analyte concentration can change over time within an individual, reflecting the random temporal variation of an analyte in homeostasis that can occur during steady state conditions (Ricos et al., 2004).

The point of biological homeostasis (estimated by the arithmetic mean value, μ) is different for each person, and it is assumed to be constant for a certain period (e.g., months, years). The biological within-subject variation is described by the standard deviation (σ), which is obtained from measurements around the mean value (Petersen, 2005). To facilitate the comparison between individuals and analytes, the coefficient of intra-individual variation ($CV_I\%$) is calculated from the following equation:

$$CV_I = \sigma/\mu \times 100 \qquad (1)$$

The Table 2 shows an example of the biological variation in the serum CK activity from samples that were collected monthly during the training/competition season of six soccer players.

Athletes	1st result	2nd result	3rd result	4th result	5th result	Individual mean (μ)	Standard deviation (σ)	CV_I (%)
1	1232	911	1239	1232	1380	1232	173	14
2	424	455	327	347	324	347	60	17
3	218	218	147	247	189	218	38	17
4	1214	1055	667	557	560	667	304	46
5	205	111	230	116	137	137	54	40
6	427	173	200	181	273	200	67	33

Table 2. Coefficient of intra-individual variation (CV_I) related to serum CK activity (U/L) of six male soccer players.

These data show that each athlete has a different point of homeostasis for CK activity (represented here as the individual mean), and this is also true for any other analyte. These individual values span different parts of the reference interval for CK activity (Lazarim et al., 2009).

Another component of biological variation is the coefficient of variation between subjects (CV_G), which is obtained via the mean and standard deviation between different subjects. For example, if ten soccer players exhibited mean serum CK values of 390 U/L with a standard deviation of 266 U/L from blood samples collected after one month of training, the calculated CV_G for these soccer players is 68%.

Both CV_I and CV_G are influenced by age, sex, weight, diet, circadian rhythm, pathologies and physical activity (Ricós et al. 2004), and it is possible to estimate them using data banks that are available in the literature for many analytes in healthy, non-exercised subjects (Ricos et al., 1999). In addition to the biological variation, pre-analytical and analytical variation can also influence the laboratory test results. The pre-analytical variation can be minimized through the adoption of standardized instructions for the patients before sample collection, handling and transportation (Banfi & Dolci, 2003). All analytical measurement techniques (manual or automatic) have some intrinsic sources of variability. This variability cannot be completely eliminated, but it can be minimized by quality laboratory practices and the choice of sound equipment, reagents and methodologies (Fraser, 2001). We can usually identify two types of analytical variation: random (precision) and systematic (bias).

The precision of one methodology or piece of equipment is measured by replicate analysis of the same sample (a control sample). The precision will be influenced by the analytical conditions. If we use the same equipment, technician, reagent lots and calibration, we will generate smaller variations than if we take replicate results over a long period, varying these components (Fraser, 2001). The precision has a Gaussian distribution, and we can calculate the coefficient of analytical variation (CV_A%) from the mean and standard deviation of control sample replicates. The International Organization for Standardization (ISO) defines bias as *the difference between the expectation of the measurement results and the true value of the measured quantity*. In practice, bias is the difference between the results that we obtain and some estimate of the true value (Fraser, 2001).

The analytical variation can be monitored by an internal quality control (IQC) program. The protocol of IQC should include control samples that simulate the matrix of the sample analysis (Westgard, 2004). The statistical analysis of the quality control can be performed through the Levey-Jennings flow chart for each analyte and the correct applications of the Westgard control rules (Westgard, 2004). In addition, the level of performance must be established. The most widely applied term is *quality specifications*. Other terms include *quality goals, quality standards, desirable standards, analytical goals,* and *analytical performance goals* (Fraser, 2001). Considering that all analytes suffer from the influence of biological variation (intra- and inter-individual), one useful quality specification is based on biology (Fraser & Petersen, 1999). In this model, the quality specification has 3 levels for judging imprecision: *desirable performance* is defined as $CV_A < 0.5 \times CV_I$; *optimum performance* is defined as $CV_A < 0.25 \times CV_I$ and the *minimum performance* is defined as $CV_A < 0.75 \times CV_I$ (Fraser & Petersen, 1999).

The analysis of consecutive samples by comparison with values from a reference population is useful mainly when $CV_I > CV_G$ (Fraser 2004). However, the majority of analytes that are quantified in the clinical laboratory have $CV_I < CV_G$. In this case, the comparison of an individual result with a population-based reference interval might not be useful in monitoring slight effects because some individuals may show significant changes in serial testing that are within the normal limits of a reference population (Petersen et al., 1999).

A proposed alternative tool to verify a significant and biologically relevant difference between two consecutive analyses is the reference change value (RCV) or critical difference calculation

(Harris & Yasaka, 1983; Ricos et al., 2004). The RCV defines the percentage of change that must be exceeded given the inherent biological and analytical variation in the test. This tool can increase the sensitivity of serial analyses due to the exclusion of false positive results.

1.3 Calculating reference change values

The total variation associated with a laboratory test result is the sum of the component variations (pre-analytical, analytical and intra-individual biological variation). The pre-analytical variation can be minimized if we standardize the conditions of patient preparation and the procedures for collecting and handling the samples. Therefore, we must consider only the biological and analytical variation when calculating the total variation (CV_T) according equation 2 (Fraser & Harris, 1989).

$$CV_T = (CV_A^2 + CV_I^2)^{\frac{1}{2}} \qquad (2)$$

The coefficient of analytical variation (CV_A) can easily be obtained from the mean and standard deviation of the control sample analytes, and the CV_I is available in the data bank for most of the analytes from healthy subjects (Ricos et al., 1999) or physically active subjects (Nunes et al., 2010).

The term RCV was introduced by Harris & Yasaka (1983) and can be calculated by the following equation (3):

$$RCV = 2^{\frac{1}{2}} \times Zp \times (CV_A^2 + CV_I^2)^{\frac{1}{2}} \qquad (3)$$

Where $2^{1/2}$ denotes the probability of bidirectional change, and Zp denotes the standard deviation corresponding to the level of statistical significance for the bidirectional change (1.96=95% and 2.58=99%) (Harris & Yasaka; 1983; Fraser & Harris, 1989).

Recently, we have established the respective $RCV_{95\%}$ for hemograms and for certain biochemical parameters from individuals who had undergone 4 months of regular and planned physical activity (Nunes el al., 2010). We showed that the RCV values for leukocytes and for all biochemical analytes were elevated as compared to the literature values of sedentary subjects, clearly indicating a training effect on these blood analytes. However, the RCV values for the red blood cell count were slightly lower in physically active than in sedentary individuals (Nunes el al., 2010).

Soccer is the most widely played sport worldwide, and it also has many different cultural, social and economic aspects. The elite soccer player must have good, but not exceptional, all-around physical strength and must be able to effectively respond to the diverse demands of the game. Several studies have determined the pattern of activities performed and the individual distance covered during a game: these values have been used as an indication of the total work performed. It is well accepted that outfield players cover 8-12 km during a game that involves many different activities, with a rapid change in the type or level of activity each 4-6 seconds (Reilly, 1997; Bangsboo, 1994). While the majority of the exercise associated with competitive soccer is at sub-maximal intensities, the intermittent efforts with higher energy demands should not be slighted during a match, and often their successful execution determines the results of a game (Bangsbo et al., 2006).

The trade of elite soccer players produces large sums of money and affects the emotional state of soccer fans all around the world. Great savings can therefore be obtained by elite soccer players and their clubs with the physical protection of athletes. Our aim in this study was to verify the applicability of the reference interval described here and the previously determined RCVs (Nunes et al., 2010) for monitoring, through hematological and biochemical analyses, the effects of training/competition on soccer players during five months of the competitive season.

2. Material and methods

2.1 Subjects
Fifty-six male soccer players (17-19 years old) participated in this study. The athletes were evaluated during four months that included both training (pre-season) and competitive periods (regional soccer championship for players under 20). The volunteers responded to a questionnaire about their use of medications and complaints of pain and injuries caused by training or competition. Those who were using medications or who were injured were not included in the study. Volunteer subjects were duly informed about the research and signed an informed consent form. This research was approved by the Human Research Ethics Committee of the University (CAAE: 0200.0.146.000-08).

2.2 Collection of blood samples
The subjects were longitudinally evaluated through five blood samples that were collected monthly [C1 = pre-competitive period of training; C2 = after 1 month (training); C3 = after 2 months (training and beginning of competitions); C4 = after 3 months (training and competitions); and C5 = after 4 months (mainly competitions)]. The blood samples were collected under standardized conditions: 2.0 mL of total venous blood was collected in vacuum tubes containing EDTA/K3 to determine the hematological parameters, and 8.0 mL of venous blood was collected in tubes with a Vacuette® (Greiner Bio-one) gel separator to obtain serum for the biochemical measurements. The blood samples were collected in the morning after 12 hours of fasting, in a seated position, and they were transported at 4°C to the laboratory within 30 minutes, centrifuged under refrigeration at 1,800 x g for 10 minutes, were immediately separated, and were protected from light. All blood samples were collected after two days of rest to avoid the effects of hemodynamic variations and the acute hemodilution that is induced by exercise (Sawka et al., 2000).

2.3 Hematological and biochemical analysis
The hematological parameters were measured with a KX-21N Sysmex® analyzer, and the biochemical analyses (CK activity, uric acid, urea and creatinine concentration) were run in an Autolab analyzer (Boehringer) using commercial kits (Wiener Lab, Rosario, Argentina). All analyses were run in parallel with commercial serum and blood controls. To minimize analytical variations, all samples were tested by the same technician without changing reagent lots, standards, or control materials.

2.4 Statistical analysis
The percent differences between the serial results were calculated for each subject using Microsoft Excel® and were compared with $RCV_{95\%}$ to detect significant changes. As the activity of CK had a value distribution that was slightly skewed to the right, we opted to transform the data using natural logarithms (Wu et al., 2009). The Matlab 7.0 software was used to generate graphs.

3. Results

Figure 1 presents, as an example, the CK values analyzed in comparison to both the upper reference limit and the RCV established from a physically active population (Nunes & Macedo, 2008; Nunes et al., 2010). Thus, Figure 1A presents the CK values (mean, minimum and maximum) for each soccer player at five time points in comparison with the reference upper limit (97.5th percentile - <1.309 U/L), and Figure 1B presents the percentage change between successive pairs of serial results of the five time points in comparison to the RCV (119.8%).

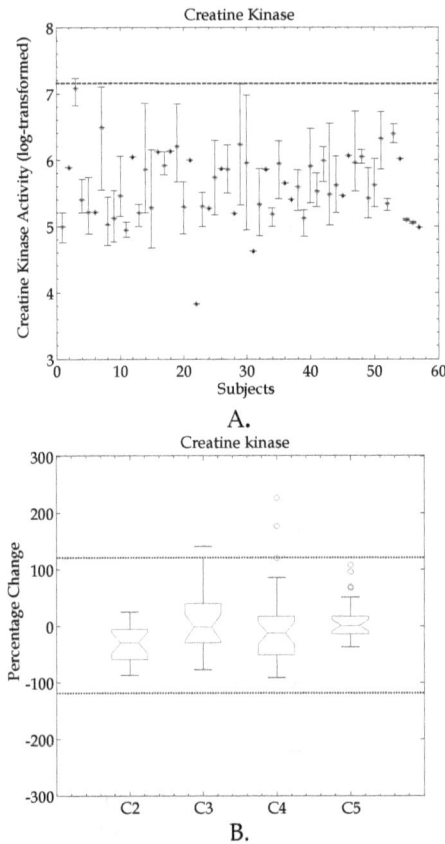

A.

B.

Fig. 1. (A.) CK values (mean, minimum and maximum) for each soccer player at five time points. The dotted horizontal lines indicate the reference interval (97.5% upper limit = 1309 U/L) from a physically active population. (B.) CK percentage change between successive pairs of serial results of the soccer players during the training/competition season. The dotted horizontal lines indicate the RCV 95% for CK = 119.3%.

We can observe that the five consecutive results for all individuals were within the reference upper values (Figure 1A). However, the comparison of the serial analytes to the RCV showed a significant increase of 119.8% in three players (Figure 1B), even though the serial results were within the upper reference limit.

It is important to point out that the behavior observed in Figure 1A and 1B was the same for all other analytes monitored. Thus, we will show only those athletes who presented at any time point a significant change, based on the RCV values, as compared to the previous analysis. The results are presented in Table 3.

Analyte	Time point	Players	Measured values current - previous (Δ)	Percentage change (%)
CK (U/L) RCV$_{95\%}$ = 119.3% RI = 1309 U/L	C3	35	535 – 223 (312)	+139.9
	C4	14	951 – 345 (606)	+175.7
		19	942 – 289 (653)	+226.0
Urea (mmol/L) RCV$_{95\%}$ = 42.5% RI = 3 – 8.5 mmol/L	C2	8	6.2– 3.7 (2.5)	+68.2
		14	4.7 – 3.2 (1.5)	+47.4
		19	7.7 – 5.0 (2.7)	+53.3
		23	4.4 – 2.7 (1.7)	+62.5
		25	3.8 – 2.6 (1.2)	+43.8
		27	5.3 – 3.5 (1.8)	+52.4
		29	4.9 – 3.4 (1.5)	+45
		32	6.4 – 3.7 (2.7)	+72.7
	C3	9	4.2 – 4.34 (1.3)	+47.1
	C4	3	4.9 – 2.9 (2)	+70.6
		32	3.3 – 6.3 (- 3)	-47.4
		38	5.8 – 4.0 (1.8)	+45.8
		42	3.8 – 2.6 (1.2)	+43.8
Creatinine (µmol/L) RCV$_{95\%}$ = 26.8% RI = 77.8 – 132.6 µmol/L	C3	4	113 – 87. 6 (25.4)	+29.3
		7	95.4 - 74.2 (21.2)	+28.6
		15	93.7 – 70.7 (23)	+32.5
		42	95.4 – 73.4 (22)	+30.1
		44	121.0 – 88.0 (33)	+37

RI= reference interval for physically active subjects; RCV = reference change value for physically active subjects; Δ = absolute difference between 2 consecutive analyses.

Table 3. Soccer players and their biochemical analytes with significant change based on RCV values.

One player at C3 and two at C4 presented CK values above 119.3%. The serum urea concentrations were significantly increased in eight subjects after the first month of training (C2). Five athletes showed creatinine values that were significantly increased at C3. Note that all of the altered analytes were inside of the reference intervals for the physically active population.

The Table 4 presents the results of the hematological parameters of those athletes that showed significant changes, based on the RCV values, as compared to the previous analysis.

Analyte	Time point	Players	Measured values current - previous (Δ)	Percentage change (%)
WBC (10^9/L) RCV$_{95\%}$ = 43.9% RI = 4.5 - 10.1 10^9/L	C2	1	7.8 – 4.5 (3.3)	+73.3
		4	6.2 – 4.0 (2.2)	+55
	C3	14	9.6 – 6.5 (3.1)	+47.7
		15	7.2 – 4.9 (2.3)	+46.9
		44	9.3 – 5.3 (4.0)	+75.5
	C4	19	10.1 – 5.4 (4.7)	+105.6
	C5	20	9.8 – 6.6 (3.2)	+48.5
		47	8.1 – 4.8 (3.3)	+68.8
		53	7.1 – 4.5 (2.6)	+57.8
Neutrophils (10^9/L) RCV$_{95\%}$ = 65.3% RI = 1.8 - 6.7 10^9/L	C2	1	5.1 – 2.3 (2.8)	+119.5
		4	4.5 – 2.4 (2.1)	+84.9
		23	4.0 – 2.4 (1.6)	+69.7
	C3	14	6.9 – 3.7 (3.2)	+86.4
		15	4.8 – 2.5 (2.3)	+92.9
		44	6.4 – 3.0 (3.4)	+113.8
	C4	19	8.6 – 3.0 (5.6)	+182.7
		42	3.9 – 2.2 (1.7)	+79.6
	C5	20	7.9 – 3.7 (4.2)	+112.2
		47	4.8 – 1.9 (2.9)	+150.8
		53	4.9 – 2.4 (2.5)	+104.6
Hemoglobin (g/dL) RCV$_{95\%}$ = 8% RI = 13 - 16 g/dL	C2	23	13.2 – 14.4 (-1.2)	-8.3
	C3	7	15.2 – 14.0 (1.2)	+8.6
		15	15.7 – 14.5 (1.2)	+8.3
		17	15.3 – 13.3 (2.0)	+15
		23	14.8 – 13.2 (1.6)	+12.1
		39	16.5 – 14.7 (1.8)	+12.2
		42	13.8 – 12.5 (1.3)	+10.4
		43	15.6 – 13.7 (1.9)	+13.9
	C4	23	13.6 – 14.8 (-1.2)	-8.1
RBC (10^{12}/L) RCV$_{95\%}$ = 8.3% RI = 4.4 - 5.6 10^{12}/L	C3	7	5.3 – 4.8 (0.5)	+10
		17	5 – 4.3 (0.7)	+15.9
		20	4.3 – 4.8 (-0.5)	-9.8
		23	5.1 – 4.6 (-0.5)	+10.3
		39	5.4 – 4.9 (0.5)	+10.4
		42	5.1 – 4.6 (0.5)	+10.4
		43	5.3 – 4.7 (0.6)	+14.1
	C4	20	5.0 – 4.3 (0.7)	+10.3

RI= reference interval for physically active subjects; RCV = reference change value; Δ = absolute difference between 2 consecutive analyses.

Table 4. Soccer players and their hematological parameters with significant changes based on RCV values.

Nine athletes were found to have elevated leukocyte counts, mainly neutrophils, at one or
more time points. We found seven athletes with hemoglobin values that were significantly
increased at C3. It is important to point out that all variations in these hematological
parameters were within the reference intervals shown here (Table 1). The exception for this
rule was the serum uric acid concentrations, as shown in Figure 2.

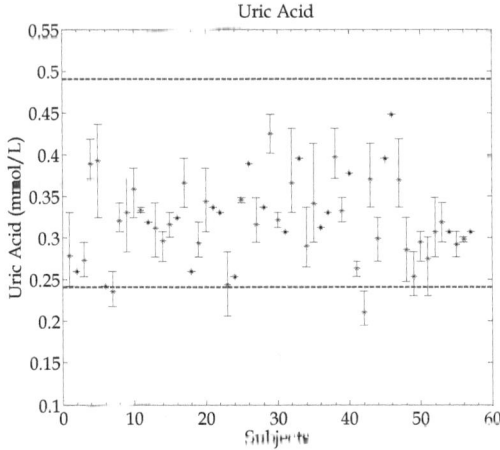

A.

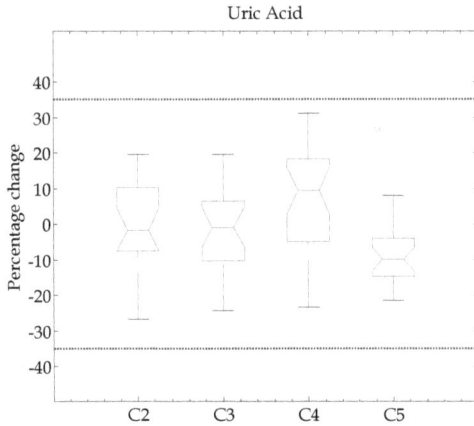

B.

Fig. 2. (A.) Uric acid concentration (mean, minimum and maximum) for each soccer player
at five time points. The dotted horizontal lines indicate the reference interval (2.5% lower
limit = 0.24 mmol/L and 97.5% upper limit = 0.49 mmol/L) from a physically active
population. (B.) Uric acid percentage change between successive pairs of serial results for
the soccer players during a season of training/competition. The dotted horizontal lines
indicate the RCV95% for uric acid = 35.0%

While there were no significant changes in the serial results during the season (Figure 2B),
three players were determined to be below the lower reference interval (Figure 2A).

4. Discussion

This study is the first to test the applicability of reference intervals and the RCV values obtained from physically active individuals (Nunes & Macedo, 2008; Nunes et al., 2010) in longitudinally monitoring the effects of training/competition on soccer players.

The players analyzed in this study were from the under-20 category. During the competition season (14 weeks), the games occurred on Saturday mornings. All players, including the outfield players, were submitted to a daily game-based training, where modified games are played on reduced pitch areas, often using adapted rules and involving a smaller number of players than in traditional soccer games. Different small-sided game designs were used during the season to improve specific physical capacities (e.g., sprint, speed, aerobic) (Hill-Haas et al., 2011). An important observation emerging from our data is that all of the soccer players supported this type of training very well for the entire season, including the competitions schedule, as the majority of the alterations shown here were within the reference interval for all of the analytes.

On the other hand, the comparison of serial analyses with RCV values increased the sensitivity and specificity of some analytes as biomarkers of individual training effects. From 56 players, only 17 and 15 exhibited significant alterations in a biochemical analyte or hemogram parameter, respectively, at any time point (Table 3 and 4). Knowledge of the RCV values permits an individual response to those subjects who exceed the percentage of alteration at one or more blood analyses as compared to previous analyses; these subjects can undergo a closer follow up daily or weekly, contributing to the individual adjustment of the training intensity, improvement of nutritional interventions and prevention of stress overload.

For example, the athletes 14 and 19 (Table 3 and 4) were submitted to the same training load and competitions and showed significant increases in the levels of their CK, leukocytes and neutrophils after three months. Although only the neutrophils showed changes that were above the reference interval, this set of changes may be related to a higher inflammatory response and muscle damage after this period of training and competitions, which can lead to an acute deterioration in performance (Ispirlidis et al., 2008). Note that athlete 35 at C3 also exhibited a ΔCK that was higher than the RCV (119.8%), but no other parameters were altered. Additionally, the absolute value was lower than that for athletes 14 and 19. It is likely that the higher ΔCK for this player merely indicated a higher participation in the training schedule. This information can therefore be useful to help the coach plan for adequate recovery time for just those athletes, especially if they are competing players. This information can also be useful to the nutritionist in individually adjusting some nutrients to improve the recovery rate between training sections and games, preserving these athletes.

An interesting point observed here is that after the first month of training, 8 athletes showed significant changes in their serum urea when compared to RCV values. This result may indicate a continuous catabolic state at the beginning of competitions (Hartmann & Mester, 2000). It is not unusual that soccer players present with an inadequate ingestion of carbohydrates because of a low energy intake or a high fat and protein intake (Garrido et al., 2007). As this macronutrient is important in preserving muscle mass, an inadequate ingestion can lead some athletes to a catabolic state that can impair their performance if not corrected. Thus, these 8 athletes could undergo a specific nutritional intervention.

The time point (C3) showed a higher number of positive training adaptations in the majority of the players. The serum creatinine values were significantly higher than the RCV values for five players, which could indicate a muscular mass gain in these subjects at the beginning of the competitions. In addition to creatinine, the hemoglobin concentrations increased significantly at C3, mainly in the athletes with levels near the lower limit of the population-based reference interval, indicating a positive training adaptation that is related to O_2 transport, such as increasing the plasma volume and the erythrocyte number (Sawka et al., 2000; Convertino, 2007). Only athlete 23 must be followed more carefully after C4 due to a significant decrease in the Hb concentration as compared to C3. This decrease can also be influenced by nutritional status, such as an inadequate intake of minerals like iron, zinc, copper, folic acid and complex B vitamins (Lukaski, 2004).

In this study we have also shown the need for a comparison of results with reference intervals that were established from a physically active population. For example, all of the players exhibited serum urate concentrations that were within the RCV values (Figure 2B), but three athletes exhibited values below the 2.5% percentile (Figure 2A). As uric acid is one of the most important plasma antioxidants (Lippi et al., 2008) this result could indicate a lower capacity of defense against ROS. The nutritionist could individually improve the antioxidant content of the diet, offering to these athletes more vegetables and fruits rich in this nutrient. This simple intervention may increase plasma antioxidant levels (Brevik et al., 2004).

5. Conclusions

The data presented here point to the Reference Interval and the RCV as important tools for the correct interpretation of the results proceeding from blood analyses related to the monitoring of athletes' training. Advances in analytical technology, such as proteomic analysis, may present new information concerning the athlete's protein and metabolic profile. These methods must also have their reference intervals and RCVs determined for effective for sport science application, providing coaches and interdisciplinary teams with the ability to make individual, punctual interventions that could make a difference in the continuous adaptive processes of all athletes throughout the season.

6. Acknowledgments

The authors thank the voluntary research subjects, Cristian Ramirez (Paulinia Futebol Clube coach) and the Commander of the Military Army, who permitted this study. We would also like to thank Ana Porto, Mauro Pascoa, Madla Adami dos Passos and Lucas Samuel Tessuti for their assessment of the given technique. This study was supported by the University Foundation (Funcamp-Conv927.7–BIO0100). Lázaro Alessandro S. Nunes and Fernanda Lorenzi Lazarim received scholarships from Brazilian agencies CNPq and CAPES, respectively.

7. References

Banfi, G. & Del Fabro, M. (2006). Relation between serum creatinine and body mass index in elite athletes of different sport disciplines. *Br J Sports Med*, Vol.40, No.8 (Aug), pp.675-678, ISSN 0306-3674.

Banfi, G. & Dolci, A. (2003). Preanalytical phase of sport biochemistry and haematology. J *Sports Med Phys Fitness*, Vol.43, No.2 (Jun), pp.223-230, ISSN 0022-4707

Banfi, G., Del Fabbro, M. & Lippi, G. (2009). Serum creatinine concentration and creatinine-based estimation of glomerular filtration rate in athletes. *Sports Med*, Vol.39, No.4, pp.331-337, ISSN 0112-1642

Bangsbo, J. (1994). The physiology of soccer—with special reference to intense intermittent exercise. *Acta Physiot Scand*, Vol.151, No.suppl 619, pp.1-156, ISSN 0302-2994

Bangsbo, J., Mohr, M. & Krustrup, P. (2006). Physical and metabolic demands of training and match-play in the elite football player. *J Sports Sci*, Vol.24, No.7 (Jul), pp.665-674, ISSN 0264-0414

Brancaccio, P., Lippi, G. & Maffulli, N. (2010). Biochemical markers of muscular damage. *Clin Chem Lab Med*, Vol.48, No.6 (Jun), pp.757-767, ISSN 1434-6621

Brancaccio, P., Maffulli, N., Buonauro, R. & Limongelli, F. M. (2008). Serum enzyme monitoring in sports medicine. *Clin Sports Med*, Vol.27, No.1 (Jan), pp.1-18, ISSN 1556-228X

Brevik, A., Andersen, L.F., Karlsen, A., Trygg, K.U., Blomhoff, R. & Drevon, C.A. (2004). Six carotenoids in plasma used to assess recommended intake of fruits and vegetables in a controlled feeding study. *Eur J Clin Nutr*, Vol.58, No.8 (Aug), pp.1166-1173, ISSN 0954-3007.

Butterfield, T.A., Best, T.M. & Merrick, M.A. (2006). The dual roles of neutrophils and macrophages in inflammation: a critical balance between tissue damage and repair. *J Athl Train*, Vol.41, No.4 (Oct-Dec), pp.457-465, ISSN 1062-6050

Carlsohn, A., Rohn, S., Bittmann F., Raila, J., Mayer, F. & Schweigert, F.J. (2008). Exercise increases the plasma antioxidant capacity of adolescent athletes. *Ann Nutr Metab*, Vol.53, No.2, pp.96-103, ISSN 1421-9697

Catanho da Silva, F.O. & Macedo, D.V. (2011). Physical exercise, inflammatory process and adaptive condition: an overview. *Braz. J. Kinanthropometry and Human Performance*. Vol.13, No.4, pp.320–328, ISSN 1415-8426.

Cervellin, G., Comelli, I. & Lippi, G. (2010). Rhabdomyolysis: historical background, clinical, diagnostic and therapeutic features. *Clin Chem Lab Med*, Vol.48, No.6 (Jun), pp.749-756, ISSN 1434-6621

Chatzinikolaou, A., Fatouros, I. G., Gourgoulis, V., Avloniti, A., Jamurtas, A. Z., Nikolaidis, M. G., Douroudos, I., Michailidis, Y., Beneka, A., Malliou, P., Tofas, T., Georgiadis, I., Mandalidis, D. & Taxildaris, K. (2010). Time course of changes in performance and inflammatory responses after acute plyometric exercise. *J Strength Cond Res*, Vol.24, No.5 (May), pp.1389-1398, ISSN 1533-4287

Clarkson, P.M. & Ebbeling, C. (1988). Investigation of serum creatine kinase variability after muscle-damaging exercise. *Clin Sci*, Vol.75, No.3 (Sep), pp.257—261, ISSN 0143-5221

Convertino, V.A. (2007). Blood volume response to physical activity and inactivity. *Am J Med Sci*, Vol.334, No.1 (Jul), pp.72-79, ISSN 0002-9629

Eliakim, A., Nemet, D. & Shenkman, L. (1995). Serum enzyme activities following long-distance running: comparison between Ethiopian and white athletes. *Isr J Med Sci*, Vol.31, No.11 (Nov), pp.657–659, ISSN 0021-2180

Fatouros, I. G., Chatzinikolaou, A., Douroudos, I. I., Nikolaidis, M. G., Kyparos, A., Margonis, K., Michailidis, Y., Vantarakis, A., Taxildaris, K., Katrabasas, I., Mandalidis, D., Kouretas, D. & Jamurtas, A. Z. (2010). Time-course of changes in oxidative stress and antioxidant status responses following a soccer game. *J Strength Cond Res*, Vol.24, No.12(Dec), pp.3278-3286, ISSN 1533-4287

Fielding, R. A., Manfredi, T. J., Ding, W., Fiatarone, M. A., Evans, W. J. & Cannon, J. G. (1993). Acute phase response in exercise. III. Neutrophil and IL-1 beta accumulation in skeletal muscle. *Am J Physiol*, Vol.265, No.1 (Jul), pp.R166-172, ISSN 0002-9513

Finaud, J., Lac, G. & Filaire, E. (2006). Oxidative Stress. Relationship with exercise and training. *Sports Med*, Vol.36, No.4, pp.327-358, ISSN 0112-1642

Fraser, C.G. & Harris, E.K. (1989). Generation and application of data on biological variation in clinical chemistry. *Crit Rev Clin Lab Sci*, Vol.27, No.5, pp.409–437, ISSN 0112-1642

Fraser, C.G. & Petersen, P.H. (1999). Analytical performance characteristics should be judged against objective quality specifications. *Clin Chem*, Vol.45, No.3 (Mar), pp.321-323, ISSN 0009-9147

Fraser, C.G. (2004). Inherent biological variation and reference values. *Clin Chem Lab Med*, Vol.42, No.7 (Jul), pp.758-764, ISSN 1434-6621

Fraser, CG. (2001). Changes in the serial results, In: *Biological variation: from principles to practice*, pp. 67-90, ISBN 1-890883-49-2, AACC Press, Washington DC

Garrido, G., Webster, A. L. & Chamorro, M. (2007). Nutritional Adequacy of different Menu Settings in Elite Spanish Adolescent Soccer Players. *Int J Sport Nutr Exerc Metab*, Vol.17, No.5(Oct), pp.421-432, ISSN 1526-484X

Gilligan, D. R., Altschule, M. D. & Katersky, E. M. (1943). Physiological intravascular hemolysis of exercise hemoglobinemia and hemoglobinuria following cross-country runs. *J Clin Invest*, Vol.22, No.6 (Nov), pp.859-869, ISSN 0021-9738

Gleeson, M. (2006). Immune system adaptation in elite athletes. *Curr Opin Clin Nutr Metab Care*, Vol.9, No.6 (Nov), pp. 659-665, ISSN 1363-1950

Gleeson, M. (2007). Immune function in sport and exercise. *J Appl Physiol*, Vol.103, No.2 (Aug), pp.693-699, ISSN 8750-7587

Gruys, E., Toussaint, M. J., Niewold, T. A. & Koopmans, S. J. (2005). Acute phase reaction and acute phase proteins. *Journal of Zhejiang University. Science. B*, Vol.6, No.11(Nov), pp. 1045-1056, ISSN 1673-1581

Harris, E.K. & Yasaka, T. (1983). On the calculation of a "reference change" or comparing two consecutive measurements. *Clin Chem*, Vol.29, No.1(Jan), pp.25–30, ISSN 0009-9147

Hartmann, U. & Mester, J. (2000). Training and overtraining markers in selected sport events. *Med. Sci. Sports Exerc*, Vol.32, No.1 (Jan), pp.209-215, ISSN 0195-9131

Hawley, J.A., Tipton, K.D. & Millard-Stafford, M.L. (2006). Promoting training adaptations through nutritional interventions. *Journal of Sports Sciences*, Vol.24, No.7 (Jul), pp.709–721, ISSN 0264-0414

Hawley, JA., Burke, LM., Phillips, SM. & Spriet, LL. (2011). Nutritional modulation of training-induced skeletal muscle adaptations. *J Appl Physiol*, Vol.110, No.3 (March), pp. 834-845.

Hill-Haas, S.V., Dawson, B., Impellizzeri, F.M. & Coutts, A.J. (2011). Physiology of small-sided games training in football: a systematic review. *Sports Med*, Vol.41, No.3 (Mar), pp.199-220, ISSN 0112-1642.

Hohl, R., Ferraresso, RLP., Oliveira, RB., Lucco, R., Brenzikofer, R., & Macedo, DV. (2009). Development and characterization of an overtraining animal model. *Med. Sci. Sports Exerc*, Vol.41, No. 5 (May), pp. 1155-1163, ISSN 1530-0315

Horn, P.S., Feng, L., Li, Y., & Pesce, A.J. (2001). Effect of outliers and nonhealthy individuals on reference interval estimation. *Clin Chem*, Vol.47, No 12 (Dec), pp. 2137-2145, ISSN 0009-9147

Ispirlidis, I., Fatouros, I. G., Jamurtas, A.Z., Nikolaidis, M.G., Michailidis, I., Douroudos, I., Margonis, K., Chatzinikolaou, A., Kalistratos, E., Katrabasas, I., Alexiou, V. & Taxildaris, K. (2008). Time-course of changes in inflammatory and performance responses following a soccer game. *Clin J Sport Med*, Vol.18, No.5 (Sep), pp. 423-31, ISSN 1536-3724

Ji, L.L. (1999). Antioxidants and oxidative stress in exercise. *Proc Soc Exp Biol Med*, Vol.222, No.3 (Dec), pp.283-292, ISSN 0037-9727

Kasapis, C. & Thompson, P. D. (2005). The effects of physical activity on serum C-reactive protein and inflammatory markers: a systematic review. *J Am Coll Cardiol*,Vol.45, No.10 (May), pp.1563-1569, ISSN 0735-1097

Kjeldsberg, C. (1992). Normal Values of blood and bone marrow in human, In: *Wintrobe's Hematology Clinical Hematology*, T.C. Bithell, J. Forester, J.W. Athens, J.N. Lukens & J. Kushner, pp.2531-2543, Lea & Febinger, Philadelphia

Lac, G. & Maso F. (2004). Biological markers for the follow-up of athletes throughout the training season. Pathol Biol, Vol.52, No.1(Feb), pp. 43-49, ISSN 0369-8114

Lazarim, F.L., Antunes-Neto, J.M.F., Oliveira da Silva, F.C., Nunes, L.A.S., Cameron, A.B., Cameron, L.C., Alves, A.A., Brenzikofer, R., & Macedo, D.V. (2009). The upper values of creatine kinase of professional soccer players during a Brazilian national championship. J Sci Med Sport. Vol.12, No. 1 (Jan), pp. 85-90, ISSN 1440-2440.

Lehmann, M., Foster, C., Dickhuth, H. H. & Gastmann, U. (1998) Autonomic imbalance hypothesis and overtraining syndrome. *Med Sci Sports Exerc*, Vol.30, No.7 (Jul), pp.1140-1145, 0195-9131

Lippi, G., Montagnana, M., Franchini M, Favaloro, E. J. & Targher, G. (2008). The paradoxical relationship between serum uric acid and cardiovascular disease. *Clin Chim Acta*, Vol.392, No.1-2 (Jun), pp.1-7, ISSN 0009-8981

Lira, F.S., Rosa J.C., Yamashita, A.S., Koyama, C.H., Batista Jr, M.L. & Seelaender M. (2009). Endurance training induces depot-specific changes in IL-10/TNF-a ratio in rat adipose tissue. *Cytokine*, Vol.45, No.2 (Feb), pp.80-85, ISSN 1096-0023

Lukaski, H.C. (2004). Vitamin and Mineral Status: Effects on Physical Performance. *Nutrition*, Vol.20, No.7-8 (Jul-Aug 2004), pp.632–644, ISSN 0899-9007

Malm, C. (2001). Exercise-induced muscle damage and inflammation: fact or fiction? *Acta Physiol Scand*, Vol.171, No.3 (Mar), pp.233–239, ISSN 0001-6772

Manfredi, T. G., Fielding, R. A., O'Reilly, K. P., Meredith, C. N., Lee, H. Y. & Evans, W. J. (1991). Plasma creatine kinase activity and exercise-induced muscle damage in older men. *Med Sci Sports Exerc*, Vol.23, No.9 (Sep), pp.1028-1034, ISSN 0195-9131

McNeil, P.L. & Khakee, R. (1992). Disruptions of muscle fiber plasma membranes. Role in exercise-induced damage. *Am J Pathol*, Vol.140, No.5 (May), pp.1097–1109, ISSN 0002-9440

Nordin, G., Mårtensson, A., Swolin, B., Sandberg, S., Christensen, N. J., Thorsteinsson, V., Franzson, L., Kairisto, V. & Savolainen, E. R. (2004). A multicentre study of reference intervals for haemoglobin, basic blood cell counts and erythrocyte indices in the adult population of the Nordic countries. *Scand J Clin Lab Invest*, Vol.64, No.4, pp. 385-98, ISSN 0036-5513

Nunes, L.A.S. & Macedo, D.V. (2008). Reference intervals for biochemical parameters in physically active young men. *Clin Chem Lab Med*, Vol.46 (Aug), pp.S1-S859, ISSN 1434-6621

Nunes, LAS., Brenzikofer, R., & Macedo, DV. (2010). Reference change values of blood analytes from physically active subjects. *Eur J Appl Physiol*, Vol. 110, No.1 (Sep), pp. 191-198, 1439-6327

Pattwell, D.M., McArdle, A., Morgan, J.E., Jackson, M. J.Patridge, T.A. (2004). Release of reactive oxygen and nitrogen species from contracting skeletal muscle cells. *Free Radic Biol Med*, Vol.37, No.7 (Oct), pp.1064-1072, 0891-5849

Peake, J.M., Suzuki, K. & Coombee JS. (2007). The influence of antioxidant supplementation on markers of inflammation and relationship to oxidative stress after exercise. *J Nutr Biochem*, Vol.18, No.6 (Jun), PP.357-371, ISSN 0955-2863

Pedersen B.K., Rohde T.M. & Ostrowski K. (1998). Recovery of the immune system after exercise. *Acta Physiol Scand*. Vol.162, pp.325-32 ISSN 0001-6772.

Pedersen, B.K. & Hoffman-Goetz, L. (2000). Exercise and the immune system: regulation, integration, and adaptation. *Physiol Rev*, Vol.80, No.3 (Jul), pp.1055-1081, ISSN 0031-9333

Pedersen, B.K., Rohde, T. & Ostrowski, K. (1998). Recovery of the immune system after exercise. *Acta Physiol Scand*, Vol.162, No.3 (Mar), pp.325-332, ISSN 0001-6772

Perrone, R.D., Madias, N.E. & Levey, A.S. (1992). Serum creatinine as an index of renal function: new insights into old concepts. *Clin Chem*. Vol.38, No.10 (Oct), pp.1933-1953, ISSN 0009-9147

Petersen, A.M.W. & Pedersen, B.K. (2005). The anti-inflammatory effect of exercise. *J Appl Physiol*, Vol.98, No.4 (Apr), pp.1154-1162, ISSN 8750-7587

Petersen, P.H. (2005). Making the most of a patient's laboratory data: optimisation of signal-to-noise ratio. *Clin Biochem Rev*, Vol.26. No.4(Nov), pp.91-96, ISSN 0159-8090

Petersen, P.H., Fraser, C.G., Sandberg, S. & Goldschmidt, H. (1999). The index of individuality is often a misinterpreted quantity characteristic. *Clin Chem Lab Med*, Vol.37, No.6 (Jun), p.655-661, ISSN 1434-6621

Pyne, D.B. (1994). Regulation of neutrophil function during exercise. *Sports Med*, Vol.17, No.4(Apr), pp.245-258, ISSN 0112-1642

Reilly, T. (1997). Energetics of high-intensity exercise (soccer) with particular reference to fatigue. *J Sports Sci*, Vol.15, No.3(Jun), pp.257-263, ISSN 0264-0414

Ricós, C., Alvarez, V., Cava, F., García-Lario, J.V., Hernández, A., Jiménez, C.V.,Minchinela, J., Perich, C. & Simón, M. (1999). Current databases on biologic variation: pros, cons and progress. *Scand J Clin Lab Invest*, Vol.59, No.7 (Nov), pp.491-500, ISSN 0036-5513

Ricós, C., Cava, F., Garcia-Lario, J.V., Hernández, A., Iglesias, N., Jiménez, C.V., Minchinela, J., Perich, C., Simón, M., Domenech, M.V. & Alvarez, V. (2004). The reference change value: a proposal to interpret laboratory reports in serial testing based on biological variation. *Scand J Clin Lab Invest*, Vol.64, No.3, pp.175-184, ISSN 0036-5513

Rowbottom, D.G. & Green, K.J. (2000). Acute exercise effects on the immune system. *Med Sci Sports Exerc*, Vol.32, No.7(Jul), pp.S396-S405, ISSN 0195-9131

Rustad, P., Felding, P., Franzson, L., Kairisto, V., Lahti, A., Mårtensson, A., Hyltoft Petersen, P., Simonsson, P., Steensland, H. & Uldall, A. (2004). The Nordic Reference Interval Project 2000: recommended reference intervals for 25 common biochemical properties. *Scand J Clin Lab Invest*, Vol.64, No.4, pp.271-284, ISSN 0036-5513

Sawka, M.N., Convertino, V.A., Eichner, R., Schinieder, S.M., & Young, A.G. (2000). Blood volume: importance and adaptations to exercise training, environmental stresses, and trauma/sickness. *Med Sci Sports Exerc*, Vol. 32, No.2 (Feb), pp. 332-348, ISSN 0195-9131

Sayers, S.P. & Clarkson, P.M.(2003). Short-term immobilization after eccentric exercise. Part II: creatine kinase and myoglobin. *Med Sci Sports Exerc*, Vol.35, No.5 (May), pp.762-768, ISSN 0195-9131

Schumacher, Y.O., Schmid, A., Grathwohl, D., Bültermann, D. & Berg, A. (2002). Hematological indices and iron status in athletes of various sports and performances. *Med. Sci. Sports Exerc*, Vol.34, No.5 (May), pp.869-875, ISSN 0195-9131

Serrão, F.V., Foerster, B., Spada, S., Morales, M.M., Monteiro-Pedro, V., Tannu's, A. & Salvini, T. F. (2003). Functional changes of human quadriceps muscle injured by eccentric exercise. *Braz J Med Biol Res*, Vol.36, No.6(Jun), pp.781–786, 0100-879X

Smith, J.A. (1995). Exercise, training and red blood cell turnover. *Sports Med*, Vol.19, No.1(Jan), pp.9-31, ISSN 0112-1642.

Smith, L.L. (2000). Cytokine hypothesis of overtraining: a physiological adaptation to excessive stress? *Med Sci Sports Exerc*, Vol. 32, No.2 (Feb), pp.317-331, ISSN 1522-1601

Solberg, H.E. (2004). The IFCC recommendations on estimation of reference intervals. The RefVal Program. *Clin Chem Lab Med*, Vol.42, No.7 (Jul), pp. 710-714, ISSN 1434-6621

Sottas, P.E., Robinson, N. & Saugy, M. (2010). The athlete's biological passport and indirect markers of blood doping. *Handb Exp Pharmacol*. Vol.195, pp305-326, ISSN 0171-2004

Steensberg, A., van Hall, G., Osada, T., Sacchetti, M., Saltin, B. & Pedersen, K.B. (2000). Production of interleukin-6 in contracting human skeletal muscles can account for the exercise-induced increase in plasma interleukin-6. *J Physiol*, Vol. 529, Pt 1 (Nov), pp.237-242, ISSN 0022-3751

Telford, R. D., Sly, G. J., Hahn, A. G., Cunningham, R. B., Bryant, C. & Smith, J. A. (2003). Footstrike is the major cause of hemolysis during running. *J Appl Physiol*, Vol.94, No.1(Jan), pp.38-42, ISSN 8750-7587

Tidball J.G. (2005a) Mechanical signal transduction in skeletal muscle growth and adaptation. *J Appl Physiol*, 98(5):1900-8.

Tidball, J.G. (2005b). Inflammatory processes in muscle injury and repair. *Am J Physiol Regul Integr Comp Physiol*, Vol.288, No.2(Feb), R345-353, ISSN 0363-6119

Tiidus, P.M. (2000). Estrogen and gender effects on muscle damage, inflammation and oxidative stress. *Can J Appl Physiol*, Vol.25, No.4 (Aug), pp274–287, ISSN 1066-7814

Toumi, H. & Best, T.M. (2003). The inflammatory response: friend or enemy for muscle injury? *Br J Sports Med*, Vol.37, No.4 (Aug), pp.284-286, ISSN 0306-3674

Urhausen, A. & Kindermann, W. (2002). Diagnosis of Overtraining. What Tools Do We Have? *Sports Med*, Vol.32, No. 2, pp.95-102, ISSN 0112-1642

Weight, L.M., Byrne, M. J. & Jacobs, P. (1991). Haemolytic effects of exercise. *Clin Sci (Lond)*, Vol.81, No.2 (Aug), pp.147-152, ISSN 0143-5221.

Westgard, J.O. (2004). Design of internal quality control for reference value studies. *Clin Chem Lab Med*, Vol.42, No.7 (Jul), pp. 863-867, ISSN 1434-6621

Wu, A.H.B., Smith, A. & Wians, F. (2009). Interpretation of creatine kinase and aldolase for statin-induced myopaty: Reliance on serial testing based on biological variation. *Clin Chim Acta*, Vol.399, No1-2(Jan), pp.109-111, ISSN 1873-3492

Youssef, H., Groussard, C., Machefer, G., Minella, O., Couillard, A., Knight, J. & Gratas-Delamarche, A. (2008). Comparison of total antioxidant capacity of salivary, capillary and venous samplings: interest of the salivary total antioxidant capacity on triathletes during training season. *J Sports Med Phys Fitness*, Vol.48, No.4 (Dec), pp.522-529, ISSN 0022-4707

Zoller, H. & Vogel, W. (2004). Iron supplementation in athletes--first do no harm. *Nutrition*, Vol.20, No.7-8 (Jul-Aug), pp.615-619, ISSN 0899-9007

5

Eccentric Exercise, Muscle Damage and Oxidative Stress

Athanasios Z. Jamurtas[1,2] and Ioannis G. Fatouros[2,3]
[1]Department of Physical Education and Sport Science,
University of Thessaly, Trikala,
[2]Institute of Human Performance and Rehabilitation,
Center for Research and Technology –Thessaly, Trikala,
[3]Department of Physical Education and Sport Science,
Democritus University of Thrace, Komotini,
Greece

1. Introduction

Participation in exercise has been linked with positive results on the cardiovascular system, metabolism, musculature etc. Some of these benefits are linked with reductions in blood pressure, increases in resting energy expenditure, changes in lipid profile, reductions in fat mass, increases in fat free mass etc. (Evans, 1999). There are different types of exercise that someone can participate in, i.e. walking, running, lifting weights, participating in organized sports which involve different muscular contractions. Isometric, concentric and eccentric muscle actions are the main muscular contractions involved in all exercise activities. Eccentric muscular contraction is this type of contraction where the length of the muscle is increased while tension is developed. Unaccustomed eccentric exercise has been linked with greater muscle damage compared to isometric or concentric muscular contractions. However this phenomenon is temporary and perturbations in functional and biochemical indices are back to normal within a week from the initiation of the trauma. Furthermore, the damage works as a protective mechanism since data indicates that the muscle damage is attenuated when a subsequent exercise bout of the same intensity is performed even a few months later. Eventhough eccentric exercise leads to greater muscle damage, recent data indicates that eccentrically induced muscle damage is related with positive changes in lipid profile that are evident for a few days following the initial event. Furthermore, the limited data from eccentric training studies indicate that this type of exercise is linked with positive changes in strength as well as in the metabolic profile of the exercise participant.

Oxidative stress indicates a condition where the cellular production of pro-oxidant molecules exceeds the ability of the antioxidant system to reduce reactive oxygen or nitrogen species (RONS). There are several studies that indicate that oxidative stress is evident following muscle damaging exercise. Its role has been related to cleaning the debris from the damaged tissue and providing the means for biochemical adaptations that lead to a stronger and more resistant to muscle damage muscular tissue. This phenomenon is transient and existing evidence suggests that oxidative stress indices are attenuated when a subsequent exercise bout is performed a few weeks after the initial damaging protocol. Finally, eccentric exercise has been linked with health benefits that are evident either after an acute bout of exercise or following a training protocol.

This review highlights muscle damage and oxidative stress adaptations as well as the health benefits associated with acute and chronic eccentric exercise.

2. Benefits from exercise

Numerous experimental and epidemiological studies have documented a large number of health benefits derived from systematic engagement with cardiovascular exercise training such as enhanced physiologic, metabolic, and psychologic adaptations, as well as reduced risk for development of many chronic diseases and premature mortality (USA, 1996; Kesaniemi et al., 2001). It is well-established that physical activity and/or chronic exercise prevent the occurrence of adverse cardiac events, decreases the incidence of hypertension, atherosclerosis, stroke, osteoporosis, obesity, insulin resistance, type 2 diabetes, cancer, and depression, causes body weight and fat loss, and delays mortality (USA, 1996; Kesaniemi et al., 2001; ACSM, 2006; Feskanich et al., 2002; Leitzmann et al., 1999; Sahi et al., 1998; Rockville, 1995). Large-scale studies have also demonstrated that systematic exercise or switching from being sedentary to a more physically active life-style reduces disease rates and premature mortality (Hein et al., 1994; Paffenbarger et al., 1993; Blair et al., 1995; Erikssen et al., 1998). In fact, exercise-induced health benefits occur even at old ages (Paffenbarger et al., 1993).

Resistance exercise training (a form of which is eccentric training) also induces substantial health benefits, especially to older individuals. Strength training increases not only muscular strength and power but also improves bone mineral density as well as cardiovascular and psychological function (Ay and Yurtkuran, 2005; Takeshima et al., 2002; Wang et al., 2007). Although, the response to resistance exercise training is individualized, there is a consensus that a properly designed and supervised program should improve not only muscular fitness parameters (strength, muscular endurance, power, balance, speed) but the quality of life as well (Evans, 1999). These adaptations are particularly evident in the elderly. Resistance exercise training has been repeatedly shown to increase muscular strength and muscle mass which in turn improve the functional status (coordination, balance etc.) and limit sarcopenia in the aged (Evans, 1999; Fatouros et al., 2006; Fiatarone et al., 1993; Frontera et al., 1991; ACSM, 1998).

3. Eccentric exercise

Daily movement involves different muscular contractions. Concentric type of contractions occurs when a muscle is activated and shortens. In contrast, eccentric contraction occurs when a skeletal muscle lengthens while it produces force. Both types of contractions occur during the day and the best example to differentiate between the two types of contraction is the ascending or descending the stairs. During the ascending of stairs leg muscles are working concentrically while during the descending of the stairs leg muscles are working eccentrically.

Eccentric exercise has been used as a means to develop muscle strength and size (Dudley et al. 1991). However, eccentric exercise training has been used lately as a novel rehabilitation modality in order to improve several conditions, i.e. tendinopathy, following anterior cruciate ligament reconstruction e.t.c. (Gerber et al. 2009) The health benefits derived from eccentric exercise training on metabolism will be discussed in a subsequent section.

4. Eccentric exercise and muscle damage

During eccentric exercise, force is generated when muscle fibers are lengthened. It is well documented that intense, unaccustomed eccentric exercise is associated with muscle damage (Clarkson et al. 1992). Evidence of damage includes morphological changes with ultrastructural damage to muscle fibers usually seen with microscopy Friden 1984), decrements in muscle force and the involved joint's range of motion (ROM) (Nosaka & Newton 2002), deterioration of running economy (Paschalis et al. 2005; 2008; Chen et al. 2007; 2009), alterations in position sense and reaction angle (Paschalis et al. 2007; 2010) elevated plasma proteins such as creatine kinase (CK) and myoglobin (Nosaka & Clarkson 1995; Jamurtas et al. 2000), elevation in inflammatory by products (Fatouros et al. 2010; McIntyre et al. 2001), connective tissue damage (Tofas et al. 2008), large increases in blood and muscle oxidative stress (Paschalis et al. 2007; Theodorou et al. 2010; 2011) and delayed onset of muscle soreness (Cheung et al. 2003). Eccentric exercises have been shown to produce the greatest amount of delayed onset muscle soreness (DOMS) and larger elevations of plasma CK compared to concentric or isometric exercises (Ebbeling & Clarkson 1989; Jamurtas et al. 2000).

Eccentric exercise results in greater muscle damage because fewer muscle fibers are recruited to exert a given amount of force as compared to concentric contractions. Since the force–velocity relationship indicates that each individual muscle fiber can exert a larger force while being stretched than it can while being shortened (Hill, 1938) and fewer fibers are activated during eccentric contractions, larger forces per muscle fiber are developed during eccentric actions thereby resulting in greater damage. Furthermore, during an eccentric contraction, some sarcomeres in muscle fibers are more resistant to stretching than others forcing weaker sarcomeres to absorb more stretch. With repeated eccentric contractions, the weaker sarcomeres first and then the stronger sarcomeres are overstretched. If the latter fail to withstand the stretching force during the relaxation phase, damage may occur. If the damage spreads to adjacent fibers, disruption of the membrane of the sarcoplasmic reticulum or sarcolemma may be seen. In that case intracellular Ca^{++} concentration increases leading to additional degradation of muscle fibers due to activation of calcium dependent proteolytic enzymes, such as the calpain mediated proteases, resulting in neutrophil infiltration to the injured site (Raj et al. 1998; Proske & Allen 2005).

Histological changes are evident following an intense bout of eccentric exercise and data indicates that approximately one third of the muscle fibers obtained from individuals who performed 300 maximal voluntary eccentric contractions of the knee extensors show intense myofibrillar disruptions, myofillament disorganization and loss of Z line integrity (Raastad et al. 2010). Changes in functional measurements are considered to be the best tool for quantifying muscle damage and monitoring exercise-induced muscle damage (Warren et al. 1999). Following eccentrically induced muscle damage, functional measurements (Maximal Voluntary Contractions, eccentric peak torque, jumping performance) demonstrate a marked deterioration reaching their lowest values approximately 72 hours post exercise and return to normal values within 7 days of recovery (Miyama & Nosaka 2004; Nikolaidis et al. 2008).

Following eccentrically induced muscle damage, changes in running economy appear to depend on the intensity of exercise used to asses this parameter. Reports indicate no changes in running economy following eccentric exercise when a moderate intensity exercise is used to assess running economy (Paschalis et al. 2005; 2008; Chen et al. 2009) whereas others report significant perturbations when higher intensities are used (Braun & Dutto 2003; Chen et al. 2007; 2009). For example, Chen et al. reported significant changes in running economy during level running when the intensity of exercise was set at 80% and 90% of VO2max but not at 70% VO_{2max} (Chen et al. 2009). When submaximal intensities (55% and 75% of VO2max) were used to assess changes in running economy following eccentrically induced muscle damage it was found that running economy indicators remained unaffected throughout recovery (24-96 hours post exercise) (Paschalis et al. 2005; 2008). Perhaps there is an impairment in the fast twitch fibers, which are the ones that are mainly affected by intense eccentric exercise thereby leading to changes in running economy and kinematic measures (Paschalis et al. 2007; Tsatalas et al. 2010).

As it was indicated earlier, eccentric exercise may cause a disruption to the plasma membrane of a muscle fiber. Disruption of the sarcolemma results in the release of intracellular proteins (CK, myoglobin) into circulation. The time frame of entry of various muscle proteins into the circulation following sarcolemma damage may depend on the size of the protein. For instance, there is a difference in the peak between CK and myoglobin (Nosaka, 2011). Small proteins such as myoglobin (the molecular weight of myoglobin is 18 kD) enter the circulation through capillaries whereas large proteins such as CK (the molecular weight of CK is 80 kD) enter the circulation via the lymph (Lindena et al. 1979).

One of the main characteristics of the unaccustomed eccentric exercise is the development of muscle soreness. Muscle soreness needs to be differentiated between the temporary soreness and DOMS. Temporary soreness is usually felt during the final stages of fatiguing exercise and is a product of metabolic waste accumulation (Friden J 1984). DOMS is characterized by a sensation of dull, aching pain that is usually felt during movement or palpation of the affected muscle (Clarkson et al. 1992). DOMS appears 24 hours after exercise and peaks 48-72 hours post-exercise. DOMS subsides and dissipates slowly and does not fully disappear until 7-10 days after exercise. The delayed response of DOMS seems to be related to an initial insult to the muscle due to mechanical reasons and this insult sets off a chain of events that leads to more damage while regeneration processes are also activated. Inflammatory responses to eccentric exercise play a role in the degeneration and regeneration of the damaged muscle (Peake et al. 2005). Following the initial insult, neutrophils are released into the circulation and enter the damaged muscle tissue within several hours (Beaton et al. 2002). Natural killer cells and lymphocytes are also released into the circulation during and after eccentric exercise. Macrophages and proinflammatory cytokines are produced in the muscle within 24 hours and can be present for several days following exercise. These responses are important for the acute phase response of the immune system and the removal of the damaged muscle tissue. Reactive oxygen and nitrogen species (RONS), such as superoxide produced by neutrophils and nitric oxide generated by macrophages, contribute to muscle damage (Close et al. 2005). The role of RONS on muscle damage will be discussed in a following section.

5. Oxidative stress

Oxidative stress may be defined as a condition in which cellular production of prooxidants exceeds the physiological ability of the system to quench reactive species. It is an imbalance between the production of reactive oxygen and nitrogen (RONS) species and antioxidant defense mechanisms. When the imbalance is in favor of RONS it can lead to biomolecular damage (Sies, 1991). RONS include several molecules such as superoxide (O_2^-), hydroxyl radical ($\cdot OH$) and nonradical derivatives of oxygen such as hydrogen peroxide (H_2O_2), nitric oxide (NO·) and nonradical derivatives of NO· such as peroxynitrite (ONOO·). These molecules have a singlet electron in the outer membrane and often are called free radicals. RONS occur as a consequence of normal cellular metabolism and have an effect on important biological processes such as gene expression (Pendyala & Natarajan 2010), signal transduction (Santos et al. 2011) and posttranslational modifications (Radak et al. 2011). Therefore, it appears that low levels of RONS are important for normal physiological function and homeostasis. RONS seem to be increased under conditions of psychological and physical stress (Sen et al. 1994). Evidence also indicates that enhanced production of RONS can lead to cardiovascular diseases and cancer due to chronic inflammation (Halliwell B, 1993).

Due to short half-life of RONS an indication of their presence is monitored by the measurement of by-products resulting from damage of various macromolecules such as proteins, lipids and nucleic acids. Oxidative damage to proteins involves the oxidation of amino acids and the most often utilized index of protein oxidation is protein carbonyls (Vincent & Taylor 2006). Lipid peroxidation markers include lipid hydroperoxides, conjugated dienes, malondialdehyde (MDA), thiobarbituric acid reactive substances (TBARS), and isoprostanes, with the level of F_2-isoprostanes in blood or urine to be widely regarded as the reference marker for the assessment of oxidative stress (Nikolaidis et al. 2011). Significant alterations to normal physiological function can be induced due to elevated lipid peroxidation and loss of membrane fluidity and cytosolic membranes are examples of this modification. Strand breaks and single base modifications of DNA are examples of RONS associated DNA damage. 8-hydroxy-2'-deoxyguanosine (8-OHdG) represents the most frequently marker used to assess DNA damage (Vincent & Taylor 2006). RONS are quenched through molecules that are called antioxidants. The main purpose of these molecules is to delay or prevent oxidative stress and damage. Antioxidants donate one of their electrons in order to reduce the formed oxidizing agent. Antioxidants are separated into the ones that have enzymatic activity and those with non-enzymatic activity. The main enzymatic antioxidants include superoxide dismutase, glutathione peroxidase and catalase. Non enzymatic compounds include vitamins (e.g. vitamin C, vitamin E), proteins (e.g. ferritin, transferrin, ceruloplasmin) or peptides (e.g. glutathione).

6. Eccentric exercise, oxidative stress and muscle damage

It was stated in a previous section that eccentric exercise leads to DOMS. At the same time numerous evidence suggests that eccentrically induced muscle damage appears concurrently with changes in oxidative stress. Paschalis et al. had 10 healthy females with no previous history of eccentric training perform five sets of 15 eccentric maximal voluntary contractions of the knee extensors and assessed indices of muscle function and muscle damage (isokinetic peak torque, ROM, CK) as well as indices of oxidative stress and the antioxidant system (glutathione, TBARS, protein carbonyls, catalase, uric acid, total antioxidant capacity) (Paschalis et al. 2007). The results showed that eccentric exercise resulted in significant loss of torque, decreases in ROM and elevation in CK concentration for several days following the exercise bout. These changes coincided with marked elevations of selected oxidative stress indices manifested in a uniform and prolonged pattern. Oxidative stress indices peaked at 48 hours of recovery and remained significantly elevated for 72 hours post exercise (Paschalis et al. 2007). The authors also report a moderate relationship between muscle damage and oxidative stress indices that may indicate a link between muscle damage and oxidative stress.

Nikolaidis et al. assessed also oxidative stress following eccentric exercise in healthy females and found significant perturbations in all assessed indices (Nikolaidis et al. 2007). Subjects had to perform five sets of 15 eccentric maximal voluntary contractions of the knee flexors and indices of muscle function and muscle damage (isokinetic peak torque, ROM, CK) and indices of oxidative stress and the antioxidant system (glutathione, TBARS, protein carbonyls, catalase, uric acid, total antioxidant capacity) were assessed before the exercise session and 1, 2, 3, 4 and 7 days post exercise. Eccentric exercise caused muscle damage and uniformly modified the levels of the selected oxidative stress indices in the blood. Oxidative stress indices peaked at 72 hours and returned toward baseline after 7 days post exercise (Nikolaidis et al. 2008).

Results from another study from our laboratory (Theodorou et al. 2010) performed in healthy males provided similar results with the aforementioned studies. In Thedorou et al. study, nine healthy males performed five sets of 15 eccentric maximal voluntary contractions of the knee extensors and indices of muscle function and muscle damage and oxidative stress were also assessed. Indices of oxidative stress in this study were assessed in plasma and erythrocyte lysate before, as well as 1, 2, 3, 4, and 5 days post-exercise in order to determine whether there was a different response between the two blood compartments (plasma and red blood cells) as well. The results showed that eccentric exercise markedly increased muscle damage, oxidative stress and hemolysis indices that peaked at 2 and 3 days post exercise (Theodorou et al. 2010).

Silva et al. reported significant elevation in lipid peroxidation (TBARS) and protein carbonylation indices following eccentric exercise (Silva et al. 2010). Subjects performed three sets of eccentric exercise of the elbow flexors at an intensity of 80% of maximum repetition until exhaustion. A point of interest is the significant elevated TBARS and protein carbonyls for 7 days after the eccentric exercise which is in contrast with previous reports indicating a return of oxidative stress indices at baseline levels within five to seven days post exercise (Nikolaidis et al. 2007; Theodorou et al. 2010). Goldfarb et al. reported significant elevations in protein carbonyls and MDA up to 72 hours post exercise in subjects that performed four sets of 12 maximal repetitions of eccentric actions at an angular velocity of $20^{o} \cdot s^{-1}$, with 60 s of rest between sets using their nondominant arm elbow flexors (Goldfarb et al. 2011). Eccentric exercise resulted also in significant changes in force and muscle damage indices. Other reports also indicate significant elevations in indices of oxidative stress (i.e. protein carbonyls) following eccentric resistance exercise (arm elbow flexors) performed by humans (Goldfarb et al. 2005; Lee et al. 2002) or downhill running (Close et al. 2004; 2005; 2006).

Eventhough the previously reported studies suggest that eccentrically induced muscle damage is accompanied with changes in oxidative stress indices for some days after exercise there are reports indicating no changes in oxidative stress following eccentric exercise. Kerksick et al. showed no changes in lipid peroxidation (F2-isoprostanes) and superoxide dismutase following eccentric exercise (10 sets of 10 repetitions at an isokinetic eccentric speed of $60^{o} \cdot s^{-1}$ on an isokinetic dynamometer) that caused muscle damage (Kerksick et al. 2010). In Goldfarb et al. study no changes in lipid hydroperoxides and glutathione levels were observed (Goldfarb et al. 2011). Saxton et al. also did not find significant changes in oxidative stress measures immediately post and two days following exercise of the forearm flexors (Saxton et al. 1994).

Taken collectively, the results from the aforementioned studies suggest that muscle damaging exercise seems to increase lipid peroxidation and protein oxidation in blood of humans. These results also indicate that disturbances in indices of blood oxidative stress may persist for several days following muscle-damaging exercise. This response is different compared to non-muscle damaging exercise where the disturbances in oxidative stress indices are not uniform and return towards baseline within hours after the end of exercise (Michailidis et al. 2007).

Direct comparisons of different studies are difficult. It has to be stated here that only human studies were presented in this section. A point of consideration relates to the mode of exercise used to cause muscle damage and the muscle groups used to perform the exercise. Eccentric exercise on an isokinetic device and downhill running are primarily the two main modes of exercise used to induce muscle damage following which oxidative stress markers were assessed. These two modes differ considerably since eccentric exercise on an isokinetic device isolates the muscle group used to perform the exercise whereas downhill running integrates the action of multiple muscle groups besides quadriceps in order to perform the exercise. In addition, the aerobic component of downhill running might be an additional confounding factor in causing oxidative stress (through electron leakage from mitochondrial respiration and other mechanisms).

Another point of consideration that relates to eccentrically induced muscle damage is the cause of the enhanced appearance of RONS following eccentric exercise. Muscle mitochondria (through electron leakage in the electron transport chain) could be one source of RONS during or shortly after muscle damaging exercise. However, that mild elevation of RONS production is unlikely to contribute to the delayed increased oxidative stress response that appears hours or days following exercise. Ischemia-reperfusion could be another cause of RONS elevation during exercise. It is well known from cardiac physiology that reperfusion in cardiac tissue following angioplasty operations leads to elevated myocardium damage that is partly attributed to elevated RONS production (Zhao et al. 2000). Blood flow redistribution during exercise is a well-known adaptation in exercise physiology and describes the vasodilation of the vascular system of the active muscle and the vasoconstriction of the vasculature of the non-active muscle tissue. The hypoxic non-active tissue receives a greater quantity of blood after exercise and enhanced formation of RONS is possible due to the xanthine oxidase mechanism (Finaud et al. 2006; Veskoukis et al. 2008). This mechanism of RONS production seems also unlikely to account for the increased oxidative stress that appears days following eccentrically-induced muscle damage. Oxidation of hemoglobin and myoglobin during exercise can also cause RONS formation (Finaud et al. 2006) but this mechanism is also unlikely to be responsible for the delayed response of oxidative stress when muscle damage is present.

Inflammatory responses to eccentric exercise play a major role in the degeneration and regeneration of the damaged muscle (Peake et al. 2005). Following the initial insult neutrophils are released into the circulation and enter the damaged muscle tissue within several hours (Beaton et al. 2002). Therefore, infiltrating white blood cells into skeletal muscle may be another source of RONS production following the insult caused to skeletal muscle due to eccentric exercise. Indeed activated neutrophils and other phagocytic cells are a major cause of RONS production leading to tissue damage and if remain unchecked can destroy adjacent healthy tissue (Close et al. 2005). Therefore, RONS can assist in repairing damaged tissue via phagocytosis and white blood cell respiratory burst activity. Production of RONS when muscle damage is present may serve a secondary role which is not other than the induction of the antioxidant activity of the damaged tissue in order to prevent harm when a subsequent exercise session is performed. Figure 1 illustrates a simplistic approach to the events that takes place following an eccentrically induced muscle damage exercise session. In brief, eccentric exercise due to mechanical stress causes injury to the sarcolemma and muscle damage is induced. The inflammatory processes that take place lead to enhanced production of RONS which serve a dual purpose: first, they clean the debris and repair the damaged tissue and secondly upregulate several transcription factors that lead to increased antioxidant activity of the remaining healthy muscle fibers that become more resistant to muscle damage when a bout of similar exercise is performed.

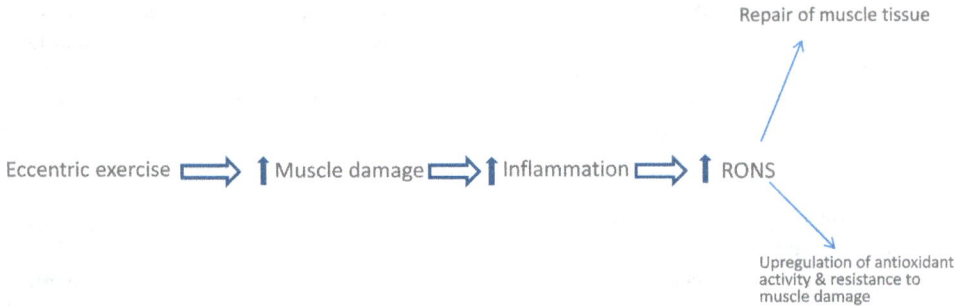

Repair of muscle tissue

Eccentric exercise ⇒ ↑ Muscle damage ⇒ ↑ Inflammation ⇒ ↑ RONS

Upregulation of antioxidant
activity & resistance to
muscle damage

7. Eccentric exercise, oxidative stress and the repeated bout effect

As it has been mentioned earlier unaccustomed eccentric exercise results in muscle damage. Furthermore, it was eluded that the initial injury to muscle tissue leads to changes in its structure that make it more resistant to a subsequent bout of exercise. This process is referred in the literature as the "repeated bout effect". Numerous studies have shown an attenuation of indices related to muscle damage due to the repeated bout effect (Chen et al. 2007; McHugh et al. 2003). In regards to oxidative stress similar changes (i.e. attenuation) to indices of muscle damage have been observed. Nikolaidis et al. had 12 females perform two sessions of eccentric exercise, separated by three weeks, and assessed muscle damage and oxidative stress indices prior to exercise and 1, 2, 3, 4, and 7 days after exercise (Nikolaidis et al. 2007). The two exercise sessions were identical in intensity and duration and consisted of five sets of 15 maximum eccentric voluntary contractions of the knee flexors. The first exercise bout changed significantly all muscle damage and oxidative stress indices indicating that severe muscle damage and increased oxidative stress had occur. Nevertheless, the second exercise bout resulted in significant attenuation in the perturbations of muscle damage and oxidative stress indices. Assessment of the increase or decrease area under the curve for the oxidative stress indices revealed a 1.8-6.1-fold less change in oxidative stress compared to the changes induced by the first bout (Nikolaidis et al. 2007). One possible explanation for the reduced oxidative stress following the second bout of exercise relates to the less muscle damage and less invasion of white blood cells in the damaged tissue. Data from animal work supports this idea since no significant changes in the concentration of ED1[+] and ED2[+] macrophages were found after a second bout of lengthening contractions (Lapointe et al. 2002) and treatment with diclofenac, a widely used non-steroidal anti-inflammatory drug (NSAID), affected in parallel the concentration of macrophage subpopulations and the adaptive response after the second bout of exercise (Lapointe et al. 2002). Therefore, inflammation plays a significant role in repair or strengthening of the muscle and might be the basis for the repeated bout effect. Results from human data are needed in order to substantiate the results obtained from the animal studies.

8. Health benefits from eccentric exercise

Participation in exercise has been linked with positive results on the cardiovascular system, metabolism, musculature etc. Some of these benefits are linked with reductions in blood pressure, increases in resting energy expenditure, changes in lipid profile, reductions in fat mass, increases in fat free mass etc. The majority of the studies that examined the positive effects of exercise have used either endurance exercise or resistance exercise with both types of exercise showing beneficial effects on health (Booth et al. 2000).

It has been mentioned previously that pure eccentric contractions lead to increased muscle damage and soreness levels. This phenomenon is transient, lasts a few days and can make the muscle more resistant to further damage when a repeated bout is performed. However, due to appearance of muscle soreness and the associated changes in muscle function eccentric exercise was viewed as the "bad guy" in the exercise physiology area. Besides the negative effects on muscular function eccentrically induced muscle damage was associated with impaired insulin action (Kirwan et al. 1992) and impaired muscle glycogen resynthesis (O'reilly et al. 1987). The transient augmented insulin responses to hyperglycaemia resulting from muscle damaging exercise seems to serve a dual purpose, i.e. to maintain glucose homeostasis and provide an anabolic environment for the damaged muscle, at least in muscles predominately composed of fast twitch fibres (Flucke et al. 2001).

Eccentric exercise has been used as means of training for several pathological conditions showing positive results in patients with Parkinson disease (Dibble et al. 2006), older cancer survivors (LaStayo et al. 2010), patients undergone anterior cruciate ligament reconstruction (Gerber et al. 2007) etc. Lately there has been an attempt to elucidate the acute and chronic effects of eccentric exercise on metabolism. Eventhough previous reports have attempted to examine the acute effects of muscle damaging exercise on blood lipids only total cholesterol was used as an index of blood lipid profile in these studies (Smith et al. 1994; Shahbazpour et al. 2004). In a study that was performed in our laboratory, the acute effects of muscle damaging exercise on time-course changes of blood lipid profile and the effect of the repeated bout on blood lipids were assessed (Nikolaidis et al. 2007). Twelve healthy females participated in this study. They performed two isokinetic eccentric exercise sessions (five sets of 15 eccentric maximal voluntary contractions at an angular velocity of $60^{\circ} \cdot s^{-1}$) during the luteal phase. The two exercise sessions were separated by 24-30 days, depending on the duration of their menstrual cycle. Markers of the lipid profile and muscle damage indices were assessed before, immediately, 1, 2, 3, 4, and 7 days after exercise. The results revealed that eccentric exercise uniformly modified the levels of the lipids and lipoproteins (triglycerides, total cholesterol, HDL and LDL). The repeated bout effect affected the assessed variables in a way that the response of lipids and lipoproteins were higher after the first session of exercise compared to those induced by the second identical session performed 4 weeks later. Those changes in the blood peaked at 2 to 4 days post exercise (Nikolaidis et al. 2007). Beneficial changes in lipid profile after eccentric exercise in overweight and lean women were observed in another study performed in our laboratory (Paschalis et al.

2010b). Subjects performed again five sets of 15 maximal voluntary contractions and energy expenditure, respiratory quotient (RQ), muscle damage and lipid and lipoprotein (triglycerides, total cholesterol, HDL and LDL) changes were assessed prior to, immediately after, 12, 24, 48 and 72 hours post exercise. The results revealed increased energy expenditure at all time-points following exercise, lower RQ at 24 hours post exercise andsignificant changes in muscle damage indices and lipids and lipoproteins at 24, 48 and 72 hours post exercise. These changes were exacerbated in the overweight group probably due to the higher muscle damage that was induced by the eccentric exercise protocol in this group of participants (Paschalis et al. 2010b). Similar results with the aforementioned studies were obtained from another study where significant lower triacylglycerol total area under the curve by approximately 12% and significantly elevated insulin incremental area under the curve, indicating transient insulin resistance, were also found 16 hours and 40 hours following an acute bout of eccentric exercise (Pafili et al. 2009).

Eccentric training seems also to improve muscle performance and diminishes the reductions in muscle performance, the elevation in muscle damage indices and the oxidative stress responses (Theodorou et al. 2011). The chronic effects of eccentric training on metabolism have been examined and show promising results in regards to this type of training. Drexel et al. had two groups of subjects hiking either upwards or downwards, three times a week, and assessed metabolic and inflammatory indices (Drexel et al. 2008). The results showed a reduction in total cholesterol (4.1%), LDL (8.4%), apolipoprotein B/apolipoprotein A1 ratio (10·9%), homeostasis model assessment of insulin resistance (26·2%) and C-reactive protein (30.0%) in the eccentric group. These results indicate favorable metabolic and anti-inflammatory results following this type of exercise. Paschalis et al. examined also the effects of a weekly bout of eccentric versus concentric exercise on health parameters of healthy women (Paschalis et al. 2011). Subjects performed an isokinetic eccentric or concentric exercise protocol once per week for eight weeks. Subjects had to complete five sets of 15 concentric or eccentric maximum voluntary contractions in each of their lower limbs with a 2-min rest between sets. The results showed that eccentric training improved the resting levels of blood lipid profile. More specifically, triglygerides, total cholesterol (TC), LDL and TC/HDL ratio decreased by 12.8%, 8.8%, 16.4% and 17%, respectively whereas HDL levels increased by 9.3%. No changes in apolipoprotein A1, apolipoprotein B and lipoprotein (α) were seen. Eccentric training resulted also in significant reductions in glucose, insulin, HOMA and glycosylated hemoglobin levels (Paschalis et al. 2011). However, Marcus et al. did not find any significant changes in insulin sensitivity in overweight or obese postmenopausal women with impaired glucose tolerance (Marcus et al. 2009). Subjects performed three exercise sessions per week for 12 weeks. The exercise was performed on a high-force eccentric ergometer and ranged from 5 minutes in the beginning to 30 minutes at the end of training. Eventhough the eccentric training resulted in significant positive changes on body composition, strength, and physical function no significant changes were found in insulin sensitivity following a hyperinsulinemic-euglycemic clamp test. The different modes of exercise (isolated isokinetic eccentric exercise vs. aerobic type eccentric exercise on an ergometer) might account for the difference in the results obtained in the latter study compared to the former studies.

9. Eccentric exercise programming

Latest research indicates that systematic eccentric exercise can lead to positive changes in physical capabilities, improved rehabilitation and health outcome measures. It has been also reported that unaccustomed eccentric exercise produces greater muscle damage and pain which subsides in a few days. Therefore, it is of great importance to develop exercise programs that incorporate eccentric actions that minimize muscle damage and the associated pain discomfort. Initial low intensity, short duration and progression are key elements in designing eccentric exercise programs. Rate of perceived exertion (RPE) is an important element that could be used in the exercise program. An example of how the aforementioned elements could be appropriately used is presented in an elegant study by Lastayo where older cancer survivors participated in an eccentric exercise intervention study (Lastayo et al. 2011). Subjects begun the intervention program participating in an exercise regimen of low intensity (7, very very light on an RPE scale) and short duration exercise (3-5 minutes per session) that progressed to a higher intensity (11-13, fairly light to somewhat hard on an RPE scale) and longer duration (16-20 minutes) after 12 weeks which was the duration of the exercise program. The program proved to be efficacious since increases in muscle size, strength and power along with improved mobility were noted. Another area where eccentric training could be applied is rehabilitation. Program designing in this area should also follow the same principles as the ones outlined previously. Lorenz & Reiman have outlined the role of eccentric training in various injuries in the athletic field and the reader is encouraged to read their review (Lorenz & Reiman 2011). In conclusion, eccentric training could be an effective means of increasing performance and lead to better health. Incorporation of basic principles in exercise program development (load, volume, intensity, frequency and progression) is essential in order to avoid unwanted outcomes (i.e. muscle damage).

10. Conclusion

Unaccustomed eccentric exercise can cause muscle damage that is evident by morphological changes of the muscle fiber, reductions in physical performance, elevation in inflammatory products and muscle soreness. These responses are significantly attenuated when a second exercise bout of the same intensity is implemented, a phenomenon known as the repeated bout effect. Oxidative stress indices follow the same pattern of response as the one previously mentioned. Significant perturbations in oxidative stress are evident following an eccentrically induced muscle damage exercise protocol that are attenuated due to the repeated bout effect. Elevation in oxidative stress seems to be related with cleaning the debris from damaged muscle fibers and upregulating the antioxidant activity of healthy fibers making them more resistant to muscle damage. Finally, strong evidence indicates that eccentric training can induce health-promoting effects.

11. References

[1] American College of Sports Medicine. Guidelines for Exercise Testing and Prescription, 7th ed., Whaley MH (ed.). Lippincott Williams & Wilkins: Baltimore, Maryland, 2006.

[2] American College of Sports Medicine. Position Stand: the recommended quantity and quality of exercise for developing and maintaining cardiorespiratory and muscular fitness, and flexibility in healthy adults. Med Sci Sports Exerc 30: 975–91, 1998.

[3] Ay A, Yurtkuran M. Influence of aquatic and weight-bearing exercises on quantitative ultrasound variables in postmenopausal women. Am J Phys Med Rehabil 84: 52–61, 2005.

[4] Beaton LJ, Tarnopolsky MA, Phillips SM. Contraction-induced muscle damage in humans following calcium channel blocker administration. J Physiol. 2002 Nov 1;544(Pt 3):849-59.

[5] Blair SN, Kohl HW 3rd, Barlow CE, et al. Changes in physical fitness and all-cause mortality. A prospective study of healthy and unhealthy men. JAMA 273: 1093–8, 1995.

[6] Booth FW, Gordon SE, Carlson CJ, Hamilton MT. Waging war on modern chronic diseases: primary prevention through exercise biology. J Appl Physiol. 2000 Feb;88(2):774-87.

[7] Braun WA, Dutto DJ. The effects of a single bout of downhill running and ensuing delayed onset of muscle soreness on running economy performed 48 h later. Eur J Appl Physiol. 2003 Sep;90(1-2):29-34.

[8] Chen TC, Nosaka K, Sacco P. Intensity of eccentric exercise, shift of optimum angle, and the magnitude of repeated-bout effect. J Appl Physiol. 2007 Mar;102(3):992-9.

[9] Chen TC, Nosaka K, Lin MJ, Chen HL, Wu CJ. Changes in running economy at different intensities following downhill running. J Sports Sci. 2009 Sep;27(11):1137-44.

[10] Cheung K, Hume P, Maxwell L. Delayed onset muscle soreness : treatment strategies and performance factors. Sports Med. 2003;33(2):145-64.

[11] Clarkson PM, Nosaka K, Braun B. Muscle function after exercise-induced muscle damage and rapid adaptation. Med Sci Sports Exerc. 1992 May;24(5):512-20.

[12] Close GL, Ashton T, McArdle A, Maclaren DP. The emerging role of free radicals in delayed onset muscle soreness and contraction-induced muscle injury. Comp Biochem Physiol A Mol Integr Physiol. 2005 Nov;142(3):257-66.

[13] Close GL, Ashton T, Cable T, Doran D, Holloway C, McArdle F, MacLaren DP. Ascorbic acid supplementation does not attenuate post-exercise muscle soreness following muscle-damaging exercise but may delay the recovery process. Br J Nutr. 2006 May;95(5):976-81.

[14] Close GL, Ashton T, Cable T, Doran D, MacLaren DP. Eccentric exercise, isokinetic muscle torque and delayed onset muscle soreness: the role of reactive oxygen species. Eur J Appl Physiol. 2004 May;91(5-6):615-21.

[15] Dibble LE, Hale T, Marcus RL, Gerber JP, Lastayo PC. The safety and feasibility of high-force eccentric resistance exercise in persons with Parkinson's disease. Arch Phys Med Rehabil. 2006 Sep;87(9):1280-2.

[16] Drexel H, Saely CH, Langer P, Loruenser G, Marte T, Risch L, Hoefle G, Aczel S. Metabolic and anti-inflammatory benefits of eccentric endurance exercise - a pilot study. Eur J Clin Invest. 2008 Apr;38(4):218-26.

[17] Dudley, G.A., Tesch P.A., Miller B.J., Buchanan P. Importance of eccentric actions in performance adaptations to resistance training. *Aviat. Space Environ. Med.* 62:543-550. 1991.

[18] Ebbeling CB, Clarkson PM. Exercise-induced muscle damage and adaptation. Sports Med. 1989 Apr;7(4):207-34.

[19] Erikssen G, Liestol K, Bjornholt J, et al. Changes in physical fitness and changes in mortality. Lancet 352: 759-62, 1998.

[20] Evans WJ. Exercise training guidelines for the elderly. Med Sci Sports Exerc 31: 12-7, 1999.

[21] Fatouros IG, Chatzinikolaou A, Douroudos II, Nikolaidis MG, Kyparos A, Margonis K, Michalllidis Y, Vantarakis A, Taxildaris K, Katrabasas I, Mandalidis D, Kouretas D, Jamurtas AZ. Time-course of changes in oxidative stress and antioxidant status responses following a soccer game. J Strength Cond Res. 2010 Dec;24(12):3278-86.

[22] Fatouros IG, Kambas A, Katrabasas I, et al. Resistance training and detraining effects on flexibility performance in the elderly are intensity-dependent. J Strength Cond Res 20: 634-42, 2006.

[23] Feskanich D, Willett W, Colditz G. Walking and leisure-time activity and risk of hip fracture in postmenopausal women. JAMA 288: 2300-6, 2002.

[24] Fiatarone MA, Evans WJ. The etiology and reversibility of muscle dysfunction in the aged. J Gerontol 48: 77-83, 1993.

[25] Finaud J, Lac G, Filaire E. Oxidative stress : relationship with exercise and training. Sports Med. 2006;36(4):327-58.

[26] Fridén J. Muscle soreness after exercise: implications of morphological changes. Int J Sports Med. 1984 Apr;5(2):57-66.

[27] Fluckey, J. D., Asp S., Enevoldsen L. H. & Galbo H.. Insulin action on rates of muscle protein synthesis following eccentric, muscle-damaging contractions. Acta Physiol Scand. 2001 Dec;173(4):379-84.

[28] Frontera WR, Hughes VA, Lutz KJ, Evans WJ. A crosssectional study of muscle strength and mass in 45- to 78-yr-old men and women. J Appl Physiol 71: 644-50, 1991.

[29] Gerber JP, Marcus RL, Dibble LE, Greis PE, Burks RT, LaStayo PC. Effects of early progressive eccentric exercise on muscle structure after anterior cruciate ligament reconstruction. J Bone Joint Surg Am. 2007 Mar;89(3):559-70.

[30] Gerber JP, Marcus RL, Dibble LE, Greis PE, Burks RT, LaStayo PC. Effects of early progressive eccentric exercise on muscle size and function after anterior cruciate ligament reconstruction: a 1-year follow-up study of a randomized clinical trial. Phys Ther. 2009 Jan;89(1):51-9.

[31] Goldfarb AH, Garten RS, Cho C, Chee PD, Chambers LA. Effects of a fruit/berry/vegetable supplement on muscle function and oxidative stress. Med Sci Sports Exerc. 2011 Mar;43(3):501-8.

[32] Goldfarb AH, Bloomer RJ, McKenzie MJ. Combined antioxidant treatment effects on blood oxidative stress after eccentric exercise. Med Sci Sports Exerc. 2005 Feb;37(2):234-9.

[33] Halliwell B. The role of oxygen radicals in human disease, with particular reference to the vascular system. Haemostasis. 1993 Mar;23 Suppl 1:118-26.

[34] Hein HO, Suadicani P, Sorensen H, et al. Changes in physical activity level and risk of ischaemic heart disease. A six-year follow-up in the Copenhagen male study. Scand J Med Sci Sports 4: 57–64, 1994.

[35] Hill, A.V. The heat of shortening and the dynamic constants of muscle. *Proc. Res. Soc. Biol.* 126:136-195. 1938.

[36] Jamurtas A, Fatouros J, Buckenmeyer P, Kokkinidis E, Taxildaris K, Kambas A, Kyriazis G (2000) Effects of plyometric exercise on muscle soreness and creatine kinase levels and its comparison to eccentric and concentric exercise. J Strength Cond Res 14: 68-74

[37] Kerksick CM, Kreider RB, Willoughby DS. Intramuscular adaptations to eccentric exercise and antioxidant supplementation. Amino Acids. 2010 Jun;39(1):219-32.

[38] Kirwan JP, Hickner RC, Yarasheski KE, Kohrt WM, Wiethop BV, Holloszy JO. Eccentric exercise induces transient insulin resistance in healthy individuals. J Appl Physiol. 1992 Jun;72(6):2197-202.

[39] Kesaniemi YK, Danforth E Jr, Jensen MD, et al. Dose-response issues concerning physical activity and health: an evidence-based symposium. Med Sci Sports Exerc 33: S351–8, 2001.

[40] Lapointe BM, Frémont P, Côté CH. Adaptation to lengthening contractions is independent of voluntary muscle recruitment but relies on inflammation. Am J Physiol Regul Integr Comp Physiol. 2002 Jan;282(1):R323-9.

[41] Lastayo PC, Larsen S, Smith S, Dibble L, Marcus R. The feasibility and efficacy of eccentric exercise with older cancer survivors: a preliminary study. J Geriatr Phys Ther. 2010 Jul-Sep;33(3):135-40.

[42] Lee J, Goldfarb AH, Rescino MH, Hegde S, Patrick S, Apperson K. Eccentric exercise effect on blood oxidative-stress markers and delayed onset of muscle soreness. Med Sci Sports Exerc. 2002 Mar;34(3):443-8.

[43] Leitzmann MF, Rimm EB, Willett WC, et al. Recreational physical activity and the risk of cholecystectomy in women. N Engl J Med 341: 777–84, 1999.

[44] Lindena J, Küpper W, Friedel R, Trautschold I. Lymphatic transport of cellular enzymes from muscle into the intravascular compartment. Enzyme. 1979;24(2):120-31.

[45] MacIntyre DL, Sorichter S, Mair J, Berg A, McKenzie DC. Markers of inflammation and myofibrillar proteins following eccentric exercise in humans. Eur J Appl Physiol. 2001 Mar;84(3):180-6.

[46] Marcus RL, Lastayo PC, Dibble LE, Hill L, McClain DA. Increased strength and physical performance with eccentric training in women with impaired glucose tolerance: a pilot study. J Womens Health (Larchmt). 2009 Feb;18(2):253-60.

[47] McHugh MP. Recent advances in the understanding of the repeated bout effect: the protective effect against muscle damage from a single bout of eccentric exercise. Scand J Med Sci Sports. 2003 Apr;13(2):88-97.

[48] Michailidis Y, Jamurtas AZ, Nikolaidis MG, Fatouros IG, Koutedakis Y, Papassotiriou I, Kouretas D. Sampling time is crucial for measurement of aerobic exercise-induced oxidative stress. Med Sci Sports Exerc. 2007 Jul;39(7):1107-13.

[49] Miyama M, Nosaka K. Influence of surface on muscle damage and soreness induced by consecutive drop jumps. J Strength Cond Res. 2004 May;18(2):206-11.

[50] Nikolaidis MG, Kyparos A, Vrabas IS. F_2-isoprostane formation, measurement and interpretation: the role of exercise. Prog Lipid Res. 2011 Jan;50(1):89-103.

[51] Nikolaidis MG, Jamurtas AZ, Paschalis V, Fatouros IG, Koutedakis Y, Kouretas D. The effect of muscle-damaging exercise on blood and skeletal muscle oxidative stress: magnitude and time-course considerations. Sports Med 2008;38(7):579 606

[52] Nikolaidis MG, Paschalis V, Giakas G, Fatouros IG, Koutedakis Y, Kouretas D, Jamurtas AZ. Decreased blood oxidative stress after repeated muscle-damaging exercise. Med Sci Sports Exerc. 2007 Jul;39(7):1080-9.

[53] Nosaka K. Exercise-induced muscle damage and delayed-onset muscle soreness (DOMS). In Strength and Conditioning: Biological Principles and Practical Apllications (Ed. Cardinale M, Newton R, Nosaka K), Wiley-Blackwell, UK, pp.179-192.

[54] Nosaka K, Clarkson PM. Muscle damage following repeated bouts of high force eccentric exercise. Med Sci Sports Exerc. 1995 Sep;27(9):1263-9.

[55] Nosaka K, Newton M. Concentric or eccentric training effect on eccentric exercise-induced muscle damage. Med Sci Sports Exerc. 2002 Jan;34(1):63-9.

[56] O'Reilly KP, Warhol MJ, Fielding RA, Frontera WR, Meredith CN, Evans WJ. Eccentric exercise-induced muscle damage impairs muscle glycogen repletion. J Appl Physiol. 1987 Jul;63(1):252-6.

[57] Paffenbarger RS Jr, Hyde RT, Wing AL, et al. The association of changes in physical-activity level and other lifestyle characteristics with mortality among men. N Engl J Med 328: 538-45, 1993.

[58] Pafili ZK, Bogdanis GC, Tsetsonis NV, Maridaki M. Postprandial lipemia 16 and 40 hours after low-volume eccentric resistance exercise. Med Sci Sports Exerc. 2009 Feb;41(2):375-82.

[59] Paschalis V, Koutedakis Y, Baltzopoulos V, Mougios V, Jamurtas AZ, Theoharis V. The effects of muscle damage on running economy in healthy males. Int J Sports Med. 2005 Dec;26(10):827-31.

[60] Paschalis Vassilis, Theoharis Vassilis,Baltzopoulos Vassilios, Karatzaferi Christina, Mougios Vassilis, Jamurtas Z. Athanasios, Koutedakis Yiannis. Isokinetic eccentric exercise of quadriceps femoris does not affect running economy. J Strength Cond Res 22: 1222-1227, 2008

[61] Paschalis V, Nikolaidis MG, Giakas G, Jamurtas AZ, Pappas A, Koutedakis Y. The effect of eccentric exercise on position sense and joint reaction angle of the lower limbs. Muscle Nerve. 2007 Apr;35(4):496-503.

[62] Paschalis V, Nikolaidis MG, Theodorou AA, Giakas G, Jamurtas AZ, Koutedakis Y. Eccentric exercise affects the upper limbs more than the lower limbs in position sense and reaction angle. J Sports Sci. 2010 Jan;28(1):33-43.

[63] Paschalis V, Nikolaidis MG, Fatouros IG, Giakas G, Koutedakis Y, Karatzaferi C, Kouretas D, Jamurtas AZ. Uniform and prolonged changes in blood oxidative stress after muscle-damaging exercise. In Vivo. 2007 Sep-Oct;21(5):877-83.

[64] Paschalis V, Nikolaidis MG, Giakas G, Theodorou AA, Sakellariou GK, Fatouros IG, Koutedakis Y, Jamurtas AZ. Beneficial changes in energy expenditure and lipid profile after eccentric exercise in overweight and lean women. Scand J Med Sci Sports. 2010 (b) Feb;20(1):e103-11.

[65] Paschalis V, Nikolaidis MG, Theodorou AA, Panayiotou G, Fatouros IG, Koutedakis Y, Jamurtas AZ. A weekly bout of eccentric exercise is sufficient to induce health-promoting effects. Med Sci Sports Exerc. 2011 Jan;43(1):64-73.

[66] Peake J, Nosaka K, Suzuki K. Characterization of inflammatory responses to eccentric exercise in humans. Exerc Immunol Rev. 2005;11:64-85.

[67] Pendyala S, Natarajan V. Redox regulation of Nox proteins. Respir Physiol Neurobiol. 2010 Dec 31;174(3):265-71.

[68] Proske U, Allen TJ. Damage to skeletal muscle from eccentric exercise. Exerc Sport Sci Rev. 2005 Apr;33(2):98-104.

[69] Raastad T, Owe SG, Paulsen G, Enns D, Overgaard K, Crameri R, Kiil S, Belcastro A, Bergersen L, Hallén J. Changes in calpain activity, muscle structure, and function after eccentric exercise. Med Sci Sports Exerc. 2010 Jan;42(1):86-95.

[70] Radak Z, Bori Z, Koltai E, Fatouros IG, Jamurtas AZ, Douroudos II, Terzis G, Nikolaidis MG, Chatzinikolaou A, Sovatzidis A, Kumagai S, Naito H, Boldogh I. Age-dependent changes in 8-oxoguanine-DNA glycosylase activity are modulated by adaptive responses to physical exercise in human skeletal muscle. Free Radic Biol Med. 2011 Jul 15;51(2):417-23.

[71] Raj DA, Booker TS, Belcastro AN. Striated muscle calcium-stimulated cysteine protease (calpain-like) activity promotes myeloperoxidase activity with exercise. Pflugers Arch. 1998 May;435(6):804-9.

[72] Rockville, MD: U.S. Department of Health and Human Services, Public Health, Agency for Health Care Policy and Research and National Heart, Lung, and Blood Institute, 1995.

[73] Sahi T, Paffenbarger RS Jr, Hsieh CC, et al. Body mass index, cigarette smoking, and other characteristics as predictors of self-reported, physician-diagnosed gallbladder disease in male college alumni. Am J Epidemiol 147: 644–51, 1998.

[74] Santos CX, Anilkumar N, Zhang M, Brewer AC, Shah AM. Redox signaling in cardiac myocytes. Free Radic Biol Med. 2011 Apr 1;50(7):777-93.

[75] Saxton JM, Donnelly AE, Roper HP. Indices of free-radical-mediated damage following maximum voluntary eccentric and concentric muscular work. Eur J Appl Physiol Occup Physiol. 1994;68(3):189-93.

[76] Sen, C.K. and Hanninen, O. 1994. Physiological Antioxidants. In *Exercise and Oxygen Toxicity*. (Ed. C.K. Sen, L. Packer, and O. Hanninen). Amsterdam: Elsevier Science Publishers B.V. 89-126.

[77] Sies H. Role of reactive oxygen species in biological processes. Klin Wochenschr. 1991 Dec 15;69(21-23):965-8.

[78] Silva LA, Pinho CA, Silveira PC, Tuon T, De Souza CT, Dal-Pizzol F, Pinho RA. Vitamin E supplementation decreases muscular and oxidative damage but not inflammatory response induced by eccentric contraction. J Physiol Sci. 2010 Jan;60(1):51-7.

[79] Shahbazpour N, Carroll TJ, Riek S, Carson RG. Early alterations in serum creatine kinase and total cholesterol following high intensity eccentric muscle actions. J Sports Med Phys Fitness. 2004 Jun;44(2):193-9.

[80] Smith LL, Fulmer MG, Holbert D, McCammon MR, Houmard JA, Frazer DD, Nsien E, Israel RG. The impact of a repeated bout of eccentric exercise on muscular strength, muscle soreness and creatine kinase. Br J Sports Med. 1994 Dec;28(4):267-71.

[81] Takeshima N, Rogers M, Watanabe E, et al. Water-based exercise improves health-related aspects of fitness in older women. Med Sci Sports Exerc 33: 544-51, 2002.

[82] United States Department of Health and Human Services. Physical activity and health: a report of the Surgeon General, 1996.

[83] Theodorou AA, Nikolaidis MG, Paschalis V, Sakellariou GK, Fatouros IG, Koutedakis Y, Jamurtas AZ. Comparison between glucose-6-phosphate dehydrogenase-deficient and normal individuals after eccentric exercise. Med Sci Sports Exerc. 2010 Jun;42(6):1113-21.

[84] Tofas T, Jamurtas AZ, Fatouros I, Nikolaidis MG, Koutedakis Y, Sinouris EA, Papageorgakopoulou N, Theocharis DA. Plyometric exercise increases serum indices of muscle damage and collagen breakdown. J Strength Cond Res 2008 Mar;22(2):190-6.

[85] Tsatalas T, Giakas G, Spyropoulos G, Paschalis V, Nikolaidis MG, Tsaopoulos DE, Theodorou AA, Jamurtas AZ, Koutedakis Y. The effects of muscle damage on walking biomechanics are speed-dependent. Eur J Appl Physiol. 2010 Nov;110(5):977-88.

[86] Veskoukis AS, Nikolaidis MG, Kyparos A, Kokkinos D, Nepka C, Barbanis S, Kouretas D. Effects of xanthine oxidase inhibition on oxidative stress and swimming performance in rats. Appl Physiol Nutr Metab. 2008 Dec;33(6):1140-54.

[87] Vincent HK, Taylor AG. Biomarkers and potential mechanisms of obesity-induced oxidant stress in humans. Int J Obes (Lond). 2006 Mar;30(3):400-18.

[88] Wang TJ, Belza B, Thompson FE, Whitney JD, Bennett K. Effects of aquatic exercise on flexibility, strength and aerobic fitness in adults with osteoarthritis of the hip or knee. J Adv Nurs 57: 141-52, 2007.

[89] Warren GL, Lowe DA, Armstrong RB. Measurement tools used in the study of eccentric contraction-induced injury. Sports Med. 1999 Jan;27(1):43-59.

[90] Zhao ZQ, Nakamura M, Wang NP, Wilcox JN, Shearer S, Ronson RS, Guyton RA, Vinten-Johansen J. Reperfusion induces myocardial apoptotic cell death. *Cardiovascular Research*. 2000;45(3):651-660.

[91] LaStayo PC, Marcus RL, Dibble LE, Smith SB, Beck SL. Eccentric exercise versus usual-care with older cancer survivors: the impact on muscle and mobility--an exploratory pilot study. *BMC Geriatr*. 2011; 11: 5. Published online 2011 January 27. doi: 10.1186/1471-2318-11-5

[92] Lorenz D, Reiman M. The role and implementation of eccentric training in athletic rehabilitation: tendinopathy, hamstring strains, and acl reconstruction. *Int J Sports Phys Ther.* 6(1):27-44, 2011.

6

Body Mass Bias in Exercise Physiology

Paul M. Vanderburgh
University of Dayton, Dayton, OH
USA

1. Introduction

Body mass bias in the field of exercise physiology has been the subject of increased focus over the past twenty years. This is based primarily on the fact that key widely held assumptions about the relationships between body mass and human performance have been challenged by theory and empirical data. The result for how we express certain variables of physical fitness has been generally two-fold: a systematic and meaningful body mass bias against larger, not fatter, individuals and spurious attribution of the effect of body mass on key dependent variables.

Physical educators, the military services, law enforcement agencies, and conditioning coaches have readily used fitness tests comprised of events that involve body mass as the primary resistance. Common tests include pushups, situps, and timed distance runs. Virtually none of these tests takes into account one's body mass in scoring because a common assumption has been that larger people have more muscle to move the heavier mass. In short, these factors are assumed to "wash out" any body mass bias. Empirical research has shown, however, that these types of tests impose a substantial and predictable bias against larger, not just fatter, body mass (Crowder & Yunker, 1996; Harman & Frykman, 1992; Jaric et al., 2005; Markovic & Jaric, 2004; Vanderburgh et al., 1995). Similarly, because maximal oxygen consumption (VO_{2max}, in L/min) and maximal strength increase with body mass, a common convention to compare individuals is to divide VO_{2max} or strength measures by body mass. Expressing these human performance indices as simple ratios this way has been scrutinized given that the numerator does not change at the same rate as the denominator (Astrand & Rodahl, 1986; Heil, 1997). Again, the result is not only a body mass bias against larger individuals but, in the case of inferential research, improper accounting for the effects of body mass on outcome variables.

In certain physically demanding occupations, especially the military, body mass bias has substantive implications. Work physiologists have determined that despite body mass bias in the common military physical fitness tests, the larger service members were often better performers of the physically demanding occupational tasks (Bilzon et al., 2002; Lyons et al., 2005; Rayson et al., 2000). That is, they could carry more, more easily evacuate casualties, and better engage in heavy materiel handling. Yet, the smaller personnel were achieving better scores on the physical fitness tests, the results of which have significant promotion and advancement implications (Vanderburgh & Mahar, 1995; Crowder & Yunker, 1996).

This chapter chronicles the fundamentals and applications of body mass bias in fitness and exercise physiology, to include the theory and empirical data used to evaluate it. It also explains the real world implications of body mass bias in the military services, and how to mitigate its undesirable or unintended effects.

2. Body mass bias and biological scaling

Body mass bias is simply the notion that larger individuals have an unfair advantage over smaller, or vice-versa, in measures of exercise performance. It is more formally defined as the correlation between a raw score (e.g., maximal weight lifted, pushups repetitions, oxygen uptake) and body mass. A non-zero correlation indicates the presence of bias; a correlation not different from zero indicates the absence of such bias. Some biases are rather intuitive. Maximal grip strength, bench press or absolute work rate on a cycle ergometer are measures that would give larger individuals an advantage since each is largely dependent on muscle yet body mass is not the source of the resistance. As a result, a sport like powerlifting employs body weight classes and maximal power is often expressed relative to body mass. Less intuitive, perhaps, are measures that advantage smaller individuals. These include those that measure the capacity to move one's body mass in exercises such as pushups or distance running. The less-than-intuitive quality is based on the common assumption that larger individuals have more muscle to move body mass so there should be no particular advantage to the smaller. A closer look, however, at laws of biological scaling and their application to military physical fitness data make a compelling case that the common fitness test events of pushups, situps and distance running, and even VO_{2max} expressed per unit of body mass, impose a bias against larger, not just fatter, personnel (Vanderburgh, 2007, 2008).

Perhaps an easy way to think of this is through the analogy of a 2 x 2 x 4 solid rectangular block (Fig. 1) of constant density. Its cross-sectional area (CSA) would be 2 x 2 or 4 sq ft and, with a density of 1.0, its weight would be 16 lbs. Imagine that the block (PRE) turned into an identical scale-model block of the same density, but with sides 25%, or 1.25 times longer (the POST block). Simple geometric principles dictate, then, that CSA would be 2.5 x 2.5, or 5.25 sq ft. This represents a 56.25% increase in CSA. Similarly, the new weight of 31.25 lbs (2.5 x 2.5 x 5 = 31.25 lbs) is a 95.3% increase.

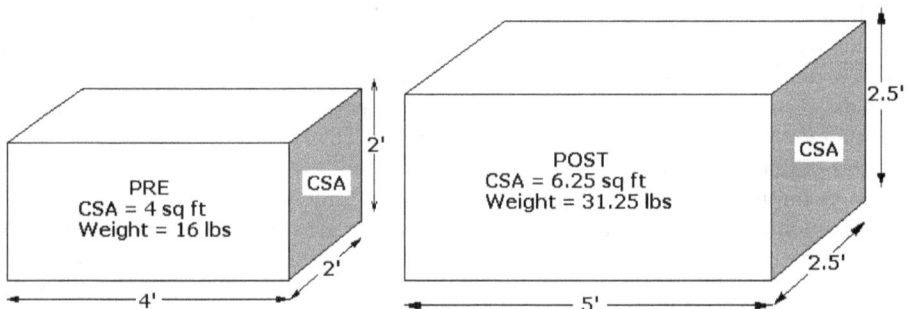

Fig. 1. Comparison of change in length, cross-sectional area (CSA) and weight

Scaling theory helps us understand why these dimensions change at different rates and biological scaling principles elucidate the relevance to human performance. As shown in

Table 1, if length increases by 1.25 (a 25% change), then CSA changes by 1.25^2 and weight changes by 1.25^3. This is because length is considered a one-dimensional variable, area is two-dimensional, and weight (just like volume) is three-dimensional. In terms of biological significance, one can think of the human body just like the block in the present example. It has its own body mass and its CSA is considered to be muscle cross sectional area, one of the prime determinants of strength. Therefore, the 95% increase in weight shown in Table 1 is accompanied by only a 56.25% increase in strength. This human performance scaling concept is critically important because it challenges the common assumption that an X% larger person should be X% stronger. Empirical evidence supports the fallacy of this assumption. Also of critical importance is the notion that "larger" assumes an exact scale model, not larger because he/she is fatter or taller.

	PRE	POST	Multiplier / % Increase	Calculation
Length	4'	5'	1.25 / 25%	$(1.25)^1 = 1.25$
CSA	4 ft²	6.25 ft²	1.5625 / 56.25%	$(1.25)^2 = 1.5625$
Weight	16 lbs	31.25 lbs	1.9531 / 95.31%	$(1.25)^3 = 1.9531$

Table 1. Calculations of Fig. 1 changes in dimensions due to scale model increase in size

3. Allometric scaling in fitness tests

Allometry, a term often associated with biological scaling, is the relationship between the size of an organism and the size of any of its parts, such as muscle or blood vessel CSA, limb length, eyeball radius, etc. Allometry provides the theoretical bases upon which empirical findings can be compared. In the case of Fig. 1 and its analogous application to the human body, strength (S) does not change proportionally to body mass (M). If it did, it would also increase by 95.3%. Instead, its 56.25% increase can be explained by the allometric relationship:

$$S \alpha M^{2/3} \tag{1}$$

This is derived from the fact that weight is a three-dimensional and CSA a two-dimensional variable (Astrand & Rodahl, 1986; Jaric, 2002). From Eq. 1 we can substitute the delta, or change on both sides such that:

$$\Delta S \alpha \Delta M^{2/3} \tag{2}$$

Indeed, 1.5625 (the change in CSA, or strength) = $1.9531^{2/3}$ (the change in mass). This exponent of 2/3, often called an allometric exponent, tells us that the proper way to express muscle strength to allow for comparisons between individuals of different body mass is: $S/M^{2/3}$. This is because both sides change at the same rate – a necessary condition for expressing ratios in physiology (Astrand & Rodahl, 1986; Vanderburgh, 1998). Though unconventional, this index should show zero correlation with body mass in a large sample of subjects. It is also very useful in understanding how other variables, such as fitness test scores, or maximal oxygen uptake, change with body size changes.

Since blood vessel CSA is also a two-dimensional variable, and oxygen delivery is associated with blood flow, then maximal oxygen uptake, VO_{2max}, would be subject to a similar relationship:

$$VO_{2max} \alpha \Delta M^{2/3} \tag{3}$$

and the following index: $VO_{2max}/M^{2/3}$. Once again, this is an unconventional index but allows for comparisons of maximal aerobic capacity between individuals of different body mass such that body mass bias is zero. This index has been validated this index in a large sample of 230 women and 210 men (Heil, 1997).

The effects of body mass changes on strength and VO_{2max} can be used to derive appropriate scaling indices for events like distance runs (DR) and maximal pushups (PU) or situps (SU) repetitions. One explanation (Jaric et al., 2002b) for its derivation is that the ability to move one's body mass is directly proportional to strength (which is directly proportional to $M^{2/3}$) and indirectly proportional to body mass (M^1). Therefore, since PU or SU $\alpha\ M^{2/3}/M^1$, then:

$$PU\ or\ SU\ \alpha\ M^{-1/3} \tag{4}$$

Interestingly, the ratio scaling that results, $PU/M^{-1/3}$, is equivalent to $PU \cdot M^{1/3}$ (same for SU). For the distance run (DR), the scaling index is derived as follows (Vanderburgh & Mahar, Vanderburgh & Crowder, 2006; Vanderburgh & Laubach, 2007): Since distance run time is indirectly proportional to VO_{2max}, expressed per unit of body mass (Nevill et al., 1992), and VO_{2max} in L/min (i.e., no adjustment for body mass) is directly proportional to $M^{2/3}$ (Eq. 3), then DR $\alpha\ M^1/M^{2/3}$, or

$$DR\ \alpha\ M^{1/3} \tag{5}$$

This means that DR time goes up as M goes up. Since low score wins in run time, the DR expression would be $DR/M^{1/3}$. This index has been empirically validated as well (Crecilius et al., 2008; Crowder & Yunker, 1996; Vanderburgh et al., in press).

4. Empirical validation of allometric modeling in fitness tests

"Empirically validated" in these cases indicates that researchers have tested the hypotheses of Eqns. 1,3-5 in reasonably large samples to determine the actual body mass exponent and compared it with the theoretical. For purposes of illustration, this can be done using real data from the sport of competitive powerlifting and the methods described in more detail by Vanderburgh (1998). Powerlifting, comprised of maximal one-repetition lifts in the squat (SQ), bench press (BP), deadlift (DL), and total (TOT) of all three, is a good choice for examining body mass exponents for several reasons. First, it is a sport of primarily muscular strength, not power, hand-eye coordination, or even complex cognition, all of which could be confounders in examining the relationship between performance and body mass. Second, at the elite level (not counting the super heavyweight division, which has no weight limit), all competitors are very lean, thus eliminating body fat as a confounder. Third, the two primary determinants of performance are strength and body mass. Therefore, a sample of powerlifting world record holders would be heterogeneous in body mass and weight lifted – almost nothing else.

The determination of the empirical exponent is done using linear regression, but on the logarithmic transformations of M and SQ, BP, DL and TOT. The procedure starts with Eq. 1, S $\alpha\ M^b$, but with SQ, BP, DL and TOT replacing S. Scatterplots of current male world record holders (as of May, 2011, http://records.powerlifting.org/world) for these four events are shown in Fig. 2. Note that the exponent is the unknown, as the purpose of empirical testing is to determine the actual M exponent for that sample. For purposes of illustrations, TOT will be chosen: TOT $\alpha\ M^b$. This really means that the best-fit curve of a scatterplot of TOT vs. M will conform to the following equation:

$$TOT = aM^b \tag{6}$$

where a and b are constants. This is an allometric, not linear relationship. For linear regression, the terms must be in the form of y = mx + b. A log transformation of both sides, then, yields the following:

$$\ln TOT = (b)\ln M + \ln(a) \tag{7}$$

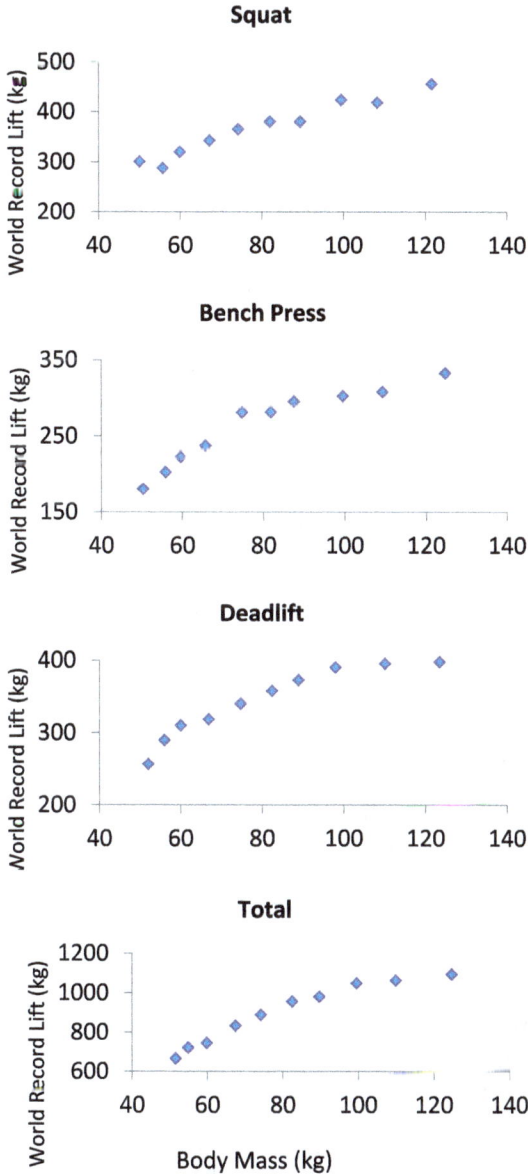

Fig. 2. World powerlifting records by body mass (as of May, 2011, http://records.powerlifting.org/world)

Now, lnTOT becomes "y," b becomes "m," and ln(a) becomes "b" in the linear equation. Regressing lnTOT on lnM will yield not only the value of b but its confidence interval (CI) as well. This is quite important since scatterplots of human performance always deviate from the best-fit curve and CIs give an indication of probability that the population's true exponent lies within it. Linear regression of the log-transformed terms for the TOT event yields an exponent of 0.58 with a 95% confidence interval of 0.48 to 0.67. Within this confidence interval (CI), an M exponent would yield zero body mass bias for TOT. Note that 2/3, or 0.667, is within (but barely) the CI. Table 2 shows the actual body mass exponents for the four different powerlifting events, along with the 95% CI ranges.

	SQ	BP	DL	TOT
Exponent	0.50	0.65	0.48	0.58
95% CI	0.42 – 0.59	0.49 – 0.80	0.37 – 0.60	0.48 – 0.67

Table 2. Body mass exponents for world record powerlifting performances (Fig.2)

This table illustrates a number of key points in evaluating empirical data for allometric scaling. First, among the world's elite, a small number of subjects (N = 10 in this case) can show the characteristic curvilinear allometric relationship between body mass and performance. Each event indicates, as body mass increases, the expected smaller and smaller increase in performance. Said differently, the relationships are clearly not linear. Second, since neither is in the CI ranges, the exponents of 0 or 1 impose a body mass bias. While an exponent of 0 yielding such bias is expected since that would be analogous to no weight classes, the exponent of 1 doing the same might be surprising. These data show that, in any of the events, dividing the performance by body mass (e.g., SQ/M^1) would also yield body mass bias. This actually conforms to the laws of biological scaling since the exponent of 1 is too large. In other words, the index SQ/M makes too much of an adjustment for M, thus penalizing larger competitors.

Third, and perhaps surprisingly, not all the exponents' CIs contain the expected value of 2/3. There are many reasons why this can, and often does happen in allometry research. With a small sample size, one case can influence the magnitude of the exponent. In the TOT, for example, removing the heaviest competitor changes the exponent from 0.58 to 0.63, the latter for which the 2/3 exponent easily fits within the 95% CI range, not barely as with all the competitors. In the case of world record holders, as others have conjectured for world class powerlifting events (Dooman & Vanderburgh, 2000; Vanderburgh & Batterham, 1999; Vanderburgh & Dooman, 2000), there are more competitors worldwide in the middle weight classes and fewer at the extremes. This would suggest that, adjusted for body mass differences, the world's best in the middle weight classes would be better than the best from the lightest and heaviest classes, thus "bumping" up the middle of the curve. This would affect goodness-of-fit with an allometric model and alter the exponent value away from the theoretical. One other worthwhile explanation in the present data is that both the squat and deadlift exercises, unlike the bench press, lift not only the barbells but a substantial percentage of the body mass as well. Since moving body mass is disadvantageous for larger individuals, this would lessen the slope of the best-fit curve for the scatterplots such as those in Fig. 2, the result would be a smaller exponent. Indeed, Table 2 indicates that the smallest exponents are for squat and deadlift. In large samples of non-world-class subjects, there are many other confounders such as body composition, effort, biomechanics, etc. Often, when deviation from theoretical is found, researchers are faced with offering reasonable explanations without the statistical control to back such claims. The best research samples, then, are those in which the subjects are heterogeneous in the dependent variable (performance score) and body mass but homogeneous in the potential confounders such as effort and body composition.

Some studies have indicated deviation from theoretical for the body mass exponent for expressing VO_{2max}. Batterham et al. (1999) found that, in a sample of 1314 adult men, although the body mass exponent was 0.65, the fat-free mass exponent was not different from 1.0. Since body fat is essentially metabolically inert, and fat-free mass is the body compartment largely responsible for generating oxygen consumption, then body composition was a confounder in leading to the spurious conclusion that the 0.65 body mass exponent matched the theoretically expected value of 2/3. Similarly, Vanderburgh et al. (1996a), in a sample of 94 adult women, determined that while ratio scaling of VO_{2max} penalized heavier women, the penalty was due to the body fatness.

Another interesting but quite common dilemma is assuming validity when the empirically derived exponent matches the theoretical, as is the case with the BP and TOT events. Indeed, these findings could be the result of confounding effects on the exponent such that the primary reason it "made the 95% CI" is that certain confounders, such as those listed above, happened to push the exponent value into the theoretical range. In other words, one can never be quite sure how the empirical did or did not match the theoretical.

As is the case with inferential statistics, however, one should always consider the totality of research evidence from multiple samples from different populations using appropriate statistical control to evaluate the overall trend for allometry's effects on human performance. Based on two extensive reviews (Jaric et al., 2005; Vanderburgh, 2008), one can make a compelling case that use of the exponents as described in Table 3 is appropriate for fitness testing, especially for adult men.

	PU (max reps)	SU (max reps)	BP (1RM)	DR (time)
Exponent	$PU \cdot M^{1/3}$	$SU \cdot M^{1/3}$	$BP/M^{2/3}$	$DR/M^{1/3}$
References	Crowder & Yunker, 2000 Markovic & Jaric, 2004 Vanderburgh et al., in press	Markovic & Jaric, 2004	Dooman & Vanderburgh, 2000 Markovic & Jaric, 2004 Vanderburgh & Dooman, 2000	Crowder & Yunker, 2000 Nevill et al., 1992 Vanderburgh & Mahar, 1995 Vanderburgh et al., in press

PU = Pushups, SU = Situps, DR = Distance run time

Table 3. Allometric indices for common fitness tests

5. The utility of allometry in fitness testing

These indices can be used to compare individual fitness scores among people of varying body weights. The results of some hypothetical examples can be illuminating. Consider two individuals, Ellen and June, with the fitness scores as shown in Table 4. Scaled scores are calculated using the indices from Table 3, maintaining the appropriate units. Clearly, body mass influences scoring with the allometric indices, which make a proper adjustment for its influence. One can interpret allometric comparisons as follows, using a Table 4 example: "Without consideration of the influence of body mass on pushups, Ellen performed 11.8% more repetitions. Considering the influence of body mass, however, June scored 4.6% better." In the case of the bench press, June's performance was 47.7% better than Ellen's for raw score but only 8.0% better when making a proper adjustment for body mass.

On a more significant scale, the effect of body mass bias among military personnel has been quantified (Vanderburgh & Crowder, 2006). For example, a 90 kg man performing at the same physiological level as a 60 kg man who achieved a maximum score on the U.S.

		Ellen	June	Comparison
Body Mass	--	50 kg	80 kg	--
Pushups	Raw	38 reps	34 reps	Ellen by 11.8%
	Scaled	140.0 reps·$M^{1/3}$	146.5 reps·$M^{1/3}$	June by 4.6%
Bench Press	Raw	44 kg	65 kg	June by 47.7%
	Scaled	3.24 kg·$M^{-0.67}$	3.50 kg·$M^{-0.67}$	June by 8.0%
2-Mile Run	Raw	13:24	15:00	Ellen by 10.7%
	Scaled	3.64 min·$M^{-1/3}$	3.48 min·$M^{-1/3}$	June by 4.4 %

Table 4. Hypothetical example of the effects of allometry in fitness testing

Army Physical Fitness Test of pushups, situps, and two-mile run, would actually receive a 15% lower score (256 vs. 300 points). In this case, "same physiological level" is the expected performance of a 90 kg man who is an exact scale model of the 60 kg man. Similarly, for a 45 kg vs. 75 kg woman, the U.S. Navy's test levies a 20% penalty. In the case of the Armed Services, there are actually two very real undesirable consequences for the larger service members. First, advancement and promotion is influenced by the fitness test scores. For the two women above, the heavier who scored physiologically equivalent 240 points compared to the lighter's 300 max points, is at a substantial promotion disadvantage, all other factors being equal. Second, occupational physiology findings suggest that larger military personnel tend to be better performers of physically demanding military tasks (Bilzon et al., 2001; Bilzon et al., 2002, Harman & Frykman, 1992; Harman et al., 2008; Lyons et al., 2005; Rayson et al., 2000). These include: heavy materiel handling, load carriage, and casualty evacuation - tasks that involve not only moving one's own weight but additional external weight. As a result, and because physical fitness test performance is linked with promotions and advancement within the services, the current physical fitness tests of the U.S. Army, Air Force, and Navy penalize the very populations that perform physically demanding military tasks better.

Body mass bias also occurs in competitive sports, most notably distance running which attracts over two million competitors in race distances of five kilometers or greater each year in the United States. The implications can be substantial. For example, a 68 kg woman's 50:00 10 km race time would be physiologically equivalent to a 50 kg woman's 45:07 10 km time. Accordingly, body weight handicap models for distance runs have been developed and validated to account for body weight differences in determining race performance (Vanderburgh & Laubach, 2007). Despite the additional credit for larger body mass, these models have also been determined to be disadvantageous for those whose larger mass is due to excess fat mass, an important health-related finding (Vanderburgh et al., in press).

In some sports, such as wrestling and power lifting, weight classes are the main method of accounting for body weight differences. One of the challenges of such a convention is that there are often few competitors in the extremes of weight and many in the middle weights. This imposes a body weight bias against the middle weight competitors who must compete against many more athletes to win or place. Recent empirical evidence suggests that allometric scaling is a technique that can be used to eliminate all weight classes for each gender and determine the best overall lifter when properly adjusting for body weight differences (Vanderburgh & Batterham, 1999). In competitive rowing, there are typically only two weight classes for each gender, light and heavy. Vanderburgh et al. (1996) developed and validated an allometric index that allows all rowers of any size within each gender, to be compared to each other while properly factoring out the influence of body mass and age. Their results suggest that rowing time multiplied by stature (or $M^{1/3}$) was the optimal index to remove body mass bias among these competitive rowers.

6. Body fatness and allometry in fitness testing

One of the main critiques of using allometric scaling in fitness testing is that giving credit for weight in the scoring is to also give credit for excess body fat. In other words, some perceive that such scoring gives advantages for being fatter. Indeed, one's denominator of $M^{1/3}$ for the distance run score computed from the DR/$M^{1/3}$ calculation would be larger for a fatter individual, thus leading to a lower (and better score, since low score wins). What is not often considered, however, is the effect of the excess fatness on the numerator – in this case, the distance run time. Vanderburgh and colleagues have modeled the effects of adding additional fat weight on the resultant distance run time for the 5 km and 2-mile runs and have shown that, in all cases, adding fat weight leads to a worse scaled score (Crecilius et al., 2008; Vanderburgh & Laubach, 2007). Recently, they tested this empirically, by adding external weight to the DR and PU events for college-age men. Results indicated that the addition of 16 kg of external weight led to 38% worse scaled PU scores and 12% worse two-mile run scaled scores (Vanderburgh et al., in press).

7. Practical techniques for using allometry in fitness testing

As shown in Table 4, allometrically scaled scores yield strange units and currency. That is, one may find the interpretation of a scaled score for a 65 kg bench press, 3.50 kg·$M^{-0.67}$, quite difficult to interpret. This is likely due to the units, kg·$M^{-0.67}$, being unlike those encountered elsewhere and the magnitude of 3.50 not being as readily evaluated as 65 kg would be. Another problem with these scores is that they require a calculator to compute. In short, though arguably proper and fair, allometrically scaled scores are not practical.

Other solutions have been proposed. The first, correction factors, are dimensionless numbers based on body weight, which are multiplied by the raw score to produce an adjusted in the same units and more easily interpretable (Vanderburgh, 2007). For example, from Table 4, Ellen's and June's correction factors would, for PU, be: 1.0 and 1.17, respectively. This is calculated based on a body mass standard - a baseline from which all ratios are computed, the individual's body mass, and the particular event. For a standard weight of 50 kg, for example, and June's body mass of 80 kg, and the PU, her correction factor would be (80 kg/50 kg)$^{1/3}$, or 1.170″ (in both cases). Multiplying her raw score of 34 pushups by 1.211 yields an adjusted score of 39.78 pushups. Using the same methodology,

Ellen's adjusted score would be 38 x 1.0 = 39.4 pushups and June's adjusted performance is exactly the same 4.6% better than Ellen using the correction factors.

Simple tables can be constructed to determine correction factors without calculators and the multiplication of raw score by correction factor can be done with pencil-and-paper. Table 5 illustrates an example from Vanderburgh (2007), applied to the distance run events of United States armed forces fitness tests. In this case, the weight standards were selected as 120 lbs. and 150 lbs. for women and men, respectively. These values were specifically chosen to allow no credit below these body weights. Though the selection of the standard is arbitrary, it must be used consistently once chosen. Also, correction factors can be less than one as well. Nonetheless, correction factors still impose a logistical challenge in developing tables for each event and their use is not intuitively obvious to users with very little exercise science background.

Women	120	130	140	150	160	170	180	190	200
0	1.00	0.99	0.96	0.94	0.92	0.90	0.89	0.87	0.85
1	1.00	0.98	0.96	0.94	0.92	0.90	0.88	0.87	0.85
2	1.00	0.98	0.96	0.94	0.92	0.90	0.88	0.87	0.85
3	1.00	0.98	0.96	0.93	0.92	0.90	0.88	0.87	0.85
4	1.00	0.98	0.95	0.93	0.91	0.90	0.88	0.86	0.85
5	1.00	0.97	0.95	0.93	0.91	0.89	0.88	0.86	0.85
6	1.00	0.97	0.95	0.93	0.91	0.89	0.88	0.86	0.85
7	0.99	0.97	0.95	0.93	0.91	0.89	0.87	0.86	0.85
8	0.99	0.97	0.95	0.92	0.91	0.89	0.87	0.86	0.84
9	0.99	0.97	0.94	0.92	0.90	0.89	0.87	0.86	0.84

Men	150	160	170	180	190	200	210	220	230	240	250
0	1.00	0.98	0.96	0.94	0.92	0.91	0.89	0.88	0.87	0.85	0.84
1	1.00	0.98	0.96	0.94	0.92	0.91	0.89	0.88	0.87	0.85	0.84
2	1.00	0.97	0.96	0.94	0.92	0.91	0.89	0.88	0.86	0.85	0.84
3	0.99	0.97	0.95	0.94	0.92	0.90	0.89	0.88	0.86	0.85	0.84
4	0.99	0.97	0.95	0.93	0.92	0.90	0.89	0.87	0.86	0.85	0.84
5	0.99	0.97	0.95	0.93	0.92	0.90	0.89	0.87	0.86	0.85	0.84
6	0.99	0.97	0.95	0.93	0.91	0.90	0.89	0.87	0.86	0.85	0.84
7	0.98	0.96	0.95	0.93	0.91	0.90	0.88	0.87	0.86	0.85	0.84
8	0.98	0.96	0.94	0.93	0.91	0.90	0.88	0.87	0.86	0.85	0.83
9	0.98	0.96	0.94	0.93	0.91	0.90	0.88	0.87	0.86	0.84	0.83

Table 5. Correction Factors for Distance Runs, Pushups, or Situps Tests. A 186 lb man with an actual score two-mile run time of 15:05, for example, would go to the "180" column and down to the row corresponding to "6" to yield the correction factor of 0.93. Since low score wins, this number would be multiplied by the actual time of 905 sec to yield an adjusted score of 841.7 sec or 14:02. For a 172 lb woman with 32 pushups, and high score wins, one would divide her raw score by the 0.90 correction factor to yield an adjusted score of 35.6 pushups (from Vanderburgh, 2007).

A third solution is the use of a balanced fitness test – one that imposes no body mass advantage. They can be single or multi-event. A backpack run is an example of a single-event balanced test, in which neither larger nor smaller personnel are disadvantaged. This test, which would require all military personnel to run a given distance with a standard-weight backpack, has been mathematically modeled and shown to eliminate body mass bias in men (Vanderburgh & Flanagan, 2000). This has occupational relevance since the standard backpack load for service members is typically the same, regardless of one's body mass. He/she must carry that load often over some considerable distance in arduous terrain. The advantage to the larger body mass of the standard weight for everyone is counterbalanced by the disadvantage of moving one's body mass. This backpack run test, along with a backpack pushups test, using the same standard weight of 16 kg, has been validated for college-age men as being free of body mass bias (Vanderburgh, in press). These types of tests, then, require no special calculations and produce raw scores that are fair and occupationally relevant. They do, however, pose a mass testing challenge in terms of the extra equipment needed.

One multi-event test that purports to be balanced is the popular "Pump & Run,"which entails a distance run and bench press event. One's final score is equal to the distance run time (in sec) minus 30 sec times each repetition of the bench press. The weight lifted, however, is based on a percentage of one's body mass. As Vanderburgh & Laubach (2008) determined empirically for 74 female and 343 male competitors of one event, the body mass bias against larger competitors was substantial, largely because both events imposed the penalty. The bench press was actually analogous to the pushup exercise which also lifts a percentage of one's weight. The researchers proposed a correction factor table but also recommended the study of a standard weight lifted for all competitors, not one based on body mass. This case study is probably the best single example of the non-intuitive nature of body mass bias; race officials were trying to level the playing field with the two events but the result had just as much body mass bias as the distance run alone.

8. Conclusion

Body mass bias is a real phenomenon in fitness testing which is based on the fundamental notion that the ability to move one's weight is not directly proportional to one's body mass. This bias, especially in large-scale testing such as the military, leads to not only an advantage for smaller service members, but a disadvantage against those who perform the physically demanding occupational tasks of the military better – the larger service members. Allometric scaling and its derivative technique of correction factors can be used to erase such biases but, while these are mathematically appropriate and valid, they impose logistical and non-intuitive challenges. Such scoring is also useful in determining the best overall performer in sports such as distance running, powerlifting, and even indoor rowing. Evidence suggests that, although allometric scaling grants a credit for being heavier, if the increased body mass is fat mass, then the resulting scaled score is worse. This is because the detriment in raw score performance is of greater magnitude than the credit granted. Balanced fitness tests like the backpack run and pushups tests, which impose no body mass bias, have been shown to be intuitive, useful and occupationally relevant but are not without their mass testing challenges with regard to equipment needed. Most importantly, exercise scientists who can exercise some level of fluency in the principles of biological scaling and allometry as they apply to fitness testing will be able to best interpret human performance scores not only sport, but in occupational fitness and health-related fitness as well.

9. Acknowledgment

I would like to acknowledge the following:

- My colleagues at the United States Military Academy at West Point, also my alma mater, where physical fitness is highly valued and excellence is a habit; your energy and passion were contagious.
- The many soldiers and USMA/ROTC cadets of the United States Army who served as subjects in our research; your compliance and cooperation were top-shelf in every way and your efforts were always maximal, a necessary condition for this type of research.
- My colleagues in the field of exercise physiology, especially Dr. Todd Crowder, Dr. Alan Batterham, Dr. Lloyd Laubach, and Dr. Tom Rowland; your friendship, enthusiasm, and collegiality were not only the key ingredients for productivity but for having fun along the way.
- The graduate students with whom I've had the pleasure to work; I hope you learned as much from our collaborations as I did.

10. References

Astrand, P. & Rodahl, K. (1986). *Textbook of Work Physiology*. McGraw Hill ISBN 0-7360-0140-9, New York, pp.399-405,

Batterham, A.; Vanderburgh, P.; Mahar, M. & Jackson, A. (1999). Modeling the influence of body size on VO_{2peak}: Effects of model choice and body composition. *Journal of Applied Physiology*, Vol.87, No.4, pp. 1317-1325, ISSN 8750-7587

Bilzon, J.; Allsopp, A. & Tipton, M. (2001). Assessment of physical fitness for occupations encompassing load-carriage tasks. *Occupational Medicine*. Vol.51, No.5, pp. 357-361, ISSN 0962-7480

Bilzon, J; Scarpello, E.; Bilzon, E. & Allsop, A. (2002) Generic task-related occupational requirements for Royal Navy personnel. *Occupational Medicine*, Vol.52, No.8, pp. 503-510, ISSN 0962-7480

Crecelius, A.; Vanderburgh, P. & Laubach, L. (2008). Contributions of body fat and effort in the 5K run age and body weight handicap model. *Journal of Strength and Conditioning*, Vol.22, No.5, pp. 1475-1480, ISSN 1064-8011

Crowder, T. & Yunker, C. (1986). Scaling of push-up, sit-up and two-mile run performances by body weight and fat-free weight in young, fit men [Abstract]. *Medicine and Science in Sports and Exercise*, Vol.28, No.5, p.S183, ISSN 0195-9131

Dooman C. & Vanderburgh, P. (2000). Allometric modeling of the bench press and squat: Who is the strongest regardless of body mass? *Journal of Strength and Conditioning Research*, Vol.14, No.1, pp. 32-36, ISSN 1064-8011

Harman, E. & Frykman, P. (1992). The relationship of body size and composition to the performance of physically demanding military tasks. In: *Body Composition and Physical Performance*. National Academy Press ISBN 0-309-0458, pp.105-18

Harman, E.; Gutekunst, D.; Frykman, P.; Sharp, M.; Nindl, B.; Alemany, J. & Mello, R. (2008). Prediction of Simulated Battlefield Physical Performance from Field-Expedient Tests. *Military Medicine*, Vol.173, No.1, pp.36-41, ISSN 0026-4075

Heil, D. (1997). Body mass scaling of peak oxygen uptake in 20- to 79-yr-old adults. *Medicine and Science in Sports and Exercise,* Vol.29, No.12, pp.1602-1608, ISSN 0195-9131

Jaric, S. (2002). Muscle strength testing – Use of normalization for body size. *Sports Medicine,* Vol.32, No.10, pp. 615-631, ISSN 0112-1642

Jaric, S.; Ugarkovic, D. & Kukolj, M. (2002). Evaluation of methods of normalizing muscle strength in elite and young athletes. *Journal of Sports Medicine and Physical Fitness,* Vol.42, No.2, pp. 141-151, ISSN 0022-4707

Jaric, S.; Radosavljevic-Jaric, S. & Johansson, H. (2002). Muscle force and muscle torque in humans require different methods when adjusting for differences in body size. *European Journal of Applied Physiology,* Vol.87, No. 3, pp. 304-7, ISSN 1439-6319

Jaric, S.; Mirkov, D. & Markovic, G. (2005). Normalizing physical performance tests for body size: A proposal for standardization. *Journal of Strength and Conditioning Research,* Vol.19, No.2, pp.467-74, ISSN 1064-8011

Lyons, J.; Allsopp, A. & Bilzon, J. (2005). Influences of body composition upon the relative metabolic and cardiovascular demands of load-carriage. *Occupational Medicine,* Vol.55, No.5., pp. 380-384, ISSN 0962-7480

Markovic, G. & Jaric, S. (2004). Movement performance and body size: The relationship for different groups of tests. *European Journal of Applied Physiology,* Vol.92, No.1, pp. 139-149, ISSN 1439-6319

Nevill, A.; Ramsbottom, R. & Williams, C. (1992). Scaling physiological measurements for individuals of different body size. *European Journal of Applied Physiology,* Vol.65, No.2, pp. 110-17, ISSN 1439-6319

Rayson, M; Holliman, D. & Belyavin, A. (2000). Development of physical selection procedures for the British Army. Phase 2: Relationship between physical performance tests and criterion tasks. *Ergonomics,* Vol.43, No.1, pp. 73-105, ISSN 0014-0139

Vanderburgh, P.; Mahar, M. & Chou, C. (1995). Allometric scaling of grip strength by body mass in college-age men and women. *Research Quarterly for Exercise and Sport,* Vol.66, No.1, pp.80-84, ISSN 0270-1367

Vanderburgh, P., & Mahar, M. (1995). Scaling of 2-mile run times by body weight and fat-free weight in college-age men. *Journal of Strength and Conditioning Research,* Vol.9, No.2, pp. 67-70, ISSN 1064-8011

Vanderburgh, P. & Katch, F. (1996). Ratio scaling of VO_{2max} penalizes women with larger percent body fat, not lean body mass. *Medicine and Science in Sports and Exercise,* Vol.28, No.9, pp. 1204-8, ISSN 0195-9131

Vanderburgh, P.; Katch, F; Schoenleber, J.; Balabinis, C. & Elliott, R. (1996). Multivariate allometric scaling of men's world indoor rowing championship performance. *Medicine and Science in Sports and Exercise,* Vol.28, No.5, pp. 626-30, ISSN 0195-9131

Vanderburgh, P. (1998). Two important cautions in the use of allometric scaling: The common exponent and group differences principles. *Measurement in Physical Education and Exercise Science,* Vol.2, No.3, pp. 153-63, ISSN 1091-367X

Vanderburgh, P. & Batterham, A. (1999). Validation of the Wilks Powerlifting formula. *Medicine and Science in Sports and Exercise,* Vol.31, No.12, pp. 1869-75, ISSN 0195-9131

Vanderburgh, P. & Dooman C. (2000). Considering body mass differences, who are the world's strongest women? *Medicine and Science in Sports and Exercise*, Vol.32, No.1, pp. 197-201, ISSN 0195-9131

Vanderburgh, P. & Flanagan, S. (2000). The Backpack Run Test: A model for a fair and occupationally relevant military fitness test. *Military Medicine*, Vol.165, No.5, pp.418-21, ISSN 0026-4075

Vanderburgh, P. & Crowder, T. (2006). Body weight penalties in the physical fitness tests of the Army, Air Force, and Navy. *Military Medicine*, Vol.171, No.8, pp. 753-756, ISSN 0026-4075

Vanderburgh, P. & Laubach, L. (2007). Derivation of an age and weight handicap for the 5K run. *Measurement in Physical Education and Exercise Science*, Vol.11, No.1, pp. 49-59, ISSN ISSN 1091-367X

Vanderburgh, P. (2007). Correction factors for body mass bias in military physical fitness tests. *Military Medicine*, Vol.172, No.7, pp. 738-742, ISSN 0026-4075

Vanderburgh, P. & Laubach, L. (2008). Body mass bias in a competition of muscle strength and aerobic power. *Journal of Strength and Conditioning Research*, Vol.22, No.2, pp. 375-382, ISSN 1064-8011

Vanderburgh, P. (2008). Occupational relevance and body mass bias of in military physical fitness tests. *Medicine and Science in Sports and Exercise*, Vol.40, No.8, pp. 1538-1545, ISSN 0195-9131

Vanderburgh, P.; Mickley, N.; Anloague, P. & Lucius K. Load carriage distance run and pushups tests: No body mass bias and occupationally relevant. *Military Medicine*, (in press), ISSN 0026-4075

7

Aging in Women Athletes

Monica C. Serra, Shawna L. McMillin and Alice S. Ryan*
VA Research Service, Department of Medicine,
Division of Gerontology and Geriatric Medicine,
University of Maryland School of Medicine,
Baltimore VA Medical Center Geriatric Research,
Education and Clinical Center (GRECC),
VA Maryland Health Care System, Baltimore,
USA

1. Introduction

Since instating Title IX of the Education Amendments of 1972, there has been a significant increase in sports participation and athletic opportunities among women (1). While it is still more common for younger than older women to engage in athletic competition, the participation of older women is growing, with over 50 countries sponsoring master athletes events (2). While aging is associated with a decrease in metabolic and physiologic function, competitive athletic women may experience more gradual declines. These declines can be slowed further, by combining adequate dietary intake with proper exercise training. Therefore, this chapter will 1) discuss how aging influences physiologic and metabolic adaptations of highly trained women athletes and 2) explore how nutrition recommendations may change with exercise and the possible benefit of supplementation of micronutrients to improve athletic performance.

2. Aging and physiological adaptations of women athletes

2.1 Endurance performance

Many master athletes are capable of performances equal to those of non-elite young athletes (3). Nevertheless, age-related alteration to functional and physiological capacities are inescapable and as a result these age-related alteration lead to a decline in performances. It is widely accepted that aerobic capacity decreases with age. The rate of decline in maximal oxygen consumption (VO_2max) varies between 5-9% per decade starting at the age of ~35 years in healthy sedentary adults (4, 5, 6). Several studies report a greater rate of decline with age in endurance-trained men and women (7, 8). Running performances decrease in a curvilinear fashion with the greatest decline after 60 years of age with women demonstrating a threefold greater decrease in performance compared to men (8, 9). Marcell et al. (10) provided evidence that a decline in VO_2max is the best predictor of age-related changes in endurance performances in female athletes. Elite endurance performances are attributed to three primary determinants: aerobic capacity, lactate threshold, and exercise economy.

---

* Corresponding Author

2.2 Aerobic capacity

A high VO_2max is an identifiable marker for a successful endurance athlete. Observed VO_2max in elite male endurance athletes can measure between 75 and 85 ml/kg/min; whereas; VO_2max is approximately 10% lower in elite women athletes (11). VO_2max is higher in athletes at any age than sedentary women (8, 7, 11). Endurance performance and aerobic capacity are strongly related across varying age groups of competitive athletes (9). Aerobic capacity, as measured by VO_2max is determined by cardiac output and arteriole-venous oxygen difference (12). Both cardiac output and arteriole-venous oxygen difference decrease with age in endurance athletes (5). Cardiac output is the product of heart rate and stroke volume and accounts for approximately 50% of oxygen consumption during exercise (12). Heart rate is the primary factor for increases in cardiac output during exercise; whereas stroke volume peaks at ~50% of max exercise then levels off or slightly decreases (12). The age-related loss in maximal heart rate is between 0.5-1 beat per year (13). Several studies have exhibited that habitual exercise status has no effect on the age-associated reductions in maximal heart rate (7, 14, 4). With maximal heart rates similar between athletes and non-athletes, the principle difference in cardiac output is stroke volume (11). Ogawa et al. (5) observed a greater rate of decline in stroke volume in female athletes compared to that observed in sedentary controls. The decrease in maximal heart rate, stroke volume, and arteriole-venous oxygen difference contributes to the decline in master athletes' endurance performances.

2.3 Lactate threshold

Lactate threshold is the fraction of VO_2max where there is a significant increase in blood lactate accumulation (12). Lactate threshold is a primary factor in determining endurance performances of both men and women (11). In sedentary subjects there is typically a rise in blood lactate concentration to ~60% VO_2max. In trained athletes this value can be 75–90% of VO_2max (14). A study by Evans et al. (7), showed that lactate threshold as a percentage of VO_2max did not change with age in female distance runners. This evidence coupled with similar findings in male distance runners (15) suggests that a reduction in VO_2max rather than a reduction in lactate threshold contribute the most to the decline in performance with age.

2.4 Exercise economy

Exercise economy is the oxygen cost of an endurance performance at a given velocity and can vary up to ~ 30-40% among individuals (11). Exercise economy is a predictor of performance in a population with similar VO_2max (11). Results in male runners suggest that exercise economy does not change with age in highly trained endurance runners (15). Older female runners have demonstrated a slight change in economy at submax speeds and yet displayed no relationship between age and economy at a 10K race pace (7). Therefore, exercise economy is unlikely to contribute to the age-related decline in endurance performances.

2.5 Physiological and training mechanisms for aging declines in VO_2 max

Both central (cardiac output and blood volume) and peripheral (muscle mass and oxygen delivery/utilization) factors contribute to the high VO_2max demonstrated in elite athletes (11). At present, it is still unclear as to the exact cause(s) of the age-related decrease in VO_2max in master athletes compared to young athletes. Stroke volume is responsible for the higher cardiac output in athletes versus healthy sedentary individuals (11). Determinates of stroke volume are cardiac preload, left-ventricular end-diastolic volume, and myocardial contractility. Blood volume plays an important role in stroke volume and decreases with normal aging in healthy sedentary females. However, total blood volume is maintained in older endurance trained female athletes (16). Master athletes demonstrate a larger left ventricular mass and left ventricular end-diastolic volume compared to healthy sedentary adults (17). Given the benefits of habitual endurance training, it is uncertain how advanced age alters stroke volume which would consequently result in a similar decrease in VO_2max in aging athletes compared to sedentary women. Peripheral adaptations with aging have also been suggested to contribute to reductions in VO_2max through changes in both oxygen delivery and utilization to active skeletal muscles (9). Arteriole-venous oxygen difference decreases slightly with age in trained athletes (5). It has been observed that enzyme activity and capillarization (expressed per muscle fiber) of skeletal muscle are preserved in older male athletes (18). Though muscle characteristics have not been examined in older female athletes, the reduced VO_2max per kilogram muscle in female athletes is similar to male athletes (19). Therefore, it is likely that the age-associated reductions in VO_2max are a result of oxygen delivery and/or muscle mass.

Changes in body weight/composition may be a second mechanism for the decline in performance with age in athletes. Regardless of age, a decrease in lean body mass and an increase in percent body fat may contribute to a decrease in VO_2max (6, 19). Endurance trained women did not demonstrate the expected relationship between changes in body composition and age-related changes in VO_2max (4). Male endurance runners who maintained their lean body mass also maintained their relative VO_2max, whereas the female runners who maintained their relative VO_2max had the greatest decrease in lean body mass (4). This finding suggests that other factors, including the maintenance of training and/or estrogen rather than body composition have a greater affect on the female age-related decline of VO_2max (4).

The training stimulus may also play a role in the performance decline with age. With advanced age there seems to be a reduction in overall exercise "stimulus" (i.e. intensity, duration, and frequency) (5, 9, 14). VO_2max is positively associated with training volume and as such, the age-related decrease in VO_2max is associated with a reduction in training volume (14). However, female endurance athletes between the ages 34-78 years who maintained or increased their training volume with age, exhibited a similar change in VO_2max compared to healthy sedentary adults (14). Training stimulus appears to be a key determinant in the decline in aerobic capacity with age. Whether the decline in training is a result of the aging-process, injury, time, or motivation, has yet to be determined.

Despite the health benefits achieved through a lifetime of participating in physical activity, it seems that diminished performances are an inevitable aspect of aging. The exact mechanism(s) for the reduction in performance with age has yet to be determined. The finding that women demonstrate a greater rate of decline in performances compared to men could be a result of fewer women participating in competitive events as they age (3). However, given that more women have been encouraged to participate in sporting events since the induction of Title IX, it will be interesting to see whether the gender difference is maintained in the future.

3. Aging and metabolic adaptations in women athletes

3.1 Body composition
Normal aging results in significant changes in body composition with increases in abdominal fat and losses of muscle mass. The increase in obesity alters the risks for type 2

diabetes, cardiovascular disease, and hypertension, whereas the decline in fat-free mass (FFM) may alter energy expenditure and resting metabolic rate. It is interesting to question whether the increase in visceral fat and decrease in FFM can be prevented in women athletes. Our study of highly trained competitive women athletes aged 18 – 69 years indicates that percent body fat by DXA (dual energy x-ray absorptiometry) was lowest in 30 – 39 year old women athletes (~16% body fat) but was not different in 18 – 69 yr, 40 – 49 yr, and >50 yr old athletes (20). Total body fat was low and averaged 21 – 23% in these groups and considerably lower than normal BMI age-matched controls who were approximately 30 - 36% fat. To address whether central fat was different with age in women athletes, we measured visceral fat and subcutaneous fat by CT (computed tomography) scans. Visceral fat was significantly lower in the youngest athletes (18 – 29 yrs vs. 30 – 39 yrs) and significantly lower in the middle-aged than older athletes (Figure 1). Thus, despite the finding that athletes prevented gains in total body fat with aging, visceral fat increased with age in women athletes. However, putting the central obesity in context, it is remarkable that the oldest athletes have similar visceral fat and lower subcutaneous abdominal fat than normal BMI control women who were one-third their age. Lastly, FFM was not significantly different among the women athlete groups suggesting that muscle mass was maintained with aging and may be, in part, explained by the competitive training of these women.

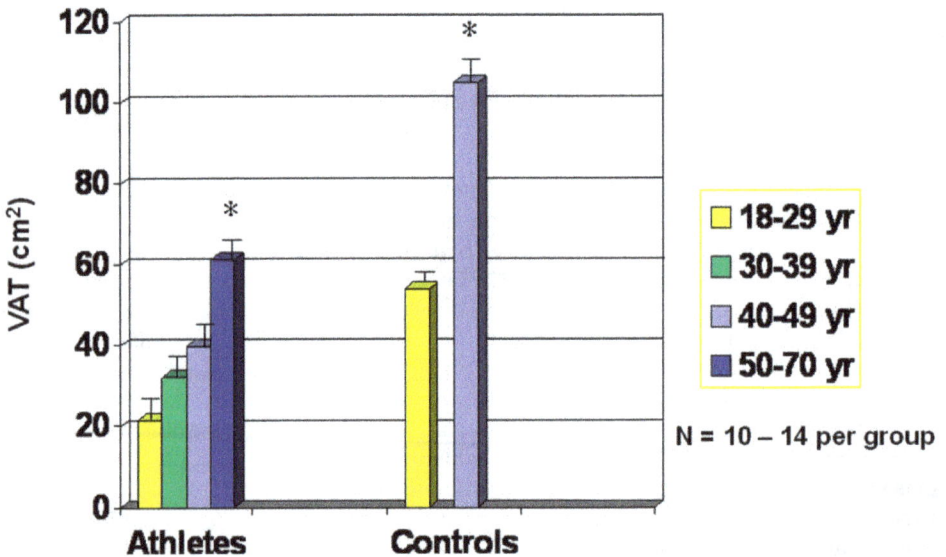

Fig. 1. Visceral adipose tissue (VAT) of women athletes and controls. Values are means ± SE. * P< 0.01

There are only a few other studies besides our own that have examined body composition in older women athletes. In agreement with our study, FFM did not differ between pre- and post-menopausal women runners (21). However, in contrast to our results, postmenopausal women athletes had higher % body fat and fat mass than the premenopausal athletes (21) but these differences were modest. More specifically, the difference was less than half that of the comparison between the healthy sedentary premenopausal and postmenopausal women. In comparison to sedentary controls, the athletes had lower % body fat, fat mass, waist circumference and trunk fat. Their results suggest that women who engage in vigorous exercise have a much smaller increase in total adiposity with advancing age (21). Two more studies (7, 22) provide some contrast as to whether age-related changes in body fat occur in women athletes. When female runners are divided into three age groups (e.g. 23-35, 37-47, 49-56 years), percent body fat by hydrostatic weighing did not differ by age and averaged 15, 14, and 18%, respectively (7). Across a continuum of age (40-77 years), body fat measured by hydrostatic weighing increased with age in women athletes, the majority of whom (90%) competed in running events (22). Thus, athletes have less total and central body fat than sedentary women (21, 23) and the vigorous training of master athletes may prevent an increase in total adiposity (7, 21).

Menstrual dysfunction in athletes could potentially alter body composition in young women. Young rowers with menstrual disorders have less subcutaneous and visceral fat by MRI compared to young controls (23). We are unaware of any studies in women athletes in the perimenopausal state. Further investigation is necessary to investigate whether the changes in hormonal status as women athletes age and go through menopause, influence body composition.

3.2 Glucose metabolism

There are two studies examining glucose metabolism in women athletes (24, 25) with one in older women athletes. We utilized a sequential clamp procedure which allowed the assessment of both ß-cell sensitivity to glucose and peripheral tissue sensitivity to insulin in a single session in young, middle-aged and older female athletes (25). Plasma insulin responses during the hyperglycemic clamp were reduced in older athletes vs. older controls and ß-cell sensitivity was maintained across the age span. First and second phase insulin response was positively correlated with body fat and negatively with VO2max suggesting that high levels of training and low body fat in women athletes across the age span predict insulin action. Rates of utilization (Rd) of glucose during the euglycemic portion of the clamp were significantly higher in athletes than controls and were not different across the age groups of athletes (Figure 2). Although some studies show a difference in insulin clearance rate with age (26), we showed that insulin clearance rate was similar across the age of 18 to 70 years in women athletes. Thus, older sedentary women had a 70% greater first-phase and 103% greater second-phase insulin response during hyperglycemia than the athletes. Moreover, older athletes utilized on average 31% more glucose than similarly aged sedentary women, suggesting an increase in insulin sensitivity due to the effects of training.

Investigators have examined the relationships between insulin sensitivity, body composition, fitness, and muscle and metabolic predictors. In younger women athletes (age 29 yrs), insulin sensitivity determined by the frequently sampled intravenous glucose tolerance test (FSIGT) was weakly correlated with VO2max and proportion of type 1 muscle fibers but not with percent body fat, fasting respiratory exchange ratio (RER) or RER during exercise, energy intake, macronutrient composition, and muscle triglyceride and glycogen content (24). In women athletes aged 18-69 years, we showed that percent body fat is associated with first-phase insulin release, whereas visceral fat and total body percent fat predict second-phase insulin release during hyperglycemic clamps (25). In addition, glucose uptake during the last hour of a hyperinsulinemic-euglycemic clamp was positively associated with FFM and VO2max, negatively associated with total fat mass, visceral fat, and subcutaneous abdominal fat (25). Thus, greater physical fitness and muscle mass and lower total and abdominal fat contribute to the enhanced tissue sensitivity observed in female athletes.

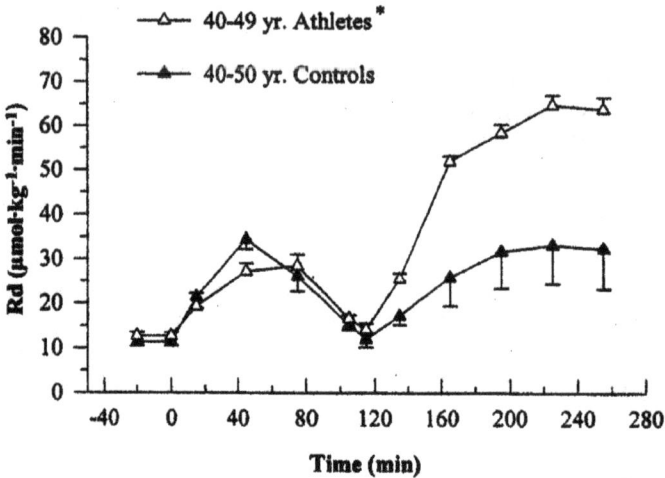

Fig. 2. Rate of utilization (Rd) of glucose during the 3-step clamp in 40- to 50 yr-old athletes and controls. Values are means ± SE. * P< 0.005

3.3 Cardiovascular risk factors

Lipid profiles are generally better in endurance trained athletes than sedentary individuals (27, 28). What occurs with aging in athletes with respect to lipid levels? We showed that total cholesterol, LDL-C (low density lipoprotein cholesterol) and triglyceride levels increased with age in women athletes (27). These relationships persisted even after adjusting for age-related declines in VO2max and increases in visceral fat. HDL-C (high density lipoprotein cholesterol) was higher in athletes than controls and LDL-C was lower in athletes than sedentary women. Regarding the lipoprotein subfractions, we also demonstrated that LDL3-C (larger LDL-C subfraction) was lower in athletes than untrained women and there was a tendency for a higher HDL5-C (the largest HDL-C subfraction) which would suggest a protective effect. Middle-aged women (n =147) who were grouped into active ex-athletes, sedentary ex-athletes, recreational exercisers, and non-exercisers did not differ in TG (triglycerides) and HDL-C (29). In another study, HDL-C was higher in master athletes than older sedentary women but LDL-C did not differ (28). These lipid differences suggest that women athletes would have a lower risk of coronary heart disease.

Intensity or the level of exercise may influence lipoprotein lipid levels. Williams (30) utilized a national survey of ~1800 female recreational runners to examine the dose-response relationship between exercise levels and HDL-C and CVD risk factors. The women were divided into groups based on weekly running mileage and were on average 40 years of age. Lipid levels were obtained from medical records. The results of the survey indicated that women who ran more than 64 km/week had significantly higher HDL-C levels than women who ran less than 48 km/week. Further analysis revealed that plasma HDL-C was 0.133 mg/dl higher for every additional kilometer run per week. The results suggest that women who exercise at greater levels have significantly greater increases in HDL-C which in turn reduced their risk for CVD (30).

Other cardiovascular risk and metabolic parameters have been examined in older athletes. Women athletes (n=94) between 13 and 77 years of age showed some cardiovascular risk factors, including hypertension that were prevalent in athletes over the age of 35 (31). In a small sample of women master athletes (n=6), coronary artery calcium which is linked to endothelial dysfunction (32) was not significantly different than age-matched sedentary women (28). In another study that also contained only six females, older endurance trained athletes with pre-hypertension had lower arterial stiffness than sedentary controls and longer travel time of pressure waves (33). In addition, the greater augmented pressure in the athletes which disappeared after controlling for resting heart rate may have contributed to the lack of difference in carotid SBP (systolic blood pressure) and carotid intima-media thickness. The authors suggest that the vascular stiffening with pre-hypertension can be modified by chronic exercise training but that chronic training is unable to compensate for age-associated increases in pressure from wave reflections (33).

4. Nutrition recommendations in women athletes

4.1 Energy and macronutrients

Most athletes strive to achieve energy balance where energy intake − energy expenditure during exercise training. Energy expenditure (EE) consists of 3 components: basal metabolic rate, thermic effect of activity, and the thermic effect of food. These generally account for 60-70%, 25-35%, and 5-10%, respectively, of total daily energy expenditure, but can be greatly altered by the type, intensity, and duration of exercise.

Typically, energy requirements decline with age; however, debate exists whether these declines are due only to decreases in physical activity patterns or if there is also an accompanying decline in basal metabolic rate. This information is difficult to obtain because environmental factors, such as work schedules and family obligations, often make maintaining vigorous intensity training difficult for older athletes. However, in older adults, matched for exercise volume, compared to younger adults, RMR is not different (34). This one study would suggest that the decline in RMR does not occur in older adults who maintain their exercise volume. Lean mass is the greatest determinant of basal metabolic rate, accounting for up to 75-80% of energy expenditure. In our study of women athletes, age and FFM were independent predictors of the decline in RMR where the oldest athletes expended approximated 965 kJ/day less than the youngest athletes (20). In middle aged women with similar BMI and fat-free mass, habitual exercisers (9 hours per week of physical activity for 10 or more years) have greater RMR than their sedentary counterparts (35).

In women athletes, decreased energy intake can result in declines in body weight, muscle mass and bone density, as well as increased menstrual dysfunction, fatigue, injury and illness. Maintaining or gaining body weight is often difficult for athletes performing large volumes of physical activity. A popular trend is for athletes to consume only extra protein which may promote greater WL, (weight loss) by increasing EE through thermogenesis (36). Ideally, extra energy should come from a combination of all three macronutrients. Caloric intake recommendations are often based upon prediction equations, which multiply a predicted resting metabolic rate by a physical activity factor, and the athlete's goal to maintain, gain, or lose weight.

While numerous studies exist examining the macronutrient requirement of athletes, a variety of variables (i.e. sport type, training status) affect nutritional requirements, resulting in broad recommendations. Current recommendations for a trained women include 45-65% (5-7 g/kg/d for general training, 7-10 g/kg/d for endurance athletes, and 11+g/kg/d for ultraendurance athletes) of energy from carbohydrates, 20-35% (~1 g/d) from fat, for general training, and 10-35% (1.2-1.4 g/kg/d for endurance trained and 1.6-1.7 g/kg/d for strength trained athletes) from protein (37). For all athletes, carbohydrates are recommended to make up the majority of energy intake, with an emphasis on whole grains, fruits, and vegetables. A diet high in carbohydrates typically results in adequate total protein intake, but may be lacking some of the essential amino acids, as well as intake of essential fatty acids and fat soluble vitamins and minerals.

Meal timing and nutrient composition recommendations surrounding athletic competition recommendations are based upon substrate utilization. Exercise intensity and duration drive these recommendations. For lower intensity activities (performed at ~25% of VO_{2max}), circulating fat provides the majority of energy during exercise. At moderate intensity (performed at ~65% VO_{2max}), fat oxidation contributes less and energy is mainly supplied from intramuscular stores of fat and glycogen. During high intensity exercise (performed at ~85% VO_{2max}), glycogen is the major energy source. At lower intensities where fat oxidation is providing the dominate source of energy, exercise can be sustained for up to a few hours; however, as intensity increases and requirements switch to glycogen, the ability to perform physical activities decline without carbohydrate repletion. Few studies have examined how macronutrient needs of women are altered by age; therefore, current macronutrient recommendations are similar between older and younger women athletes. During endurance based activities, depletion of plasma and muscle glycogen results in reduced exercise performance and fatigue. Prior to endurance exercise, it is recommended that 1 g/kg of carbohydrates be consumed for each hour prior to exercise (i.e. 1 g/kg if 1 hour prior and 4 g/kg if 4 hours prior) (37). Also, the meal should be low in fat and fiber and moderate in protein to facilitate gastric emptying and minimize gastrointestinal distress. During exercise, 30-60 g should be consumed every hour. If longer than 90 minutes, 6-20 g of protein should also be consumed during exercise and 1.5 g/kg carbohydrates with a small amount of protein immediately following exercise, with an additional 1.5 g/kg of carbohydrates consumed 2 hours later (37). Ensuring adequate fat intake during aerobic training is important since fat oxidation results in sparing of glycogen. Very low fat diets reduce intramuscular fat stores, impeding endurance. For strength based activities, protein intake has been suggested to maximize muscle synthesis by enhance amino acid uptake into skeletal muscle, providing substrate for hypertrophy if consumed immediate after the strength training bout. However, protein intake greater than 1.7-1.8 g/kg/d results in oxidation of the excess amino acids and is not incorporation into greater muscle mass, even when coupled with vigorous resistance training (38).

4.2 Micronutrients

Exercise and micronutrient activity work synergistically to ensure maximal performance of the body; therefore, if micronutrient deficiencies exist, there is a subsequent risk for declines in metabolic and physical function. Studies of dietary intake in women endurance athletes shown low intakes of calcium, vitamin D, vitamin E and zinc (39, 40). However, numerous other nutrients should be monitored for insufficient intake in women master athletes, including B_{12}, folate, riboflavin, pyridoxine, and magnesium (41). Additionally, the Dietary Reference Intakes (DRIs) acknowledge a decreased need for iron in older women (http://www.iom.edu/Activities/Nutrition/ SummaryDRIs.pdf). Because specific recommendation regarding micronutrient intake for older women have not been established, women athletes should consume at least the recommended dietary allowance (RDA) for all micronutrients to avoid nutrient deficiencies. In female master athletes partaking in nutritional supplementation, the supplemented group had significantly greater intakes of calcium, magnesium, vitamin C, and vitamin E than non supplemented women, indicating that female master athletes may rely on supplements to assist achieving micronutrient intake goals (40). If women consume a variety of foods in their diets and meet caloric requirements, vitamin and mineral supplementation typically is not necessary. Women greater than 60 years of age may want to consider a synthetic form of vitamin D and B_{12} because of altered absorption and nutrient action occurring with age. If a nutrient-balanced diet is not consumed, athletes should consider taking a multivitamin and mineral supplement. Too little data exists to recommend micronutrient supplementation above the RDA to improve athletic performance.

Free radicals produce oxidative damage during aging, as well as following strenuous exercise. During an intense endurance competition, master athletes experience elevations in reactive oxygen metabolites and biological antioxidant potentials, which continue at least 48 hours after completion of competition (43). Antioxidant supplementation may improve athletic performance, recovery time, and overall health by reducing oxidative damage. In endurance trained master athletes supplemented with antioxidants 21 days prior to intense cycling, antioxidant supplementation resulted in improved cycling efficiency (44). Unfortunately, most over the counter antioxidant supplements are not regulated by the FDA, and are not subject to thorough safety and effectiveness tests. One should heed caution not to consume vitamin intakes beyond the recommended upper limit (i.e. 2,000 mg for vitamin C and 1,000 mg for vitamin E).

The injury rate for master athletes is higher than younger athletes, making a balanced dietary intake especially important to support tissue healing (45). Ensuring adequate protein intake is important during all phases of tissue repair. Insufficient protein intake can inhibit wound healing and increase inflammation (46). It appears that several amino acids, including leucine, arginine, and glutamine, play a role in tissue repair mainly through amelioration of muscle atrophy (47) and/or stimulation of collagen formation (48). Current recommendations do not include supplementing with a specific amino acid as limited research exists research exists. While it is possible to consume all essential amino acids from plant based sources, it is easier to consume the essential amino acids from animal based protein sources. Omega-3 fatty acids modulate inflammation, resulting in reduced wound healing time (49). Unless the athlete encounters excessive inflammation following an injury, supplementation is not necessary. A diet high in omega-3 rich foods, such as salmon, walnuts, and flaxseeds would be effective. Several micronutrients also act to enhance tissue healing. For example, vitamin A is required for epithelial and bone formation, cellular differentiation, and immune function, vitamin C for collagen formation, proper immune function, and as a tissue antioxidant. Vitamin E is the major lipid-soluble antioxidant in the skin (50). Although not enough information exists to warrant supplementation to promote wound healing above RDA recommendations, nutritional intake should be assessed to ensure recommended dietary intake of all micronutrients.

4.3 Fluid

Dehydration can have serious health consequences to all athletes, but older athletes are more susceptible than younger ones. During periods of heat stress, older individuals typically respond with attenuated sweat gland output, decreased skin blood flow, reduced cardiac outputs, and smaller distribution of blood flow from the splanchnic and renal circulation (51). Kenney et al. (52) compared the effects of fluid restriction while exercising under different environmental stimuli in older versus younger women. They found that the percent decrease in sweat rate and plasma volume is greater in older versus younger women, indicating that older women have a greater propensity to develop dehydration associated with lack of fluid replacement. Additionally, older individuals are more likely to have altered thirst and kidney function placing them at increased risk for consequences of dehydration. However, if older women athletes are well conditioned and acclimatized to exercising in warm environments, a tolerance to heat stress can be developed. Athletes should drink 16 oz of fluid 30-40 minutes prior to exercise to ensure enough time to optimize hydration status and excrete excess fluid (37). During exercise, athletes should attempt to match their sweat rate with fluids following the guideline to consume 6-12 fl oz every 15-20 minutes (37). Sports drinks containing 6% to 8% carbohydrates and electrolytes are recommended for events lasting greater than 1 hour (41). One needs to compare post exercise weight to pre exercise weight and replace 16-24 fl oz of a fluid for every 0.5 kg of weight lost during exercise. This should supply ample fluid for rehydration following exercise (41). Additionally, consuming foods with high water content will aid rehydration following exercise.

Prior to and during exercise, nutrition intake should be aimed at maintaining hydration, while providing carbohydrates to maintain blood glucose concentrations during exercise. After exercise, meals should provide adequate fluids, electrolytes, energy, protein, and carbohydrates to replace nutrients lost during exercise and promote recovery. More research is needed before nutritional supplementation to improve performance, promote tissue healing, and optimize aging are recommended to women master athletes. However, encouraging a varied diet with balanced energy intake will help to ensure adequate macro- and micronutrient intakes.

5. Summary

Competitive athletic women may experience successful aging. Older trained women athletes can have a 30-50% higher VO$_2$max than sedentary women but may have a greater age-related decline per decade than the normal population. Factors such as a decrease in cardiac output due to a decrease in maximal heart rate and stroke volume, altered pulmonary function, changes in arteriole compliance, and a decrease and change in skeletal muscle fibers may play a role in the age associated decrease in aerobic capacity in the normal population as well as in athletes. Women athletes also confer a favorable body composition coincident with enhanced glucose and lipid metabolism. Highly trained women athletes maintain a low percentage of total and central body fat compared to healthy sedentary women. The reduced body fat and maintenance of muscle mass may contribute to enhanced glucose uptake and insulin action observed in highly trained women athletes. Proper nutrition is essential for maximizing athletic performance and general health in older women athletes. Specific needs are highly individualized and depend upon the athlete's mode of exercise, stage of training, and recovery time, as well as the intensity, duration, and frequency of each exercise session. Athletes may want to consider taking a multivitamin and mineral supplement, pay attention to fluid requirements and consume a nutrient-balanced diet.

6. Acknowledgements

This research was supported by VA Research Career Scientist Award, Veterans Affairs Merit Award, the Baltimore Veterans Affairs Medical Center Geriatric Research, Education and Clinical Center (GRECC), T32-AG-00219, NIH grant RO1 AG030075, NORC of Maryland (DK072488), and the University of Maryland Claude D. Pepper Center (P30-AG-12583).

7. References

[1] Kaestner R, Xin, X 2010 Title IX, girls' sports participation, and adult female physical activity and weight. Eval Rev 34:52-78.

[2] Rosenbloom C, Bahns M 2006 What can we learn about diet and physical activity from master athletes? Holist Nurs Pract 20:161-166; quiz 167-168

[3] Ransdall L VJ, and Huberty J 2009 Masters athletes: an analysis of running, swimming, and cycling performance by age and gender. J Exerc Sci Fit 7:S61-S73

[4] Hawkins S, Wiswell R 2003 Rate and mechanism of maximal oxygen consumption decline with aging: implications for exercise training. Sports Med 33:877-888

[5] Ogawa T, Spina RJ, Martin WH, 3rd, Kohrt WM, Schechtman KB, Holloszy JO, Ehsani AA 1992 Effects of aging, sex, and physical training on cardiovascular responses to exercise. Circulation 86:494-503

[6] Pollock ML, Foster C, Knapp D, Rod JL, Schmidt DH 1987 Effect of age and training on aerobic capacity and body composition of master athletes. J Appl Physiol 62:725-731

[7] Evans SL, Davy KP, Stevenson ET, Seals DR 1995 Physiological determinants of 10-km performance in highly trained female runners of different ages. J Appl Physiol 78:1931-1941

[8] Tanaka H, Desouza CA, Jones PP, Stevenson ET, Davy KP, Seals DR 1997 Greater rate of decline in maximal aerobic capacity with age in physically active vs. sedentary healthy women. J Appl Physiol 83:1947-1953

[9] Tanaka H, Seals DR 2008 Endurance exercise performance in Masters athletes: age-associated changes and underlying physiological mechanisms. J Physiol 586:55-63

[10] Marcell TJ, Hawkins SA, Tarpenning KM, Hyslop DM, Wiswell RA 2003 Longitudinal analysis of lactate threshold in male and female master athletes. Med Sci Sports Exerc 35:810-817

[11] Joyner MJ, Coyle EF 2008 Endurance exercise performance: the physiology of champions. J Physiol 586:35-44

[12] Brooks G, Fahey, T., and Baldwin, K 2005 Exercise Physiology: Human Bioienergetics and its Applications: McGraw-Hill Higher Educations.

[13] Pollock ML, Mengelkoch LJ, Graves JE, Lowenthal DT, Limacher MC, Foster C, Wilmore JH 1997 Twenty-year follow-up of aerobic power and body composition of older track athletes. J Appl Physiol 82:1508-1516

[14] Eskurza I, Donato AJ, Moreau KL, Seals DR, Tanaka H 2002 Changes in maximal aerobic capacity with age in endurance-trained women: 7-yr follow-up. J Appl Physiol 92:2303-2308

[15] Allen WK, Seals DR, Hurley BF, Ehsani AA, Hagberg JM 1985 Lactate threshold and distance-running performance in young and older endurance athletes. J Appl Physiol 58:1281-1284

[16] Jones PP, Davy KP, DeSouza CA, van Pelt RE, Seals DR 1997 Absence of age-related decline in total blood volume in physically active females. Am J Physiol 272:H2534-2540

[17] Fujimoto N, Prasad A, Hastings JL, Arbab-Zadeh A, Bhella PS, Shibata S, Palmer D, Levine BD 2010 Cardiovascular effects of 1 year of progressive and vigorous exercise training in previously sedentary individuals older than 65 years of age. Circulation 122:1797-1805

[18] Proctor DN, Sinning WE, Walro JM, Sieck GC, Lemon PW 1995 Oxidative capacity of human muscle fiber types: effects of age and training status. JApplPhysiol 78:2033-2038

[19] Proctor DN, Joyner MJ 1997 Skeletal muscle mass and the reduction of VO2max in trained older subjects. J Appl Physiol 82:1411-1415

[20] Ryan AS, Nicklas BJ, Elahi D 1996 A cross-sectional study on body composition and energy expenditure in women athletes during aging. AmJPhysiol 271:E916-E921

[21] Van Pelt RE, Davy KP, Stevenson ET, Wilson TM, Jones PP, Desouza CA, Seals DR 1998 Smaller differences in total and regional adiposity with age in women who regularly perform endurance exercise. Am J Physiol 275:E626-634

[22] Wiswell RA, Hawkins SA, Jaque SV, Hyslop D, Constantino N, Tarpenning K, Marcell T, Schroeder ET 2001 Relationship between physiological loss, performance decrement, and age in master athletes. J Gerontol A Biol Sci Med Sci 56:M618-626

[23] Frisch RE, Snow RC, Johnson LA, Gerard B, Barbieri R, Rosen B 1993 Magnetic resonance imaging of overall and regional body fat, estrogen metabolism, and ovulation of athletes compared to controls. J Clin Endocrinol Metab 77:471-477

[24] Goedecke JH, Levitt NS, St Clair Gibson A, Grobler L, Noakes TD, Lambert EV 2001 Insulin sensitivity measured by the minimal model: no associations with fasting respiratory exchange ratio in trained athletes. Metabolism 50:1286-1293

[25] Ryan AS, Muller DC, Elahi D 2001 Sequential hyperglycemic-euglycemic clamp to assess beta-cell and peripheral tissue: studies in female athletes. JApplPhysiol 91:872-881

[26] Rowe JW, Minaker KL, Pallotta JA 1983 Characterization of the insulin resistance of aging. J Clin Invest 71:1581-1587

[27] Nicklas BJ, Ryan AS, Katzel LI 1999 Lipoprotein subfractions in women athletes: effects of age, visceral obesity and aerobic fitness. Int J Obes Relat Metab Disord 23:41-47

[28] Wilund KR, Tomayko EJ, Evans EM, Kim K, Ishaque MR, Fernhall B 2008 Physical activity, coronary artery calcium, and bone mineral density in elderly men and women: a preliminary investigation. Metabolism 57:584-591

[29] Pihl E, Jurimae T, Kaasik T 1998 Coronary heart disease risk factors in middle-aged former top-level athletes. Scand J Med Sci Sports 8:229-235

[30] Williams PT 1996 High-density lipoprotein cholesterol and other risk factors for coronary heart disease in female runners. N Engl J Med 334:1298-1303

[31] LD DEM, Caldeira ND, Perlingeiro PD, Dos Santos IL, Negrao CE, Azevedo LF 2011 Cardiovascular Risk and Clinical Factors in Athletes: 10 Years of Evaluation. Med Sci Sports Exerc 43:943-950

[32] Ghiadoni L, Cupisti A, Huang Y, Mattei P, Cardinal H, Favilla S, Rindi P, Barsotti G, Taddei S, Salvetti A 2004 Endothelial dysfunction and oxidative stress in chronic renal failure. J Nephrol 17:512-519

[33] Heffernan KS, Jae SY, Tomayko E, Ishaque MR, Fernhall B, Wilund KR 2009 Influence of arterial wave reflection on carotid blood pressure and intima-media thickness in older endurance trained men and women with pre-hypertension. Clin Physiol Funct Imaging 29:193-200

[34] van Pelt RE, Dinneno FA, Seals DR, Jones PP 2001 Age-related decline in RMR in physically active men: relation to exercise volume and energy intake. Am J Physiol Endocrinol Metab 281:E633-639

[35] Gilliat-Wimberly M, Manore MM, Woolf K, Swan PD, Carroll SS 2001 Effects of habitual physical activity on the resting metabolic rates and body compositions of women aged 35 to 50 years. J Am Diet Assoc 101:1181-1188

[36] Weigle DS, Breen PA, Matthys CC, Callahan HS, Meeuws KE, Burden VR, Purnell JQ 2005 A high-protein diet induces sustained reductions in appetite, ad libitum caloric intake, and body weight despite compensatory changes in diurnal plasma leptin and ghrelin concentrations. Am J Clin Nutr 82:41-48

[37] Sports, Cardiovascular, and Wellness Nutritionists Dietetic Practice Group 2006 Sports nutrition: a practice manual for professionals Diana Faulhaber

[38] Tipton KD, Wolfe RR 2004 Protein and amino acids for athletes. J Sports Sci 22:65-79

[39] Nieman DC, Butler JV, Pollett LM, Dietrich SJ, Lutz RD 1989 Nutrient intake of marathon runners. J Am Diet Assoc 89:1273-1278

[40] Beshgetoor D, Nichols JF 2003 Dietary intake and supplement use in female master cyclists and runners. Int J Sport Nutr Exerc Metab 13:166-172

[41] Rodriguez NR, Di Marco NM, Langley S 2009 American College of Sports Medicine position stand. Nutrition and athletic performance. Med Sci Sports Exerc 41:709-731

[42] Amati F, Dube JJ, Coen PM, Stefanovic-Racic M, Toledo FG, Goodpaster BH 2009 Physical inactivity and obesity underlie the insulin resistance of aging. Diabetes Care 32:1547-1549

[43] Martarelli D, Pompei P 2009 Oxidative stress and antioxidant changes during a 24-hours mountain bike endurance exercise in master athletes. J Sports Med Phys Fitness 49:122-127

[44] Louis J, Hausswirth C, Bieuzen F, Brisswalter J 2010 Vitamin and mineral supplementation effect on muscular activity and cycling efficiency in master athletes. Appl Physiol Nutr Metab 35:251-260

[45] McKean KA, Manson NA, Stanish WD 2006 Musculoskeletal injury in the masters runners. Clin J Sport Med 16:149-154

[46] Demling RH 2009 Nutrition, anabolism, and the wound healing process: an overview. Eplasty 9:e9

[47] Tipton KD 2010 Nutrition for acute exercise-induced injuries. Ann Nutr Metab 57 Suppl 2:43-53

[48] Stechmiller JK 2010 Understanding the role of nutrition and wound healing. Nutr Clin Pract 25:61-68

[49] McDaniel JC, Belury M, Ahijevych K, Blakely W 2008 Omega-3 fatty acids effect on wound healing. Wound Repair Regen 16:337-345

[50] MacKay D, Miller AL 2003 Nutritional support for wound healing. Altern Med Rev 8:359-377

[51] Kenney WL, Munce TA 2003 Invited review: aging and human temperature regulation. J Appl Physiol 95:2598-2603

[52] Kenney WL, Anderson RK 1988 Responses of older and younger women to exercise in dry and humid heat without fluid replacement. Med Sci Sports Exerc 20:155-160

8

Physical Activity, Physical Fitness and Metabolic Syndrome

Xiaolin Yang

LIKES-Research Center for Sport and Health Sciences, Jyväskylä, Finland

1. Introduction

The metabolic syndrome is recognized as one of the leading worldwide health problems, which is a constellation of metabolic risk factors that is associated with increased risk for developing cardiovascular disease, type 2 diabetes mellitus and myocardial infarction. Clustered metabolic risk factors include abdominal obesity, dyslipidemia, elevated blood pressure, glucose intolerance, and insulin resistance, as standardized by the international criteria [1]. Evidence from observational epidemiological studies indicates that the metabolic risk factors begin early in life [2,3]. Childhood overweight and obesity are closely associated with insulin resistance, in which result the development of metabolic syndrome. The overall prevalence of metabolic syndrome can be identified in children and adolescents. Obesity and insulin resistance may develop the metabolic syndrome during the early years of life and throughout in adulthood. In Finland, the prevalence of metabolic syndrome has increased dramatically over the past decades [4,5].

The benefits of physical activity and physical fitness on the health of the general population have been attested beyond dispute [6]. There is overwhelming evidence that participation in regular, moderate-intensity physical activity may be a preventive intervention of the metabolic syndrome and that activity of greater intensity may provide even greater benefit [7]. Remarkably, supervised exercise training in either aerobic exercise or resistance training may be an effective adjunctive treatment and produce significant functional benefits for individuals with the metabolic syndrome [8]. Physical activity and exercise are thus uniquely positioned to improve physical and psychosocial health and function by reducing the clustered metabolic risk and, in turn, by delaying or avoiding the onset of diabetes and cardiovascular diseases. However, most of the studies have been cross-sectional, but a few have been longitudinal.

The aim of this chapter is to outline physical activity and fitness to prevent or reduce the prevalence or incidence of metabolic syndrome among youth and adults. I start with the definition of physical activity, cardiorespiratory fitness and muscular strength and proceed to a discussion of the role of physical activity and fitness on the metabolic syndrome. I will discuss the importance of physical activity and fitness as their primary sources of health information that affect the metabolic syndrome in both youth and adults. Special emphasis is given to the use of long-term physical activity as a possible means of effectively reducing the prevalence of metabolic syndrome.

2. Rationale of physical activity and fitness in the prevention of metabolic syndrome

2.1 Definitions

The terms 'physical activity', 'exercise' and 'physical fitness' have been described in detail by Caspersen et al. [9]. Although these terms are related and have similar meanings, they aren't identical in meaning. Physical activity is defined as any bodily movement produced by skeletal muscles that result in energy expenditure. Exercise is a subset of physical activity that is planned, structured, and repetitive and has as a final or an intermediate objective the improvement or maintenance of physical fitness. Physical fitness is a set of attributes that are either health-related (i.e. cardiorespiratory endurance, muscular strength and endurance, body composition, and flexibility) or skill-related (i.e. agility, balance, coordination, speed, power, and reaction time). Physical fitness is also referred to almost exclusively as cardiorespiratory fitness (also called cardiovascular fitness or maximal aerobic power), which relates very closely to maximal capacity for oxygen consumption. An important distinction between physical activity and fitness is the intraindividual day-to-day variability; physical activity will undoubtedly vary on a daily basis, whereas cardiorespiratory fitness will remain relatively static, taking time to change. This variability will impact on the ability to measure these two quantities and consequently will influence the ability to demonstrate their relationship with metabolic outcomes. In this chapter physical activity will be used as a generic term, whereas cardiorespiratory fitness and muscular strength will be used in their specific meanings. Based on previous studies of assessments of physical activity and physical fitness, the main methods of these standard measures have been summarized and presented in Table 1.

The term 'metabolic syndrome' is generally defined as the clustering risk factors associated with medical disorders that increase the risk of developing atherosclerotic and insulin resistance, i.e. elevated levels of central adiposity, hypertension, dyslipidemia, impaired glucose metabolism, and a low level of high-density lipoprotein cholesterol [10]. Table 2 summarizes five international criteria in the following: World Health Organization [11], European Group for the Study of Insulin Resistance [12], American College of Endocrinology/American Association of Clinical Endocrinologists [13], International Diabetes Federation [14], and National Cholesterol Education Program Adult Treatment Panel III [10].

The World Health Organization criteria requires the presence of impaired glucose tolerance, impaired fasting glucose, type 2 diabetes, and insulin resistance in top quartile of non-diabetic population and at least two of the following: waist:hip ratio > 0.9 in men and > 0.85 in women, serum triglycerides ≥ 1.7 mmol/L, systolic/diastolic blood pressure ≥ 140/90 mmHg or medication, high-density lipoprotein cholesterol ≤ 0.9 mmol/L in men and ≤ 1.0 mmol/L in women, and microalbuminuria: urinary albumin excretion ratio ≥ 20 μg/min or albumin:creatinine ratio ≥ 30 mg/g. The European Group for the Study of Insulin Resistance criteria includes the presence of hyperinsulinemia (defined as nondiabetic subjects having fasting insulin level in the highest quartile) and at least two of the following abnormalities: fasting plasma glucose ≥ 6.1 mmol/L (110 mg/dL), triglycerides > 2.0 mmol/L, high-density lipoprotein cholesterol < 1.0 mmol/L or medication, systolic/diastolic blood pressure ≥ 140/90 mmHg or current use of antihypertensive medication, and waist circumference ≥ 94 cm in men and ≥ 80 cm in women. The American College of Endocrinology/American

Physical activity	Children and adolescents	Adults
Questionnaire	Physical activity at school Organized sport Non-organized sport Commuting to school Leisure activities Time spent sitting	Sports Occupation Household/Caregiving Transportation Conditioning Leisure/Recreation activities Time spent sitting
Interview	Face to face	Face to fact Telephone
Instrument	Heart rate monitoring Pedometer Accelerometer	Heart rate monitoring Pedometer Accelerometer
Physical fitness	Laboratory	Epidemiologic
Cardiorespiratory	Maximum oxygen uptake on treadmill or cycle ergometer	12-minutes run 1-mile walk Bench (30 cm high) step
Body composition	Underwater weighing Near infrared Bioelectrical impedance analysis	Waist girth / waist-to-hip ratio Body mass index (kg/m²) Skinfolds (biceps, triceps, abdomen, suprailium, subscapula and thigh)
Muscular strength and endurance	Dynomometer Cable tensiometer Load cells Strain gauges	Handgrip Chin ups Push ups Sit / Curl ups
Flexibility	Leighton flexometer	Sit-and-reach flexometer

Table 1. Main assessment of physical activity and physical fitness

Association of Clinical Endocrinologists criteria requires the presence of abdominal obesity (waist circumference ≥ 102 cm in men and ≥ 88 cm in women) and at least two of the following abnormalities: fasting plasma glucose ≥ 5.6 mmol/L (100mg/dL), systolic/diastolic blood pressure ≥130/85mmHg or medication, triglycerides ≥1.7 mmol/L (150 mg/dL) or medication. The International Diabetes Federation criteria includes the presence of abdominal obesity (waist circumference ≥ 94 cm in men and ≥ 80 cm in women) and ≥ 2 of the following four indicators: fasting plasma glucose ≥ 5.6 mmol/L (100 mg/dL), triglycerides ≥ 1.7 mmol/L (150 mg/dL), high-density lipoprotein cholesterol < 40 mg/dL (1.03 mmol/L) in men and < 50 mg/dL (1.29 mmol/L) in women, and systolic/diastolic blood pressure ≥130/85 mmHg or treatment for hypertension. The National Cholesterol Education Program Adult Treatment Panel III criteria includes the presence of at least three of the following: waist circumference ≥ 102 cm in men and ≥ 88 cm in women, triglycerides ≥ 150 mg/dL, high-density lipoprotein cholesterol < 40 mg/dL in men and < 50 mg/dL in women, systolic/diastolic blood pressure ≥130/85 mm Hg or use of medication for hypertension, and fasting plasma glucose ≥ 5.6 mmol/L (100 mg/dL) or medication.

	WHO (1999)	EGIR (1999)	ACE/AACE (2003)	IDF (2006)	NCEP-ATP III (2005)
Required criteria	IGT, IFG, T2D, insulin resistance in top quartile of non-diabetic population	Insulin resistance in top quartile of non-diabetic population	High risk[1], WC > 102 cm (M) or > 88 cm (F)	WC ≥ 94 cm (M) or ≥ 80 cm (F), and WC with ethnicity specific values, or BMI > 30 kg/m²	
Other criteria	plus ≥ 2 of the following:				
Waist circumference (WC)	WHR > 0.9(M), or >0.85 (F); or BMI > 30 kg/m²	≥ 94 cm (M) or ≥ 80 cm (F)			≥102 cm (M) or ≥ 88 cm (F)
Triglyceride	≥ 1.7 mmol/L	≥ 2.0 mmol/L	≥ 1.7 mmol/L (150 mg/dL)	≥ 1.7 mmol/l (150 mg/dL) or medication	≥ 150 mg/dL
High-density lipoprotein cholesterol	≤ 0.9 mmol/L (M) or ≤ 1.0 mmol/L (F) or medication	< 1.0 mmol/L or medication	< 40 mg/dL (M) or < 50 mg/dL (F)	< 40 mg/dL (1.03 mmol/L) (M) or < 50 mg/dL (1.29 mmol/L) (F)	<40 mg/dL (M) or <50 mg/dL (F)
Blood pressure	≥ 140/90 mmHg or medication	≥ 140/90 mmHg or medication	≥ 130/85 mmHg or medication	≥ 130/85 mmHg or medication	≥130/85 mmHg or medication
Glucose		≥ 6.1 mmol/L (110 mg/dL)	≥ 5.6 mmol/L (100 mg/dL)	≥ 5.6 mmol/L (100 mg/dL)	≥5.6 mmol/L (100 mg/dL) or medication
Other	Microalbuminuria; UAER ≥ 20 µg/min or ACR ≥ 30 mg/g				

WHO, World Health Organization, EGIR, European Group for the Study of Insulin Resistance; ACE/AACE, American College of Endocrinology/American Association of Clinical Endocrinologists; IDF, International Diabetes Federation; NCEP-ATP III, National Cholesterol Education Program- Adult Treatment Panel III; IGT, impaired glucose tolerance; IFG, impaired fasting glucose, T2D, type 2 diabetes; WHR, waist:hip ratio; BMI, body mass index; UAER, urinary albumin excretion ratio; ACR, albumin:creatinine ratio.

[1]High risk: family history of type 2 or gestational diabetes, known cardiovascular disease, polycystic ovary syndrome, physically inactive lifestyle, >40 years of age, and ethnic populations at high risk for type 2 diabetes. M = male, F = female.

Table 2. Metabolic syndrome definitions and diagnosis issued by international criteria

It has been noted that these definitions overlap but differ in the points of emphasis of the components. Using the above definitions of the metabolic syndrome, there are quantitatively significant differences in sample sizes, age groups and rates of healthy participants as well. For example, the International Diabetes Federation definition identifies a high degree of overlap among the participants with the metabolic syndrome using the

National Cholesterol Education Program Adult Treatment Panel III criteria. The two definitions similarly classified approximately 93% in 3601 American adults aged ≥ 20 years [15], 85% in 2182 Finnish young adults aged 24–39 years [4], and only about 16% in 5047 Swedish adults aged 46–68 years [16].

2.2 Systemic mechanisms

In general, leisure-time physical activity and aerobic exercise may provide an advantage in helping reducing the metabolic syndrome in middle-aged and elderly population. The potential mechanisms are often proposed by which physical activity and fitness can reduce the risk of the metabolic syndrome in response to insulin resistance and abdominal obesity. From a psychosocial standpoint, physical activity and fitness have a beneficial effect that can improve psychosocial well-being, leading to better mood, higher self-efficacy and stronger social motives for exercise [17,18]. Participation in regular physical activity or aerobic exercise is an effective way to establish lifelong habits for reducing the increased risk of insulin resistance and obesity. Individuals who want to maintain physical abilities may have better awareness of other health-related habits such as diet, smoking and sedentary lifestyle, all of which have been found to be related to the risk for the metabolic syndrome [19,20]. Increased physical activity and fitness may also lead to enhanced overall cardiovascular function and muscular endurance which, in turn, delay the onset or help prevent the development of metabolic syndrome. These psychosocial effects may then interact with biological processes that may result in reduction of subclinical inflammation involving cytokines derived from adipose tissue and modulation of various adipocytokines that lead to reduce the prevalence of metabolic syndrome [21]. The benefit of increased and maintained physical activity and physical fitness may be directly or indirectly associated with reduced incidence of the metabolic syndrome.

However, the relationship between physical activity or physical fitness and the metabolic syndrome may also be bidirectional. The prevalence of metabolic syndrome may lead to declining levels of physical activity and fitness as symptoms of metabolic syndrome may increase sedentary lifestyle, unhealthy diet, low energy level and lack of exercise and physical activity. Therefore, the precise mechanisms underlying the effect of physical activity and fitness on the metabolic syndrome still need further clarification.

3. Effect of physical activity and fitness on metabolic syndrome in adults

A number of cross-sectional epidemiological studies have been conducted to examine the effect of leisure-time physical activity and cardiorespiratory fitness on the metabolic syndrome in adult population over the last decade. Several studies have only focused on the association in men. An English cohort of 711 employed middle-aged men demonstrated a dose-relationship between both leisure-time physical activity and cardiorespiratory fitness and the clustering of the metabolic syndrome including fasting glucose, triglycerides, high-density lipoprotein cholesterol, blood pressure, and body mass index [22]. Men with higher physical activity, as defined by a physical activity index, were found to be less likely to have the metabolic syndrome when compared with the inactive ones. The age-adjusted odds ratios and their 95% confidence intervals for having the clustering of metabolic syndrome were 0.56 (0.33-0.96) for occasional/light physical activity, 0.37 (0.19-0.71) for moderate/moderately vigorous physical activity, and 0.12 (0.03-0.50) for vigorous physical activity. Men with moderate to high levels of the fitness were also found to be less likely to develop the metabolic syndrome when compared with those with unfit. The corresponding age-adjusted odds ratios and 95% confidence intervals were 0.27 (0.15-0.46) in the moderate fitness category and 0.18 (0.09-0.33) in the high fitness category compared to the unfit group. A similar study design and analysis was performed in a Finnish study of 1 069 middle-aged men [23]. Leisure-time physical activity, as measured by metabolic equivalent hours per week (MET h·wk-¹), was divided into three levels of intensity: low, moderate and high. The each level was grouped again into three categories from low to high. Men who engaged in moderate-intensity physical activity (<1.0 h·wk-¹) were 60% more likely to have the metabolic syndrome than those engaging in physical activity (≥ 3.0 h·wk-¹). Men with low fitness (VO$_{2max}$ ≤ 29.1 ml·kg^{-1}·min^{-1}) were approximately seven times more likely to have the metabolic syndrome than those with high fitness (VO$_{2max}$ ≥35.5 ml·kg^{-1}·min^{-1}). The relationships remained significant after adjustment for confounders.

In the Whitehall II study, which assessed a dose-response relationship between leisure-time physical activity and metabolic syndrome in 5 153 Caucasian civil servants (ages 45-68 years) from 20 departments in the London offices, showed that the odds ratios and their 95% confidence intervals for having the metabolic syndrome were 0.52 (0.40–0.67) in vigorous (≥12.5 MET h/wk) activity and 0.78 (0.63–0.96) in moderate (≥24 MET h/wk) activity than in low activity, when controlling for confounders, e.g., age, smoking, alcohol intake, socioeconomic status, and other activity [24]. Katzmarzyk et al. [25] carried out a cohort study of 19 223 men (ages 20–83 years), who were selected randomly from a general population in Canada. Cardiorespiratory fitness was used to classify each subject into two fitness exposure categories. Men with the metabolic syndrome had 1.29-fold higher all-cause mortality and 1.89-fold higher cardiovascular disease (CVD) mortality compared with healthy men. However, the associations were no longer significant after accounting for cardiorespiratory fitness. The relative risks comparing unfit vs. fit men for all-cause mortality was similar in healthy men and men with the metabolic syndrome (2.18 vs. 2.01), whereas the relative risks for CVD mortality for unfit vs. fit men were 3.21 in healthy men and 2.25 in men with the metabolic syndrome. Also, a significant dose-response relationship between cardiorespiratory fitness and mortality was observed in men with the metabolic syndrome. It was concluded that exercise provided a protective effect against the risk of all-cause and CVD mortality in healthy men and men with the metabolic syndrome.

Although there is a consistent inverse association between leisure-time physical activity and metabolic syndrome and its components in men, the association is not as consistent in women. For example, results from the Quebec family study (158 men and 198 women aged 20-60 years) found that cardiorespiratory fitness was independently related to the metabolic syndrome among both men and women. Cardiorespiratory fitness was inversely related to plasma insulin only for men, while cardiorespiratory fitness was only positively related to high-density lipoprotein cholesterol for women. However, cardiorespiratory fitness was not independently related to the components of metabolic syndrome in both sexes after accounting for total and abdominal adiposity [26]. As in another Canadian population-based study (6 406 men and 6 475 women aged 18-64 years) [27], the odds ratios and their 95% confidence intervals for having the metabolic syndrome in physically active men was 0.45 (0.29-0.69) than their physically inactive counterparts, after consideration of covariates including age, smoking, alcohol consumption, and income adequacy. The association disappeared in women after adjusting for the covariates. Sex differences were also found for the association of the metabolic syndrome with leisure-time physical activity in the Fels Longitudinal Study [28], investigating a sample of US young adults (249 women and 237 men aged 18–40 years). Among men, the odds ratios for having the metabolic syndrome risk were independently reduced with increases in both total physical activity (OR = 0.65, 95% CI = 0.47–0.90) and sport activity (OR = 0.40, 95% CI = 0.23–0.70). The components of metabolic syndrome such as abdominal circumference, triglycerides and high-density lipoprotein cholesterol also improved with total and sport physical activity. Among women, the associations of types of physical activity, i.e., leisure, sport, work, and total with the metabolic syndrome were marginal. Only high-density lipoprotein cholesterol was increased by both total physical activity (OR = 0.79, 95% CI = 0.63–0.98) and sport physical activity (OR = 0.54, 95% CI = 0.35–0.84) after controlling for age, smoking and body mass index. These differences may be partly explained by race, age and sex hormone differences, varying patterns of fat distribution, and differences in types and intensity of physical activity.

Two studies have reported an inverse association between leisure-time physical activity and metabolic syndrome in women. A cohort study [29] of a tri-ethnic sample of women (49 African-American, 46 Native-American, and 51 white) aged 40–83 years in the USA demonstrated that the odds ratios and their 95% confidence intervals for having the metabolic syndrome were 0.18 (0.03–0.90) for women in the highest category of moderate-intensity physical activity (≥491 MET min/d) compared with those in the lowest category (<216 MET min/d). The odds ratios for having the metabolic syndrome was 0.07 (0.02–0.35) for women in the highest quartile of maximal treadmill duration (>16 minutes) compared with women in the lowest quartile (≤10 minutes). Although the study population is relatively small, the increased physical activity has important implications in the prevention of metabolic syndrome independently of potential confounding variables. Similar results were found in another study [30] of 7 104 US women, which showed that prevalence of the metabolic syndrome was significantly lower across cardiorespiratory fitness quintiles, with the prevalence ranging from 19.0% in the lowest fit quintile to 2.3% in the highest fit quintile. Also, the prevalence of metabolic syndrome in the different age groups for women who achieved a maximal MET level of 11 or higher was one-third to one-fourth that of women who achieved lower maximal MET levels.

Most studies found that physical activity and fitness was related to the metabolic syndrome in both sexes. An early cohort study [31] of 15 537 men and 3 899 women in the adult US population found that the least-fit men had 3.0- and 10.1-fold higher risk factors for the metabolic clusters (elevated systolic blood pressure, serum triglycerides, fasting blood glucose, and central adiposity) compared with moderately-fit and the most-fit men, respectively. Similarly, the least-fit women had 2.7- and 4.9-fold higher risk factors for the metabolic clusters compared with moderately-fit and the most-fit women, respectively. Data from a cohort of 874 healthy Caucasian participants from the Medical Research Council Ely Study indicated that there was a strong and significant inverse association between physical activity energy expenditure and the metabolic syndrome, while the association between cardiorespiratory fitness and the metabolic syndrome was attenuated after adjusting for age, sex, physical activity, and measurement error. However, cardiorespiratory fitness modified the relationship between physical activity and metabolic syndrome [32]. Thus, prevention of the metabolic syndrome may be most effective in the subset of unfit inactive people.

An Australian study by Dunstan et al. [33] examined the associations of television viewing and physical activity with the metabolic syndrome in 6 241 adults aged ≥ 35 years. They found that the adjusted odds ratios and their 95% confidence intervals for having the metabolic syndrome were 2.07 (1.49-2.88) in women and 1.48 (0.95-2.31) in men who watched TV for >14 hrs/wk compared with those who watched ≤ 7.0 hrs/wk. Compared with those who were less active (<2.5 hrs/wk), the odds ratios for having the metabolic syndrome were 0.72 (0.58-0.90) in men and 0.53 (0.38-0.74) in women who were active (≥2.5 hrs/wk). Additionally, increased TV viewing time or physical activity was also associated with individual components of the metabolic risk in both sexes. Recently, a Swedish study by Halldin et al. [34] included 3 864 60-year-old men and women in the Stockholm region. The results showed that, compared with the low physical activity group, the odds ratios for having the metabolic syndrome in the high physical activity groups (i.e. intensive regular activity more than 2 times/week, at least 30 min each time) was 0.33 (0.22-0.51) after adjustment for covariates.

Based on a nationally representative population-based sample of US adults aged 20 years and older from the National Health and Nutrition Examination Survey (NHANES), several studies have utilized the NHANES to explore the relationship between leisure-time physical activity and metabolic syndrome. However, the results are inconsistent. Park et al. [35] used a physical activity intensity score to examine the association between physical activity and metabolic syndrome. The score was calculated as a dichotomized variable based on the frequency and intensity of leisure-time physical activity. Participants with the total density rating score > 3.5 were active and those with a total density rating score of ≤ 3.5 were inactive. When compared to the active group, the odds ratios for having the metabolic syndrome were significantly higher (OR = 1.4, 95% CI = 1.0-2.0) among inactive men, but not among inactive women. Similar findings have been reported by Zhu et al. [20], although these participants were grouped into 3 categories: active (score > 15.0), moderately activity (score > 3.6 to 14.9) and inactive (≤ 3.5). Men with the active group were found to be 42% less likely (OR = 0.58, 95% CI = 0.39-0.85) to have the metabolic syndrome compared to those with the inactive group, even after controlling for age, race, education, income levels, and other modifiable factors. In women, the association disappeared after adjusting for the confounders. These finding were also supported by a study reported by DuBose et al. [36]. Leisure-time physical activity was classified as regularly active (≥ 5 d/wk moderate- and/or ≥ 3 d/wk vigorous-intensity physical activity), irregularly active (some physical activity), and inactive (no physical activity). Regularly active represented that the participants met the recommendations of the Centres for Disease Control and Prevention and the American College of Sports Medicine [37]. The results indicated that the odd ratios for having the metabolic syndrome were only higher in men with the irregular activity (OR = 1.52, 95% CI = 1.11-1.23) and inactivity (OR = 1.60, 95% CI = 1.18-1.98) groups than those with the regularly active group after adjustment for age, race, smoking status, and educational attainment.

However, to continue to expand this field, the duration of physical activity, in addition to the frequency and intensity of physical activity, is required to examine a more precise measure of physical activity dose. In the study of examining the interaction between time spent in physical activity and sedentary behaviour on the metabolic syndrome [38], participants were asked about their moderate/vigorous intensity physical activity patterns and moderate intensity household activity, designating these activities in minutes per week (min/wk^{-1}) based on frequency, duration, and intensity of each activity. These participants were then grouped into three categories: 0, < 150, and ≥150 min/wk^{-1} of moderate/vigorous physical activity. However, after adjustment for covariates, the cross-sectional association between physical activity and metabolic syndrome was attenuated for both sexes. In a recent study [39], leisure-time physical activity was measured in two ways: (1) a six-level measure based upon participants reporting no physical activity and quintiles of physical activity (0, >

0 to ≤156.24, >156.24 to ≤393.10, >393.10 to ≤736.55, >736.55 to ≤1360.15, and >1360.15 MET·min·wk⁻¹) based on the compendium of physical activities for adults [40,41] and (2) a three level categorical measure (inactive, insufficiently active, and met physical activity recommendation) based on the recent physical activity public health recommendation of the American College of Sports Medicine/American Heart Association (ACSM/AHA) [42]. When compared to the no physical activity group, adults with physical activity between 736 and 1360 MET·min·wk⁻¹ were found to be 35% less likely (OR– 0.65, 95% CI = 0.48–0.88) to have the metabolic syndrome using the National Cholesterol education Program-Adult Treatment Panel III criteria, while adults with physical activity between 393–737 MET·min·wk⁻¹ were found to be 30% less likely (OR = 0.70, 95% CI = 0.51–0.96) to have the metabolic syndrome using the World Health Organization criteria. Additionally, adults with physical activity met the ACSM/AHA guidelines were found to be 45% (OR = 0.54, 95% CI = 0.44–0.66 for the World Health Organization criteria) and 39% (OR = 0.61, 95% CI = 0.48–0.77 for the American College of Endocrinology/American Association of Clinical Endocrinologists criteria) less likely to have the metabolic syndrome compared with those who were inactive. In addition, cardiorespiratory fitness was first measured by using a submaximal treadmill test in both healthy men (n = 692) and women (n = 608) aged 18–49 years in the 1999-2002 NHANES [43]. Participants were divided into low, moderate, and high fitness tertiles based on the age-adjusted VO$_{2max}$ values. It was showed that the odds ratios for having the metabolic syndrome in men but not women were significantly lower in moderate and high fitness categories compared with the low fitness category, after controlling for confounding variables such as age, ethnicity, poverty-income ratio, alcohol consumption, smoking and fat consumption. These inconsistent findings may be caused by different assessments of physical activity and fitness and different criteria of metabolic syndrome in different age and samples. Also, it remains unknown whether menopausal or hormonal status in women contributes to this observation.

Only two studies have addressed the relationship between muscle strength and metabolic syndrome in adult men. An American study followed 8 570 men aged 20–75 years from 1981 to 1989 [44]. Muscular strength score was computed by combining body weight-adjusted one-repetition maximal measures for leg and bench presses and then divided into strength quartile (Q) from Q1 (low strength) to Q4 (high strength). Men with high levels of muscular strength were found to be less likely to have the metabolic syndrome than those with low strength after adjusting for age and smoking. Similar results were found in an average of 6.7 years follow-up study by Jurca et al. [45]. They stated that men with more muscular strength were also less likely to develop the metabolic syndrome, even after adjusting for smoking, alcohol intake, number of baseline metabolic syndrome risk factors, family history of diabetes, hypertension, and premature coronary disease. However, these associations were partially explained by cardiorespiratory fitness. To our knowledge, only one study has explored the combined effects of muscular strength and aerobic fitness on the metabolic syndrome in both Flemish adult men (n =571) and women (n = 448) aged 18–75 years [46]. Muscular strength was evaluated by measuring isometric knee extension and flexion peak torque, using a Biodex System Pro 3 dynamometer. The relationship between muscular strength, aerobic fitness and the metabolic syndrome score was analyzed as continuous variables using a multiple linear regression. The risk of metabolic syndrome was inversely associated with muscular strength, independently of aerobic fitness and other confounding factors in women, whereas the association was attenuated when controlling for aerobic fitness in men. Thus, strength training in addition to aerobic exercise may provide additional effects in reducing the prevalence of metabolic syndrome, particularly for women. These findings are inconsistent that may be partially explained by socio-cultural differences of the samples and the methodological issues including different measures, methods of analysis and sample size.

In summary, these findings imply that leisure-time physical activity, cardiorespiratory fitness and muscular strength may be an important determinant of the overall prevalence of metabolic syndrome independent of several other confounding factors. Accumulating evidence suggests that regular physical activity which increases aerobic capacity and cardiovascular fitness and maintain muscular strength has a beneficial effect on the metabolic syndrome. However, the relationship between physical activity and metabolic syndrome is still somewhat controversial, particularly for women. Such studies have varied in assessments of physical activity (subjective vs. objective), cardiorespiratory fitness (ergometer cycle vs. treadmill tests) and muscular strength (1-repetition maximum vs. isometric dynamometry), as well as criteria or risks to define the metabolic syndrome. In addition, the cross-sectional nature of most of these studies does not allow inference of causality. Further studies examining sex differences in the relation between physical activity and metabolic syndrome that address confounding factors such as menopausal status and concurrent medical conditions are needed. A longitudinal study design is also needed to examine the causal relationship between physical activity and metabolic syndrome.

4. Effect of physical activity and fitness on metabolic syndrome in children and adolescents

The beneficial effect of leisure-time physical activity on the metabolic syndrome in children and adolescents has been assessed within the contemporary reviews [47–50]. Froberg and Andersen [47] have authored a review on the linking physical inactivity and low fitness to metabolic disorders including CVD risk factors and obesity in European children. The authors concluded that there was only weak evidence of the association between physical activity or physical fitness and CVD risk factors in children when risk factors were analyzed isolated, but the clustering of risk factors was strongly associated with low physical activity or physical fitness among children. They also stated that participation in regular physical activity was one of the key determinants of lifestyle-related health. Furthermore, the relationship between aerobic fitness, fatness and the metabolic syndrome in children and adolescents was reviewed [48]. It was concluded that the relationship between fatness and the metabolic syndrome remained significant after controlling for fitness, whereas the relationship between fitness and metabolic syndrome disappeared after controlling for fatness. The author also reviewed four studies [51–54] of the combined influence of fatness and fitness on the metabolic syndrome and concluded that fitness attenuated the metabolic syndrome score among fat children and adolescents when they were cross-tabulated into categories (fat-fit, etc.), it might be possible to involve genetics, adipocytokines and mitochondrial function.

A recent review by Steele et al. [49], outlined the evidence from 6 studies [55–60] on objectively measured physical activity (i.e. accelerometer) and 11 studies [51–54, 59–65] on cardiorespiratory fitness, identifying the influence of physical activity and fitness on the clustered metabolic risk in youth. They concluded that physical activity and fitness were separately and independently related to metabolic risk factors in children and adolescents, possibly through different causal pathways. Among more recent studies, findings have been mixed. In a population-based sample of 3 193 10- and 15-year-old youth from three European countries (Estonia, Denmark, and Portugal), Ekelund et al. [66] further found that both cardiorespiratory fitness (OR = 0.33, 95% CI = 0.15-0.75) and objectively measured physical activity (OR = 0.40, 95% CI = 0.18-0.88) were significantly and independently associated with being categorized as having the metabolic syndrome. Relatively small increases in physical activity might significantly reduce the risk of metabolic syndrome in healthy youth. Conversely, Martínez-Gómez et al. [67] did not find the same association between physical activity and metabolic syndrome in 202 adolescents (99 girls) aged 13-17 years after controlling for age, sex and maturation status, and suggested that cardiorespiratory fitness appeared to have a pivotal role in the metabolic syndrome and in the association of physical activity with the metabolic risk.

There were only few studies have reported on the effect of diet and physical activity on prevention of the metabolic syndrome in adolescents. For example, Pan and Pratt [68] investigated a sample of 4 450 US adolescents aged 12 to 19 years from the National Health and Nutrition Examination Survey 1999-2002. They reported that although there was not significant relationship between physical activity and the overall prevalence of metabolic syndrome, the differences in some metabolic syndrome components among groups were statistically significant. Adolescents with low physical activity had higher levels of triglycerides and blood pressure than those with moderate or high physical activity. In addition, the prevalence of metabolic syndrome was a 16-fold higher in overweight adolescents (BMI $\geq$ 95th percentile) compared with their normal weight peers (BMI $\leq$ 85th percentile). Higher overall healthy eating index and fruit scores were also associated with lower risk of the metabolic syndrome. The authors concluded that unhealthy lifestyle behaviours might be the major underlying cause for the metabolic syndrome in adolescents. The primary means for preventing the metabolic syndrome was needed to engage adolescents in regular physical activity and healthful dietary practices to prevent excessive weight gain.

However, these studies have not addressed issues specific to population subgroups or intervention-delivery modalities. In a very recent review of the literature on the relationship between physical activity and metabolic syndrome in youth, Brambilla et al. [50] provided an overview of 11 studies [69-79] on physical activity intervention, focusing on a subsample of obese youth and intervention modalities and concluded that the different physical activity programs, relatively short duration and small sample size of these studies likely contributed to the inconsistent results. Although there were some controversies regarding the risk of insulin resistance, fat mass and body mass index for certain subgroups of children and adolescents with obesity, regular vigorous intensity physical activity on blood pressure and lipid levels did much to alleviate concerns that physical activity programs could have positive effect in these metabolic risk parameters. Furthermore, the authors suggested that the effect of low-intensity physical activity (e.g., playing at home, walking to school, dancing, and downstairs) on the metabolic risk in a large sample of overweight and obese children and adolescents should be taken into consideration in future study.

To summarize, several studies have shown that metabolic risk factors are readily detectable in children and adolescents because obesity is closely associated with insulin resistance in youth. It seems that physical activity intervention strategies may be most effective in childhood and adolescence before the development of metabolic syndrome. The main question to be asked is whether the positive effects of physical activity seen in adults will occur in children and adolescents. Most studies have found that objectively measured physical activity and cardiorespiratory fitness are inversely associated with clustered metabolic risk score in children and adolescents, while some have shown that physical activity in adolescents does not result in significantly reduce the prevalence of metabolic syndrome when cardiorespiratory fitness is adjusted for in the analysis. A question which remains unanswered, however, is how much physical activity is needed to prevent the metabolic syndrome and the diseases with which it is associated. Also, the clustered metabolic risk score has been applied in these studies, but no clear definition of the metabolic syndrome has been formally established for either children or adolescents. Attention to these questions with further research is needed.

5. Early physical activity and fitness as a predictor of metabolic syndrome in adulthood

The mechanism behind the relationship between physical activity in childhood and adolescence and adult risk for the metabolic syndrome has been explored. Referring to the model including three possible paths from childhood physical activity to adulthood health presented by Blair et al. [80], one of the hypothetical paths is a direct connection from physical activity or physical fitness in youth to cardiovascular and metabolic health in adult life. In the Cardiovascular Risk in Young Finns Study [19], 961 participants aged 12-18 years from five cities of Finland were included and followed from 1980 to 1983 and 1986. Physical activity was assessed with a standardized questionnaire and then summed a physical activity index from its intensity, frequency and duration. The results showed that the change in physical activity over 6 years was inversely associated with changes in insulin and triglycerides among boys. Among girls, the change in physical activity did not make any independent contribution to the models for serum lipoproteins. It was concluded that participation in regular leisure-time physical activity should be encouraged among adolescents in order to improve coronary risk profiles. Similar observations have been reported in other European studies. In the Amsterdam Growth and Health Study [81], 181 13-year-old Dutch adolescents were followed over a 15 years. The daily physical activity and fitness (both cardiopulmonary and neuromotor fitness) have been measured with six repeated times during the period. They found that daily physical activity was positively related to high-density lipoprotein cholesterol, and inversely to the total cholesterol/high-density lipoprotein ratio and to the sum of four skinfolds. Additionally, cardiopulmonary fitness was inversely associated with the total cholesterol. Neuromotor fitness was inversely associated with the sum of four skinfolds, and positively to systolic blood pressure. The authors stated that during adolescence and young adulthood both daily physical activity and fitness were related to a healthy coronary heart disease risk profile.

There are two recent studies for extending the Cardiovascular Risk in Young Finns Study. Yang et al. [82] followed 1 319 boys and girls (ages 9–18 years) from five Finnish university towns and their rural surroundings from 1980 to 2001. Leisure-time physical activity was assessed by a short self-report questionnaire. The results indicated that youth physical activity predicted adult physical activity in men ($R^2 = 0.10$) and women ($R^2 = 0.03$), which, in turn, predicted waist circumference in adulthood. Youth body mass index was directly related to waist circumference in adulthood in both sexes. The models were significant explaining 19% of variance of abdominal obesity in men and 13% in women. Also, youth physical activity was indirectly associated with waist circumference in adulthood through both the maintenance of physical activity in adulthood and reducing body weight in youth. The path from youth physical activity to adult obesity through youth obesity seemed to be stronger than the path through adult physical activity. However, the level of youth physical activity did not predict adult abdominal obesity in either men or women (Figure 1). The authors concluded that the prevalence of abdominal obesity as defined by waist circumference during adulthood was directly related to adult physical activity and youth overall obesity in both sexes. Youth physical activity had an indirect effect on abdominal obesity through both the maintenance of physical activity in adulthood and reduction in body weight in youth. Participation in and maintaining physical activity from youth into adulthood might play an important role in reducing obesity in adulthood.

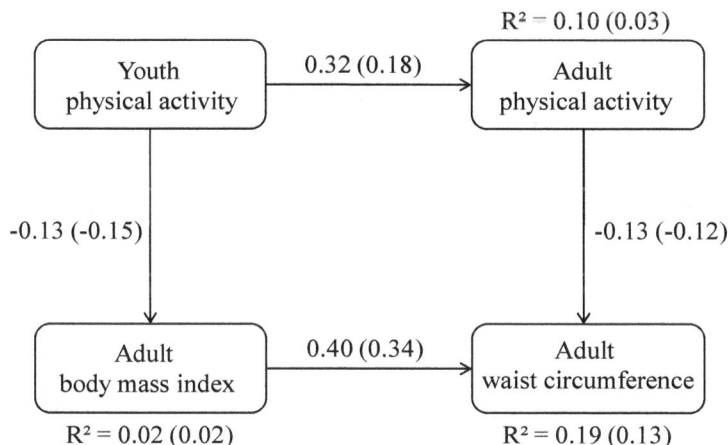

$$R^2 = 0.10 \ (0.03)$$

Youth physical activity →[0.32 (0.18)]→ Adult physical activity

-0.13 (-0.15) ↓   -0.13 (-0.12) ↓

Adult body mass index →[0.40 (0.34)]→ Adult waist circumference

$$R^2 = 0.02 \ (0.02) \qquad R^2 = 0.19 \ (0.13)$$

Fig. 1. Estimadtd parameters (stan dardized solution) in structural equation for males (females)

In another study by Yang et al. [83], 1 493 Finnish children and adolescents aged 3 to 18 years were followed over a 21-year period. Participation in sport-club training and competitions were assessed by use of a self-report physical activity questionnaire. Participants were divided into athletes and non-athletes at each measurement point (1980 and 1983), and then classified into four groups: persistent athlete, starter, leaver and non-athlete. A mean score of youth sport was assessed by calculating the average of four consecutive measurements (1980-1989). The metabolic syndrome in adulthood was defined as a categorical variable based on the guidelines of the European Group for the Study of Insulin resistance and as a continuous metabolic syndrome risk score by summing the z-scores of individual metabolic variables. The results indicated that the mean score of youth sport across the four time points and covariate variables were simultaneously entered as predictors for the adult metabolic syndrome risk score. Mean youth sport level emerged as a significant predictor of the metabolic syndrome in men (β = -0.149, P = 0.001) and women (β = -0.118, P = 0.005). Furthermore, non-athletic males and females had a significantly higher prevalence of the metabolic syndrome in adulthood than persistent athletes (Table 3). The relationships remained significant after adjustment for age and baseline clustered metabolic risk scores. The adds ratios and 95% confidence intervals for non-athletic males and females were 2.94 (1.01–8.99) and 4.04 (1.18–13.85), respectively. After additional adjustment for adult leisure-time physical activity, the trend of the associations was the same but significant difference between persistent athletic and non-athletic males disappeared. Those males who dropped out from organized sport during the 3 years had higher prevalence of the metabolic syndrome compared with persistently athletic counterparts. The difference remained significant after adjustment for age, baseline clustered metabolic risk scores and adult leisure-time physical activity (OR = 4.52, 95% CI = 1.29–15.84).

The mechanisms explaining the relationship between sport participation in youth and the prevalence of metabolic syndrome in adulthood are not well understood. One of the more obvious explanations can be that youth sport may reduce the risk of metabolic syndrome in youth, which then tracks into adulthood. However, the explanation is not clear because adjustment for youth clustered metabolic risk does not change the result. In addition, sustained youth sport seems to predict low prevalence of the metabolic syndrome in adulthood 21 years later independently of adult physical activity. It is possible that participation in organized youth sport may establish lifelong habits for good health that in turn reduces risk for the metabolic syndrome. Participation in sustained youth sport may also lead to improved cardiovascular function and physical fitness that carries over into adulthood. Furthermore, children and adolescents who want to maintain their athletic abilities may have better awareness of other health related habits such as diet, smoking and sedentary lifestyle, all of which have been found to be related to risk for the metabolic syndrome. Finally, self-selection and genetic factors shall be taken into account as possible explanations for the direct relationship between youth sport and adult health. Thus, intensive and sustained participation in youth sport may benefit adult cardiovascular health and prevent the development of metabolic syndrome. Organizers of youth sport may have a significant impact on public health by paying attention to the factors that increase adherence in youth sport.

Group	Unadjusted OR (CI)		Adjusted OR (CI) [2]		Adjusted OR (CI) [3]	
Boys						
Persistent athlete	1.00		1.00		1.00	
Starter	1.62	0.45 – 5.80	1.49	0.39 – 5.71	1.55	0.41 – 5.85
Leaver	4.55	1.39 – 14.87*	4.70	1.31 – 16.91*	4.52	1.29 – 15.84*
Non-athlete	3.06	1.08 – 8.64*	2.94	1.01 – 8.99*	2.72	0.90 – 8.17
Girls						
Persistent athlete	1.00		1.00		1.00	
Starter	1.67	0.38 – 7.27	1.63	0.35 – 7.64	1.66	0.36 – 7.69
Leaver	2.24	0.60 – 8.35	1.98	0.47 – 8.30	1.57	0.38 – 6.44
Non-athlete	3.54	1.08 – 11.55*	4.04	1.18 – 13.85*	3.46	1.03 – 11.66*

[1] 3-year follow-up youth sport: persistently athlete (did between 1980 and 1983); starter (did not in 1980 but did in 1983); leaver (did in 1980 but did not in 1983); and non-athlete (did in neither 1980 nor 1983).
[2] Adjusted for baseline age, smoking, total caloric intake and baseline-clustered risk for metabolic syndrome.
[3] Additionally adjusted for adult leisure-time physical activity. * $p < 0.05$.

Table 3. Odds ratios for the prevalence of metabolic syndrome (European Group for the Study of Insulin Resistance) according to organized youth sport [1] over 3 years in boys and girls

Contrary to the expected beneficial effect, no association between the level of physical activity and the risk of metabolic syndrome was found. In the Leuven Longitudinal Study on Lifestyle, Fitness and Health [84], 166 Belgian adolescent boys aged 13–18 years were followed over a 28-year period. Physical activity was assessed by means of a sports participation inventory in youth and the Tecumseh community health study questionnaire in adulthood. The results found that sports participation during adolescence was not related to levels of cardiovascular risk factors at 40 years of age. In the Danish Youth and Sport Study [85], 101 adolescents aged 15–19 years were followed over an 8-year period. Physical activity was assessed by a questionnaire including the number of hours per week of sports participation and physical education lessons. Physical fitness in terms of aerobic fitness was calculated as VO_{2max} relative to body weight (ml/min/kg). It was showed that the relationships between the absolute levels of physical fitness and activity in adolescence and the subsequent level of CVD risk factors were generally weak. However, the changes in physical fitness and physical activity were related to the absolute levels of CVD risk factors in young adulthood, especially in men. A subsequent study conducted by the same investigators [86] reported similar results when a physical activity index was constructed from the intensity and duration of the organized and unorganized sports activities. The results showed that the youth sports activities and fitness were not associated with clustered risk in adulthood. The lack of significant associations could be due to methodological limitations such as small samples and assessment of physical activity based on self-reported minutes spent on sports activities rather than objective measure to physical activity.

Moreover, future study is indicated in distinguishing between active and inactive on the adulthood risk of developing the metabolic syndrome. Future research is also need to develop and evaluate objective measures of physical activity (e.g., pedometers, accelerometers) in youth, define and measure the criteria of metabolic syndrome and clarify whether long-lasting changes in physical activity decrease the metabolic risk for different lifespan.

6. Effect of change in physical activity and fitness on metabolic syndrome in adulthood

According to the model [80], the most probable path is from childhood physical activity to adult physical activity and further to adult metabolic health. This supported by the studies on tracking of physical activity [87–90], and also studies on the relationship between physical activity and metabolic syndrome in either youth or adults as has just been mentioned above. Another potential path is physical activity in youth through youth clustered metabolic risk to adult metabolic syndrome. This path is supported by the finding that physical activity and physical fitness correlate negatively with the metabolic risk in youth [49]. Further, metabolic risk variables, especially obesity, likely track rather well from childhood to adulthood [82,91]. Only a few prospective population-based studies have reported long-term physical activity in predicting the prevalence of metabolic syndrome over time and especially of changes in physical activity in association with adulthood metabolic syndrome.

Laaksonen et al. [92] followed a cohort of 612 middle-aged men in the Kuopio Ischemic Heart Disease Risk Factor Study over a 4-year follow-up period. Leisure-time physical activity was measured by a questionnaire with the dose calculated as MET-minutes per week. Physical activity was then grouped into three levels: low-intensity (< 4.5 METs-min/wk), moderate- and high intensity (≥ 4.5 METs-min/wk) and high-intensity physical activity (≥ 7.5 METs-min/wk). Cardiorespiratory fitness (VO_{2max}, ml·kg^{-1}·min^{-1}) was divided into three levels: low (≤ 28.9), moderate (29.0–35.6) and high (≥ 35.7). Men with moderate and vigorous physical activity were significant lower prevalence of the metabolic syndrome than those with low physical activity. The odds ratios were 0.60 (0.37–0.99) for physical activity ≥ 4.5 METs (>3 h/wk vs. ≤60 min/wk) and 0.48 (0.29–0.77) for physical activity ≥ 7.5

METs after adjustment for major confounding variables (age, body mass index, smoking, alcohol, and socioeconomic status) or potentially mediating variables (insulin, glucose, lipids, and blood pressure), especially in high-risk men. Vigorous physical activity had an even stronger inverse association, particularly in unfit men. Men in the highest tertile of cardiorespiratory fitness were 75% less likely to develop the metabolic syndrome than men in the lowest tertile of cardiorespiratory fitness after adjustment for major confounders, but the association was attenuated after adjustment for possible mediating variables. it was included that physical activity and cardiorespiratory fitness predicted directly or indirectly the development of metabolic syndrome.

A randomized controlled trial was used to investigate the effectiveness of supervised aerobic exercise training in 105 participants with the metabolic syndrome before and after 20 weeks [93]. 30.5% (32 participants) of the participants were no longer classified as having the metabolic syndrome following exposure to a standardized 20-week exercise program. It was suggested that aerobic exercise training showed prolonged vigorous exercise programs and reduced substantially in those with the metabolic syndrome. Although limited by lack of a control group, this study supported that the effectiveness of aerobic exercise training could be useful as a treatment strategy in prevention of the metabolic syndrome. In their further study of the impact of cardiorespiratory fitness on the risk of metabolic syndrome, obesity and mortality among 19 173 American men aged 20–83 years, Katzmarzyk et al. [94] reported that the odds ratios and their 95% confidence intervals for having risks of all-cause mortality were 1.11 (0.75-1.17) in normal weight, 1.09 (0.82-1.47) in overweight, and 1.55 (1.14-2.11) in obese men with the metabolic syndrome, compared with normal weight healthy men. The corresponding risks for cardiovascular disease mortality were 2.06 (0.92-4.63) in normal weight, 1.80 (1.10-2.97) in overweight, and 2.83 (1.70-4.72) in obese men with the metabolic syndrome, compared with normal weight healthy men. However, the risks of all-cause mortality associated with obesity and metabolic syndrome were no longer significant after adjustment for cardiorespiratory fitness, which suggested that these risks were largely explained by overall physical fitness levels.

In the Medical Research Council Ely Study [95], 605 (249 males) middle-aged adults in England were followed over the past 5.6 years. Physical activity energy expenditure was measured objectively by individually calibrated heart rate against energy expenditure and was then divided into quartiles: < 44 kJ/kgFFM/d, 44-70 kJ/kgFFM/d, 71-100 kJ/kgFFM/d, and > 100 kJ/kgFFM/d. Aerobic fitness was predicted from a submaximal exercise stress test. Physical activity energy expenditure predicted progression toward the metabolic syndrome after adjusting for sex, baseline age, smoking, socioeconomic status, follow-up time, and baseline phenotypes. The associations remained significant after additional adjustment for aerobic fitness. While the relationship between aerobic fitness and metabolic syndrome was attenuated after adjusting for physical activity. In a cohort of the Oslo study, Holme et al. [96] followed 6 410 Norwegian middle-aged men from 1972/3 to 2000 in the city of Oslo. Leisure-time physical activity was measured by a questionnaire to classify men into four groups as follows: sedentary/light (usually reading, watching television or other sedentary occupations at leisure), moderate (walking, bicycling or other forms of physical activity including walking or bicycling to and from the place of work and a Sunday walk totalling at least four hours a week), moderately vigorous (exercise, sports, heavy gardening and similar activities totalling at least 4 hours a week), and vigorous (hard training or competition sports regularly several times a week). Physical activity was a significant predictor of the prevalence of metabolic syndrome (OR = 0.65, 95%CI = 0.54–0.80) and diabetes (OR = 0.68, 95%CI = 0.52–0.91) over 28 years when adjusted for age and educational attendance. However, these associations were markedly attenuated when additional adjusted for baseline clustered metabolic risks.

Yang et al. [97] followed six cohorts of 2 060 (961 males) young adults aged 24–39 years in the Young Finns Study. Leisure-time physical activity was assessed using a self-report questionnaire completed in connection with a medical examination at two consecutive measurements in 1992 and 2001. By summing the physical activity items, a physical activity index was formed for both measurement points according to which the participants were divided into tracking groups: persistently active, increasingly active, decreasingly active, and persistently inactive. The prevalence of the metabolic syndrome on all three definitions was significantly lower in men and women who were persistently active during the 9 yr of follow-up compared with persistently inactive ones. In men, the odds ratios and their 95% confidence intervals were 0.23 (0.11–0.49) for the European Group for the Study of Insulin Resistance (EGIR) criteria, 0.54 (0.31–0.93) for the National Cholesterol Education Program-Adult Treatment Panel III (NCEP) criteria, and 0.49 (0.29–0.83) for the International Diabetes Federation (IDF) criteria. In women, the odds ratios were 0.33 (0.12–0.94) for EGIR, 0.21 (0.06–0.67) for NCEP, and 0.27 (0.11–0.63) for IDF. Also, women who were increasingly active were less likely on all definitions to have the metabolic syndrome than their persistently inactive counterparts. The associations remained significant for EGIR (OR = 0.28, 95% CI = 0.09–0.92), NCEP (OR = 0.22, 95% CI = 0.07–0.73), and IDF (OR = 0.42, 95% CI = 0.19–0.94). All of these associations remained significant after adjustment for potential confounders such as age, smoking and education (Table 4). The authors concluded that

Group	EGIR Adjusted OR (CI) [2]		NCEP-ATP III Adjusted OR (CI)		IDF Adjusted OR (CI)	
Men						
Persistently inactive	1.00		1.00		1.00	
Decreasingly active	0.69	0.41 – 1.15	0.99	0.62 – 1.57	1.07	0.69 – 1.65
Increasingly active	0.73	0.30 – 1.79	0.58	0.22 – 1.52	0.48	0.19 – 1.27
Persistently active	0.23	0.11 – 0.49***	0.54	0.31 – 0.93*	0.49	0.29 – 0.83**
Women						
Persistently inactive	1.00		1.00		1.00	
Decreasingly active	0.68	0.35 – 1.34	0.65	0.35 – 1.21	0.59	0.33 – 1.05
Increasingly active	0.28	0.09 – 0.92*	0.22	0.07 – 0.73*	0.42	0.19 – 0.94*
Persistently active	0.33	0.12 – 0.94*	0.21	0.06 – 0.67**	0.27	0.11 – 0.63**

EGIR, European Group for the Study of Insulin Resistance; NCEP-ATP III, National Cholesterol education Program-Adult Treatment Panel III; IDF, International Diabetes Federation.
[1]Physical activity groups: persistently inactive (inactive both in 1992 and 2001); decreasingly active (change 1992-2001 from active to inactive); increasingly active (change 1992-2001 from inactive to active); and persistently active (active both 1992 and 2001).
[2] Adjusted for age, smoking and education. * $p < 0.05$, ** $p < 0.01$, *** $p < 0.001$.

Table 4. Adjusted odds ratios for three definitions of metabolic syndrome according to change in physical activity groups [1] over a 9-yr period

maintaining a high level of physical activity across the life span might decrease the prevalence of the metabolic syndrome not only in the short term but also in the long term. Individuals should be encouraged to participate in regular physical activity as early as possible to prevent the risk of developing the metabolic syndrome and related adult-onset diabetes and cardiovascular diseases.

7. Conclusion

Outlined in this chapter is a brief overview of leisure-time physical activity, cardiorespiratory fitness and muscular strength which focus is on prevention and intervention of the prevalence of the metabolic syndrome in youth and adulthood. In addition, there is a brief summarizes on maintaining regular physical activity and aerobic exercise over time focused on the metabolic syndrome in adulthood.

It is worth highlighting that regular leisure-time physical activity, endurance training, and strength training are critically important for prevention of the metabolic syndrome and its components in both early life and later life. Evidence is beginning to accumulate in the epidemiological literature which suggests that participation in regular aerobic and strength exercises, particularly when combined with moderate- or vigorous-intensity activity may alter all metabolic risk factors. Leisure-time physical activity is an effective intervention or modulation to improve cardiovascular functional capacity and prevent or delay the development of metabolic syndrome, which in turn maintains health status and reduces the incidence of diabetes and cardiovascular diseases. According to the recommendations of the American College of Sports medicine and the American Heart Association, all adults shall participate in accumulated moderate-intensity physical activity during leisure time for a minimum of 30 minutes or more on 5 days per week or vigorous intensity activity for a minimum of 20 minutes on 3 days per week [42]. It may be that the combination of reductions in energy intake and increases in energy expenditure, through structured exercise and other forms of physical activity, is one of the most effective way to prevent or delay the development of metabolic syndrome over time. This chapter focuses mainly on physical activity and aerobic exercise during leisure time related the prevalence of metabolic syndrome, however there is limited literature relating to specific sport activities, work-related physical activity, commuting physical activity and household physical activity. Emphasis will be placed on the impact of these activities in the future.

8. Acknowledgments

This study was financially supported by the Academy of Finland (grants no. 77841, 210283, 123621 [L.P.-R.], 121584, 124282), Social Insurance Institution of Finland, Ministry of Education, Turku University Foundation, Special Federal Grants for Turku University Hospital, Research Funds of the University of Helsinki (project no 2106012 [L.P.-R.], Juho Vainio Foundation, Finnish Foundation of Cardiovascular Research, Emil Aaltonen Foundation (M.H.), Finnish Medical Foundation, Finnish Cultural Foundation, Yrjö Jahnsson Foundation, and Signe and Ane Gyllenberg Foundation (M.H.).

9. References

[1] E.S. Ford, "Risks for all-cause mortality, cardiovascular disease, and diabetes associated with the metabolic syndrome: a summary of the evidence," *Diabetes Care*. vol. 28, no. 7, pp. 1769.–1778, Jul. 2005.

[2] J.C. Eisenmann, "Secular trends in variables associated with the metabolic syndrome of North American children and adolescent: a review and synthesis," *Am. J. Hum. Biol.* vol. 15, no. 6, pp. 786.–794, Nov-Dec. 2003.

[3] M.L. Cruz and M.I. Goran, "The metabolic syndrome in children and adolescents," *Curr. Diab. Rep.* vol. 4, no.1, pp. 53.–62, Feb. 2004.

[4] N. Mattsson, T. Rönnemaa, M. Juonala, J.S. Viikari and O.T. Raitakari, "The prevalence of the metabolic syndrome in young adults. The Cardiovascular Risk in Young Finns Study," *J. Intern. Med.* vol. 261, no. 2, pp. 159.–169, Feb. 2007.

[5] G. Hu, J. Lindström, P. Jousilahti, M. Peltonen, L. Sjöberg, R. Kaaja, J. Sundvall and J. Tuomilehto, "The increasing prevalence of metabolic syndrome among Finnish men and women over a decade," *J. Clin. Endocrinol. Metab.* vol. 93, no. 3, pp. 832.–836, Mar. 2008.

[6] C.G. Spain and B.D. Franks, "Healthy people 2010: Physical activity and fitness. President's Council Physical Fitness Sport," *President's Council on Physical Fitness and Sport Research Digest.* vol. 3, no. 13, pp. 1.–16, Mar. 2001.

[7] J.R. Churilla and R.F. Zoeller Jr, "Physical activity and the metabolic syndrome: A review of the evidence," *Am. J. Lifestyle Med.* vol. 2, no. 2, pp. 118.–125, Mar/Apr. 2008.

[8] S. Carroll and M. Dudfield, "What is the relationship between exercise and metabolic abnormalities? A review of the metabolic syndrome," *Sports Med.* vol. 34, no. 6, pp. 371.–418, 2004.

[9] C. J. Caspersen, K. E. Powell, and G. M. Christenson, "Physical activity, exercise, and physical fitness: definitions and distinctions for health-related research," *Public health Rep.* vol. 100, no. 2, pp. 126.–131, Mar-Apr. 1985.

[10] "Third report of the National Cholesterol Education Program (NCEP) Expert Panel on Detection, Evaluation, and Treatment of High Blood Cholesterol in Adults (Adult Treatment Panel III): Final report", *National Cholesterol Education Program, National Heart, Lung, and Blood Institute, National Institutes of Health.* NIH publication No. 02-5215, Sep. 2002. Available at: http://www.nhlbi.nih.gov/guidelines/cholesterol/atp3full.pdf.

[11] World Health Organization, "Definition diagnosis and classification of diabetes mellitus and its complications. Report of a WHO Consultation. Part 1: diagnosis and classification of diabetes mellitus," World Health Organization, Department of Noncommunicable Disease Surveillance, Geneva, 1999. Available at: http://www.staff.ncl.ac.uk/philip.home/who_dmg.pdf.

[12] B. Balkau, M.A. Charles, T. Drivsholm, K. Borch-Johnsen, N. Wareham, J.S. Yudkin, R. Morris, I. Zavaroni, R. van Dam, E. Feskins, R. Gabriel, M. Diet, P. Nilsson and B. Hedblad, "Frequency of the WHO metabolic syndrome in European cohorts, and an alternative definition of an insulin resistance syndrome. European Group for the Study of Insulin Resistance (EGIR)," *Diabetes Metab.* 28, pp. 364.–376, 2002.

[13] S.M. Grundy, J.I. Cleeman, S.R. Daniels, K.A. Donato, R.H. Eckel, B.A. Franklin, D.J. Gordon, R.M. Krauss, P.J. Savage, S.C. Smith Jr, J.A. Spertus and F. Costa, "Diagnosis and management of the metabolic syndrome: an American Heart Association/National Heart, Lung, and Blood Institute scientific statement," *Curr. Opin Cardiol.* vol. 21, no. 1, pp. 1.–6, Jan. 2006.

[14] G. Alberti Sir, P. Zimmet, J. Shaw and S.M. Grundy, "The IDF consensus worldwide definition of the metabolic syndrome," Available at:

http://www.idf.org/webdata/docs/IDF_Meta_def_final.pdf. International Diabetes Federation, 2006.

[15] E.S. Ford, "Prevalence of the metabolic syndrome defined by the International Diabetes Federation among adults in the U.S.," *Diabetes Care*. vol. 28, no. 11, pp. 2745.–2749, Nov. 2005.

[16] P.M. Nilsson, G. Engström and B. Hedblad, "The metabolic syndrome and incidence of cardiovascular disease in non-diabetic subjects--a population-based study comparing three different definitions," *Diabet. Med*. vol. 24, no. 5, pp. 464.–472, May. 2007.

[17] S.A. Paluska and T.L. Schwenk, "Physical activity and mental health: current concepts," *Sports Med*. vol. 29, no. 3, pp. 167.–180, Mar. 2000.

[18] P. Ekkekakis, E.E. Hall and S.J. Petruzzello, "Variation and homogeneity in affective responses to physical activity of varying intensities: an alternative perspective on dose-response based on evolutionary considerations," *J. Sport Sci*. vol. 23, no. 5, pp. 477.–500, May. 2005.

[19] O.T. Raitakari, K.V. Porkka, S. Taimela, R. Telama, L. Räsänen and J.S. Viikari, "Effects of persistent physical activity and inactivity on coronary risk factors in children and young adults. The Cardiovascular Risk in Young Finns Study". *Am. J. Epidemiol*. vol. 140, no. 3, pp. 195.–205, Aug. 1994.

[20] S. Zhu, M.P. St-Onge, S. Heshka and S.B. Heymsfield, "Lifestyle behaviors associated with lower risk of having the metabolic syndrome," *Metabolism*. vol. 53, no. 11, pp. 1503.–1511, Nov. 2004.

[21] L.E. Robinson and T.E. Graham, "Metabolic syndrome, a cardiovascular disease risk factor: role of adipocytokines and impact of diet and physical activity," *Can. J. Appl. Physiol*. vol. 29, no. 6, pp. 808.–829, Dec. 2004.

[22] S. Carroll, C.B. Cooke and R.J. Butterly, "Metabolic clustering, physical activity and fitness in nonsmoking, middle-aged men," *Med. Sci. Sports Exerc*. vol. 32, no. 12, pp. 2079.–2086, Dec. 2000.

[23] T.A. Lakka, D.E. Laaksonen, H.M. Lakka, N. Männikkö, L.K. Niskanen, R. Rauramaa and J.T. Salonen, "Sedentary lifestyle, poor cardiorespiratory fitness, and the metabolic syndrome," *Med. Sci. Sports Exerc*. vol. 35, no. 8, pp. 1279.–1286, Aug. 2003.

[24] K.L. Rennie, N. McCarthy, S. Yazdgerdi, M. Marmot and E. Brunner, "Association of the metabolic syndrome with both vigorous and moderate physical activity," *Int. J. Epidemiol*. vol. 32, no. 4, pp. 600.–606, Aug. 2003.

[25] P.T. Katzmarzyk, T.S. Church and S.N. Blair, "Cardiorespiratory fitness attenuates the effects of the metabolic syndrome on all-cause and cardiovascular disease mortality in men," *Arch. Intern. Med*. vol. 164, no. 10, pp. 1092.–1097, May. 2004.

[26] N.G. Boule, C. Bouchard and A. Tremblay, "Physical fitness and the metabolic syndrome in adults from the Quebec family study," *Can. J. Appl. Physiol*. vol. 30, no. 2, pp. 140.–156, Apr. 2005.

[27] S.E. Brien and P.T. Katzmarzyk, "Physical activity and the metabolic syndrome in Canada," *Appl. Physiol. Nutr. Metab*. vol. 31, no. 1, pp. 40.–47, Feb. 2006.

[28] K.E. Remsberg, N.L. Rogers, E.W. Demerath, S.A. Czerwinski, A.C. Choh, M. Lee, W.C. Chumlea, S.S. Sun, B. Towne and R.M. Siervogel, "Sex differences in young

adulthood metabolic syndrome and physical activity: the Fels longitudinal study," *Am. J. Hum. Biol.* vol. 19, no. 4, pp. 544.–550, Jul-Aug. 2007.

[29] M.L. Irwin, B.E. Ainsworth, E.J. Mayer-Davis, C.L. Addy, R.R. Pate and J.L. Durstine, "Physical activity and the metabolic syndrome in a tri-ethnic sample of women," *Obes. Res.* vol. 10, no. 10, pp. 1030.–1037, Oct. 2002.

[30] S.W. Farrell, Y.J. Cheng and S.N. Blair, "Prevalence of the metabolic syndrome across cardiorespiratory fitness levels in women," *Obes. Res.* vol. 12, no. 5, pp. 821.–830, May. 2004.

[31] M.H. Whaley, J.B. Kampert, H.W. 3rd, Kohl and S.N. Blair, "Physical fitness and clustering of risk factors associated with the metabolic syndrome," *Med. Sci. Sports Exerc.* vol. 31, no. 2, pp. 287.–293, Feb. 1999.

[32] P.W. Franks, U. Ekelund, S. Brage, M.Y. Wong and N.J. Wareham, "Does the association of habitual physical activity with the metabolic syndrome differ by level of cardiorespiratory fitness?" *Diabetes Care.* vol. 27, no. 5, pp. 1187.–1193, May. 2004.

[33] D.W. Dunstan, J. Salmon, N. Owen, T. Armstrong, P.Z. Zimmet, T.A. Welborn, A.J. Cameron, T. Dwyer, D. Jolley, J.E. Shaw and AusDiab Steering Committee, "Associations of TV viewing and physical activity with the metabolic syndrome in Australian adults," *Diabetologia.* vol. 48, no. 11, pp. 2254.–2261, Oct. 2005.

[34] M. Halldin, M. Rosell, U. de Faire, M.L. Hellenius, "The metabolic syndrome: prevalence and association to leisure-time and work-related physical activity in 60-year-old men and women," *Nutr. Metab. Cardiovasc. Dis.* vol. 17, no. 5, pp. 349.–357, Mar. 2007.

[35] Y.W. Park, S. Zhu, L. Palaniappan, S. Heshka, M.R. Carnethon and S.B. Heymsfield, "The metabolic syndrome: Prevalence and associated risk factor findings in the US population from the Third National Health and Nutrition Examination Survey, 1988-1994," *Arch. Intern. Med.* vol. 163, no. 4, pp. 427.–436, Feb. 2003.

[36] K.D. DuBose, C.L. Addy, B.E. Ainsworth, G.A. Hand and J.L. Durstine, "The relationship between leisure-time physical activity and the metabolic syndrome: an examination of NHANES III, 1988-1994," *Journal of Physical Activity & Health.* vol. 2, no. 4, pp. 470.–487, Oct. 2005.

[37] R.R. Pate, M. Pratt, S.N. Blair, W.L. Haskell, C.A. Macera, C. Bouchard, D. Buchner, W. Ettinger, G.W. Heath, A.C. King, et al., "Physical activity and public health. A recommendation from the Centers for Disease Control and Prevention and the American College of Sports Medicine," *JAMA.* vol. 273, no. 5, pp. 402.–407, Feb. 1995.

[38] E.S. Ford, H.W. 3rd Kohl, A.H. Mokdad, U.A. Ajani, "Sedentary behavior, physical activity, and the metabolic syndrome among U.S. adults," *Obes. Res.* vol. 13, no. 3, pp. 608.–614, Mar. 2005.

[39] J.R. Churilla and E.C. Fitzhugh, "Relationship between leisure-time physical activity and metabolic syndrome using varying definitions: 1999-2004 NHANES," *Diab. Vasc. Dis. Res.* vol. 6, no. 2, pp. 100.–109, Apr. 2009.

[40] B.E. Ainsworth BE, W.L. Haskell, M.C. Whitt, M.L. Irwin, A.M. Swartz, S.J. Strath, W.L. O'Brien, D.R. Bassett Jr, K.H. Schmitz, P.O. Emplaincourt, D.R. Jacobs Jr and A.S. Leon, "Compendium of physical activities: an update of activity codes and MET intensities," *Med. Sci. Sports Exerc.*, vol. 32, Suppl 9, pp. S498.–S504, Sep. 2000.

[41] E.T. Howley, "Type of activity: resistance, aerobic and leisure versus occupational physical activity," *Med. Sci. Sports Exerc.* vol. 33, Suppl 6, pp. S364.-S369, Jun. 2001 (discussion S419.-S420).

[42] W.L. Haskell, I.M. Lee, R.R. Pate, K.E. Powell, S.N. Blair, B.A. Franklin, C.A. Macera, G.W. Heath, P.D. Thompson, A. Bauman, American College of Sports Medicine and American Heart Association, "Physical activity and public health: updated recommendation for adults form the American College of Sports medicine and the American Heart Association," *Circulation.* vol. 116, no. 9, pp. 1081.-1093, Aug. 2007.

[43] S.E. Brien, I. Janssen and P.T. Katzmarzyk, "Cardiorespiratory fitness and metabolic syndrome: US National Health and Nutrition Examination Survey 1999-2002," *Appl. Physiol. Nutr. Metab.* vol. 32, no. 1, pp. 143.-147, Feb. 2007.

[44] R. Jurca, M.J. Lamonte, T.S. Church, C.P. Earnest, S.J. Fitzgerald, C.E. Barlow, A.N. Jordan, J.B. Kampert and S.N. Blair, "Associations of muscle strength and aerobic fitness with metabolic syndrome in men," *Med. Sci. Sports Exerc.* vol. 36, no. 8, pp. 1301.-1307, Aug. 2004.

[45] R. Jurca, M.J. Lamonte, C.E. Barlow, J.B. Kampert, T.S. Church and S.N. Blair, "Associations of muscle strength with incidence of metabolic syndrome in men," *Med. Sci. Sports Exerc.* vol. 37, no. 11, pp. 1849.-1855, Nov. 2005.

[46] K. Wijndaele, N. Duvigneaud, L. Matton, W. Duquet, M. Thomis, G. Beunen, J. Lefevre and R.M. Philippaerts, "Muscular strength, aerobic fitness, and metabolic syndrome risk in Flemish adults," *Med. Sci. Sports Exerc.* vol. 39, no. 2, pp. 233.-240, Feb. 2007.

[47] K. Froberg and L.B. Andersen, "Mini review: Physical activity and fitness and its relation to cardiovascular disease risk factors in children," *Int. J. Obes.* vol. 29, Suppl 2, pp. S34.-S39, Sep. 2005.

[48] J.C. Eisenmann, "Aerobic fitness, fatness and the metabolic syndrome in children and adolescents," *Acta Pediatric.* vol. 96, no. 12, pp. 1723.-1729, Oct. 2007.

[49] R.M. Steele, S. Brage, K. Corder, N.J. Wareham and U. Ekelund, "Physical activity, cardiorespiratory fitness, and the metabolic syndrome in youth," *J. Appl. Physiol.* vol. 105, no. 1, pp. 342.-351, Jul. 2008.

[50] P. Brambilla, G. Pozzobon and A. Pietrobelli, "Physical activity as the main therapeutic tool for metabolic syndrome in childhood," *Int. J. Obes.* vol. 35, pp. 16.-28, 2011; published online 7 Dec. 2010.

[51] J.C. Eisenmann, P.T. Katzmarzyk, L. Perusse, A. Tremblay, J.P. Despres and C. Bouchard, "Aerobic fitness, body mass index and CVD risk factors among adolescents: the Quebec Family Study," *Int. J. Obes.* vol. 29, no. 9, pp. 1077.-1083, Sep. 2005.

[52] J.C. Eisenmann, G.J. Welk, E.E. Wickel and S.N. Blair, "Combined influence of cardiorespiratory fitness and body mass index on cardiovascular disease risk factors among 8-18 year old youth: The Aerobics Center Longitudinal Study," *Int. J. Pediatr. Obes.* vol. 2, no. 2, pp. 66.-72, 2007.

[53] J.C. Eisenmann, G.J. Welk, M.A. Ihmel and J. Dollman, "Fitness, fatness and cardiovascular disease risk factors in children and adolescents," *Med. Sci. Sports Exerc.* vol. 39, no. 8, pp. 1251.-1256, Aug. 2007.

[54] K.D. DuBose, J.C. Eisenmann and J.E. Donnelly, "Aerobic fitness attenuates the metabolic syndrome score in normal-weight, at-risk-for-overweight, and overweight children," *Pediatrics.* vol. 120, no. 5, pp. e1262.-e1268, Nov. 2007.

[55] L.B. Andersen, M. Harro, L.B. Sardinha, K. Froberg, U. Ekelund, S. Brage and S.A. Anderssen, "Physical activity and clustered cardiovascular risk in children: a cross-sectional study (The European Youth Heart Study)," *Lancet.* vol. 22, no. 368(9532), pp. 299.–304, Jul. 2006.

[56] S. Brage, N. Wedderkopp, U. Ekelund, P.W. Franks, N.J. Wareham, L.B. Andersen and F. Froberg, "Objectively measured physical activity correlates with indices of insulin resistance in Danish children. The European Youth Heart Study (EYHS)," *Int. J. Obes. Relat. Metab. Disord.* vol. 28, no. 11, pp. 1503.–1508, Nov. 2004.

[57] N.F. Butte, M.R. Puyau, A.L. Adolph, F.A. Vohra and I. Zakeri, "Physical activity in nonoverweight and overweight Hispanic children and adolescents," *Med. Sci. Sport Exerc.* vol. 39, no. 8, pp. 1257.–1266, Aug. 2007.

[58] U. Ekelund, S. Brage, P.W. Froberg, M. Harro, S.A. Anderssen, L.B. Sardinha, C. Riddoch and L.B. Andersen, "TV viewing and physical activity are independently associated with metabolic risk in children: the European Youth Heart Study," *PLoS Med.* vol. 3, no. 12, pp. e488, Dec. 2006.

[59] U. Ekelund, S.A. Anderssen, K. Froberg, L.B. Sardinha, L.B. Andersen, S. Brage and European Youth Heart Study Group, "Independent associations of physical activity and cardiorespiratory fitness with metabolic risk factors in children: the European youth heart study," *Diabetologia.* vol. 50, no. 9, pp. 1832.–1840, Jul. 2007.

[60] N.S. Rizzo, J.R. Ruiz, A. Hurtig-Wennlof, F.B. Ortega and M. Sjöström, "Relationship of physical activity, fitness, and fatness with clustered metabolic risk in children and adolescents: the European youth heart study," *J. Pediatr.* vol. 150, no. 4, pp. 388.–394, Apr. 2007.

[61] S.A. Anderssen, A.R. Cooper, C. Riddoch, L.B. Sardinha, M. Harro, S. Brage and L.B. Andersen, "Low cardiorespiratory fitness is a strong predictor for clustering of cardiovascular disease risk factors in children independent of country, age and sex," *Eur. J. Cardiovasc. Prev. Rehabil.* vol. 14, no. 4, pp. 526.–531, Aug. 2007.

[62] E. Garcia-Artero, F.B. Ortega, J.R. Ruiz, J.L. Mesa, M. Delgado, M. González-Gross, M. García-Fuentes, G. Vicente-Rodríguez, A. Gutiérrez and M.J. Castillo, "Lipid and metabolic profiles in adolescents are affected more by physical fitness than physical activity (AVENA study)," *Rev. Esp. Cardiol.* vol. 60, no. 6, pp. 581.–588, 2007.

[63] I. Janssen and W.C. Cramp, "Cardiorespiratory fitness is strongly related to the metabolic syndrome in adolescents," *Diabetes Care.* vol. 30, no. 8, pp. 2143.–2144, Aug. 2007.

[64] J.R. Ruiz, F.B. Ortega, N.S. Rizzo, I. Villa, A. Hurtig-Wennlöf, L. Oja and M. Sjöström, "High cardiovascular fitness is associated with low metabolic risk score in children: the European Youth Heart Study," *Pediatr. Res.* vol. 61, no. 3, pp. 350.–355, Mar. 2007.

[65] G.Q. Shaibi, M.I. Cruz, G.D. Ball, M.J. Weigensberg, H.A. Kobaissi, G.J. Salem and M.I. Goran, "Cardiovascular fitness and the metabolic syndrome in overweight latino youths," *Med. Sci. Sports Exerc.* vol. 37, no. 6, pp. 922.–928, Jun. 2005.

[66] U. Ekelund, S. Anderssen, L.B. Andersen, C.J. Riddoch, L.B. Sardinha, J. Luan, K. Froberg and S. Brage, "Prevalence and correlates of the metabolic syndrome in a population-based sample of European youth," *Am. J. Clin. Nutr.* vol. 89, no. 1, pp. 90.–96, Jan. 2009.

[67] D. Martinez-Gómez, J.C. Eisenmann, J.M. Moya, S. Gómez-Martínez, A. Marcos and O.L. Veiga, "The role of physical activity and fitness on the metabolic syndrome in adolescents: effect of different scores. The AFINOS Study," *J. Physiol. Biochem.* vol. 65, no. 3, pp. 277.-289, Sep. 2009.

[68] Y. Pan and C.A. Pratt, "Metabolic syndrome and its association with diet and physical activity in US adolescents," *J. Am. Diet Assoc.* vol. 108, no. 2, pp. 276.-286, Feb. 2008.

[69] M.A. Ferguson, B. Gutin, N.A. Le, W. Karp, M. Litaker, M. Humphries, T. Okuyama, S. Riggs and S. Owens, "Effects of exercise training and its cessation on components of the insulin resistance syndrome in obese children," *Int. J. Obes.* Relat. Metab. Disord. vol. 23, no. 8, pp. 889.-895, Aug. 1999.

[70] H.S. Kang, B. Gutin, P. Barbeau, S. Owens, C.R. Lemmon, J. Allison, M.S. Litaker and N.A. Le, "Physical training improves insulin resistance syndrome markers in obese adolescents," *Med. Sci. Sports Exerc.* vol. 34, no. 12, pp. 1920.-1927, Dec. 2002.

[71] R.Y. Sung, C.W. Yu, S.K. Chang, S.W. Mo, K.S. Woo and C.W. Lam, "Effects of dietary intervention and strength training on blood lipid level in obese children," *Arch. Dis. Child.* vol. 86, no. 6. pp. 407.-410, Jun. 2002.

[72] J.X. Jiang, X.L. Xia, T. Greiner, G.L. Lian and U. Rosengvist, "A two year family based behaviour treatment for obese children," *Arch. Dis. Child.* vol. 90, no. 12, pp. 1235.-1238, Dec. 2005.

[73] D. Nemet, S. Barkan, Y. Epstein, O. Friedland, G. Kowen and A. Eliakim, "Short- and long-term beneficial effects of a combined dietary behavioural- physical activity intervention for the treatment of childhood obesity," *Pediatrics.* vol. 115, no. 4, pp. e443.-e449, Apr. 2005.

[74] A.L. Carrel, R.R. Clark, S.E. Peterson, B.A. Nemeth, J. Sullivan and D.B. Allen, "Improvement of fitness, body composition, and insulin sensitivity in overweight children in a school-based exercise program: a randomized, controlled study," *Arch. Pediatr. Adolesc. Med.* vol. 159, no. 10, pp. 963.-968, Oct. 2005.

[75] A.A. Meyer, G. Kundt, U. Lenschow, P. Schuff-Werner and W. Kienast, "Improvement of early vascular changes and cardiovascular risk factors in obese children after a six-month exercise program," *J. Am. Coll. Cardiol.* vol. 48, no. 9, pp. 1865.-1870, Nov. 2006.

[76] G.Q. Shaibi, M.L. Cruz, G.D. Ball, M.J. Weigensberg, G.J. Salem, N.C. Crespo and M.I. Goran, "Effects of resistance training on insulin sensitivity in overweight Latino adolescent males," *Med. Sci. Sports Exerc.* vol. 38, no. 7, pp. 1208.-1215, Jul. 2006.

[77] G.A. Kelley and K.S. Kelley, "Aerobic exercise and lipids and lipoproteins in children and adolescents: a meta-analysis of randomized controlled trials," *Atherosclerosis.* vol. 191, no. 2, pp. 447.-453, Apr. 2007.

[78] N.J. Farpour-Lambert, Y. Aggoun, L.M. Marchand, X.E. Martin, F.R. Herrmann and M. Beghetti, "Physical activity reduces systemic blood pressure and improves early markers of atherosclerosis in prepubertal obese children," *J. Am. Coll. Cardiol.* vol. 54, no. 25, pp. 2396.-2406, Dec. 2009.

[79] E.C. Murphy, L. Carson, W. Neal, C. Baylis, D. Donley and R. Yeater, "Effects of an exercise intervention using Dance Dance Revolution on endothelial function and other risk factors in overweight children," *Int. J. Pediatr. Obes.* vol. 4, no. 4, pp. 205.-214, Apr. 2009.

[80] S.N. Blair, G.G. Clark and K.J. Cureton, "Exercise and fitness in childhood: implications for a lifetime health," In *Perspectives in Exercise Science and Sport Medicine, Vol 2. Youth Exercise and Sport*, C.V. Gisolfi and D.L. Lamb Eds. Indianapolis: Benchmark Press, 1989, pp. 401.–430.

[81] J.W.R. Twisk, H.C.G. Kemper and W. van Mechelen, "Tracking of activity and fitness and the relationship with cardiovascular disease risk factors," *Med. Sci. Sports Exerc.* vol. 32, no. 8, pp. 1455.–1461, Aug. 2000.

[82] X. Yang, R. Telama, E. Leskinen, K. Mansikkaniemi, J. Viikari and O.T. Raitakari, "Testing a model of physical activity and obesity tracking from youth to adulthood: the cardiovascular risk in young Finns study," *Int. J. Obes.* vol. 31, no. 3, pp. 521.–527, Mar. 2007.

[83] X. Yang, R. Telama, M. Hirvensalo, J.S. Viikari and O.T. Raitakari, "Sustained participation in youth sport decreases metabolic syndrome in adulthood," *Int. J. Obes.* vol. 33, no. 11, pp. 1219.–1226, Sep. 2009.

[84] J. Lefevre, R. Philippaerts, K. Delvaux, M. Thomis, A.L. Claessens, R. Lysens, R. Renson, B. Vanden Eynde, B. Vanreusel and G. Beunen, "Relation between cardiovascular risk factors at adult age, and physical activity during youth and adulthood: the Leuven longitudinal study on lifestyle, fitness and health," *Int. J. Sports Med.* vol. 23, Suppl 1, pp. S32.–S38, May. 2002.

[85] H. Hasselstrom, S.E. Hansen, K. Froberg, L.B. Andersen, "Physical fitness and physical activity during adolescence as predictors of cardiovascular disease risk in young adulthood. Danish Youth and Sports Study. An eight-year follow-up study," *Int. J. Sport Med.* vol. 23, Suppl 1, pp. S27.–S31, May. 2002.

[86] L.B. Andersen, H. Hasselstrøm, V. Grønfeldt, S.E. Hansen and F. Karsten, "The relationship between physical fitness and clustered risk, and tracking of clustered risk from adolescence to young adulthood: eight years follow-up in the Danish Youth and Sport Study," *Int. J. Behav. Nutr. Phys. Act.* vol. 8, no. 1, pp. 6, Mar. 2004.

[87] X. Yang, R. Telama, M. Leino and J. Viikari, "Factors explaining the physical activity of young adults: the importance of early socialization," *Scand. J. Med. Sci. Sports* vol. 9, no. 2, pp. 120.–127, Apr. 1999.

[88] R.M. Malina, "Adherence to physical activity from childhood to adulthood: a perspective from tracking studies," *Quest.* vol. 53, no. 3, pp. 346.–355, Aug. 2001.

[89] T. Temmelin, S. Näyhä, A.P. Hills and M.R. Järvelin, "Adolescent participation in sports and adult physical activity," *Am. J. Prev. Med.* vol. 24, no. 1, pp. 22.–28, Jan. 2003.

[90] R. Telama, X. Yang, J. Viikari, I. Välimäki, O. Wanne and O. Raitakari, "Physical activity from childhood to adulthood – A 21-year tracking study," *Am. J. Prev. Med.* vol. 28, no. 3, pp. 267.–273, Apr. 2005.

[91] Y.B. Cheung, D. Machin, J. Karlberg and K.S. Khoo, "A longitudinal study of pediatric body mass index values predicted health in middle age," *J. Clin. Epidemiol.* vol. 57, no. 12, pp. 1316.–1322, Dec. 2004.

[92] D.E. Laaksonen, H.M. Lakka, J.T. Salonen, L.K. Niskanen, R. Rauramaa and T.A. Lakka, "Low Levels of Leisure-Time Physical Activity and Cardiorespiratory Fitness Predict Development of the Metabolic Syndrome," *Diabetes Care.* vol. 25, no. 9, pp. 1612.–1618, Sep. 2002.

[93] P.T. Katzmarzyk, A.S. Leon, J.H. Wilmore, J.S. Skinner, D.C. Rao, T. Rankinen and C. Bouchard, "Targeting the metabolic syndrome with exercise: evidence from the

HERITAGE Family Study," *Med. Sci. Sports Exerc.* vol. 35, no. 10, pp. 1703.–1709, Oct. 2003.

[94] P.T. Katzmarzyk, T.S. Church, I. Janssen, R. Ross and S.N. Blair, "Metabolic syndrome, obesity, and mortality: impact of cardiorespiratory fitness," *Diabetes Care.* vol. 28, no. 2, pp. 391.–397, Feb. 2005.

[95] U. Ekelund, S. Brage, P.W. Franks, S. Hennings, S. Emms and N.J. Wareham, "Physical activity energy expenditure predicts progression toward the metabolic syndrome independently of aerobic fitness in middle-aged healthy Caucasians: the Medical Research Council Ely Study," *Diabetes Care.* vol. 28, no. 5, pp. 1195.–1200, May. 2005.

[96] I. Holme, S. Tonstad, A.J. Sogaard, P.G. Larsen and L.L. Haheim, "Leisure time physical activity in middle age predicts the metabolic syndrome in old age: results of a 28-year follow-up of men in the Oslo study," *BMC Public Health.* vol. 7, pp. 154, Jul. 2007.

[97] X. Yang, R. Telama, M. Hirvensalo, N. Mattsson, J.S. Viikari and O.T. Raitakari, "The longitudinal effects of physical activity history on metabolic syndrome," *Med. Sci. Sports Exerc.* vol. 40, no. 8, pp. 1424.–1431, Aug. 2008.

9

Exercise and the Immune System – Focusing on the Effect of Exercise on Neutrophil Functions

Baruch Wolach

The Sackler School of Medicine, Tel Aviv University,
Israel

1. Introduction

A relationship between intense exercise, leukocytosis and susceptibility to illness was already reported at the beginning of the past century (1-3). Today there is a consensus among researchers and clinicians that exercise have effects on various aspects of the immune function (4). The complexity of the underlying mechanisms and the clinical implications and directions need continuous evaluation. Investigators face challenges associated with immune measures and the interpretation of their changes. They should bear in mind that there is inter-individual variability of the exercise capacity, recovery, stress tolerance and immunocompetence. Short exposure to exercise could promote beneficial and apropriate physiological response of the immune system, while heavy exertion could be detrimental to health. In recent years, the development of advanced laboratory techniques contributed to enrich our knowledge and deepened the understanding of the mechanisms underlying the immune system in sports medicine. The development of fluorescent antibodies techniques allow identifying cell sub-types and receptors. Molecular technology and new cytokine methods of identification have permitted the detection of humoral factors present in the body at low concentrations, for short periods of time and to study the effect of exercise on gene expression profiles (5,6).
Studies on recreational and elite athletes should be systematic and well controlled in order to formulate evidence-based guidelines to preserve a balanced immune function.

2. The immune system

The immune response can be divided into innate, natural-non-adaptive immunity and acquired-adaptive immunity. Innate immunity is the first response to physical or chemical foreign agents and it occurs naturally and immediately, providing the first line of defense in early stages of the infection. The innate immunity is comprised of phagocyte cells, natural killer cells, soluble factors as the complement and acute phase proteins, as well as the mucosal immune responses. The acquired immunity occurs after an adaptive, specific response to a pathogen and involves the antigen-antibody response. It includes B and T lymphocytes and the immunoglobulines (7).

In the innate immunity phagocytes can recognize and act immediately against the foreign agent without prior exposure, while the adaptive immunity is characterized by a specific response to the infectious agent, becoming fully activated after a lag period. The innate mucosal defenses are the first line of defense against pathogens present at the mucosal surfaces. The 'Common Mucosal Immune System' is a network of organized structures that protect the oral cavity, the respiratory, thegastrointestinal and the urogenital systems. The major effector function of this system is the secretory IgA (8,9).

The adaptive immunity involves the action of specialized immune cells, as are the lymphocytes, which generate antibodies against specific microorganisms, killing them directly or activating other cells through the secretion of cytokines. This adaptive response generates memory which is the basis of the preventive immunization. Both systems of immunity, the innate and the acquired, work synergistically and are essential for an optimal function of the immune response. Phagocytes play an important role in the initiation of the adaptive response by presenting antigens and secreting cytokines that stimulate cells of the adaptive system.

Neutrophils (55-65% of blood leukocytes) and monocytes (5-10%) play an important role in innate immunity and provide a major defense system against microorganisms. They act as the first line of defense against infectious agents and are involve in the muscle tissue inflammatory response to exercise-induced injury (10). The multi-step phagocytic process is activated in response to invasion of foreign microorganisms and includes the rolling and adherence of neutrophils to the blood vessel endothelium, the diapedesis and chemotaxis towards the invading organism, the ingestion, degranulation and the oxidative burst, ending with killing of the pathogen (11). Experienced and well equipped laboratories in this specific field, have established the normal range values, based on a large number of subjects examined, in health and disease. Today it is possible to assess the different steps of the phagocytic process and to detect dysfunctions at each level (11-13).

3. Exercise and the immune response – Clinical implications

The potential influence of exercise on the immune system could be beneficial, detrimental or neutral. The immune response depends on the type of the particular exercise, its intensity, volume and duration. While mild or moderate exercise was shown to be beneficial, acute intense or prolonged exercise elicits depression of several aspects of the immune response. The fitness level of the performers could also exert influence in their immunological response. It seems that there is a combination of physiological and psychological factors, known to exert their influences on the immune system. Appropriate interpretation of the immune response is vital for determining the clinical directions and the integral training program for each athlete.

The physical activity could affect one or all three arms of the immune system, the humoral, the phagocytic and the cellular arm. Eventually, dysfunction of one or more arms of the immune system could lead to the outburst of an infection. In general, the etiology of infections is usually of bacterial origin when the humoral or phagocytic arm is affected, while viral–parasitic infections are usually originated when the cellular arm is involved. Excessive, prolonged training and major competitions have been long considered factors affecting the susceptibility to infections in athletes (14-16), however, in shorter and less competitive events infections are less common (7). Frequent illness has been associated with the overtraining syndrome in athletes (17-19). During heavy exertion could be an immune suppression that creates an 'open window' of decreased host protection. Bacteria or viruses may gain a foothold, increasing the risk of subclinical and clinical infections (17, 20). In team sports or in other sports where participants are in close physical contact before, during or after the sporting event, both the infected individual and the fellow sportsmen may become infected. Some infections may appear in clusters in the sports setting, such as gastroenteritis, herpes simplex, meningitis, viral hepatitis, skin infections, tonsillo-pharyngitis (21,22). A large number of viruses and bacteria can give rise of myocarditis that can be aggravated by physical exertion (15).

There is consistent data suggesting that male endurance athletes may develop after 1 to 2-wk period increased rates of Upper Respiratory Tract Infection (URTI), following marathon or ultramarathon race events (16,23,24). URTI appears to be the most common minor viral infection in athletes. The current consensus is that the cause of URTI in athletes is uncertain (4). There is today disagreement whether 'sore throats', frequently reported by athletes, are caused by infections or are a reflexion of other inflammatory stimuli mimicking URTI (25,26). Cytokines play an important role in modulating the immune function, inducing changes that increase the risk of infection or the appearance of inflammatory symptoms (27). The physician diagnosis of URTI is based on clinical symptoms and signs, rather than by determining the infectious etiology. In few studies the pathogen was identified as the usual respiratory pathogens associated with URTI in the general population (4). The salivary IgA concentrations and secretion rates have been shown to be significantly decreased in athletes with prolong high intensity exercise (28,29). We could hypothesize that their immunity is reduced with an increase tendency to develop URTI. Other markers of infection as antimicrobial proteins in saliva (α-amylase, lactoferrin, and lysozyme) have been identified (26,30). Further, viral infections as URTI may lead to a debilitating state and an unexplained deterioration in athletic performance. Viral infections could run a protracted course of easy fatigability, myalgia and lethargy for weeks or even months (31). Additionally, it seems that athletes are more susceptible to develop Infectious Mononucleosis (32).

Infections of non-viral origin, as bacterial pneumonia, mycoplasma and Chlamydia myocarditis, sinusitis, etc., although uncommonly reported in athletes, could also develop following intense exercise (2,15,33). Athletes could aggravate the course of the disease during incubation periods of infections (34,35).

Neutrophils comprise the majority of circulating leukocytes and represent the early body's response in the battle against bacterial and fungal infections. Multi-factorial elements could be involved in the neutrophil behavior and in the immune responses to exercise, as neuro-endocrine mediators (36), corticosteroid release, interleukin production (37) and oxy-reduction processes associated with free radical production (38). Most studies show that of all subsets of circulating leukocytes, mainly neutrophils and lymphocytes, increase dramatically during exercise (39,40). The magnitude is related to the exercise intensity and duration, being more persistent with intense, prolonged exercise (40, 41). Neutrophil count may exhibit a biphasic response, characterized by an initial small increase, followed by a decline to resting values 30-60 minutes after the cessation of exercise. A delayed larger increase in neutrophil numbers could be observed

2 to 4 hours post-exercise (42). This leukocyte trafficking reflect recruitment into the circulation of neutrophils and could be related to hemodynamic changes as increased cardiac output, hyperthermia or could reflect changes in circulating stress hormones, particularly epinephrine and cortisol, released during exercise (42). Resting leukocyte number is generally normal in athletes, although long periods of high-volume training may be associated with long lasting suppression of circulating cell numbers, which may persist low over weeks (43). This may be attributed to migration of leukocytes out of the circulation to possible damaged skeletal muscle (44).

Disproportionate changes in lymphocyte subsets occur during exercise. Usually, during prolonged exercise the NK and CD8 T- cells increase far more than B cells and CD4 T- cells counts (40). Significant decline in the CD4:CD8 ratio was reported after 60 min of treadmill running. Although neutrophil counts may remain elevated for several hours after exercise cessation, lymphocyte number may decline bellow baseline values for up to 6 hours post exercise (7). Following vigorous exercise it was reported a transient fall of circulating natural killer (NK) cell count (45).

In summary, exercise increases neutrophil numbers and may reflect an appropriate response to exercise-induced stress rather than an impaired immunocompromised state. In contrast, the post-exercise decrease in the absolute lymphocyte counts, the NK decrease and the inversion of the CD4 to CD8 ratio, could indicate immunosuppresion.

It is remarkable that no significant changes were reported in B-cell circulating lymphocytes and only local salivary IgA reduction was shown following intense, prolonged exercise. The relationship between the leukocyte dynamics and the clinical implications is still unclear.

4. Immunological studies – Our experience

Scant information exists on exercise-induced changes in the immune system among children. We investigated the effect of aerobic exercise on several aspects of cellular and humoral functions among 10-12 year-old highly trained female gymnasts and untrained girls (46). All girls were pre-pubertal. Venous blood samples were drawn before, immediately after and 24 h following 20 min of treadmill running (heart rate 170-180 beats.min-1). White blood cells' number rose significantly following exercise and remained elevated for 24 h. The increase in leukocyte number was due to an increase in granulocytes as well as an increase in lymphocytes and monocytes. While neutrophil count returned to basal values after 24 h, lymphocytes and monocytes number remained elevated 24 h following exercise. Exercise resulted in a significant elevation of T cell lymphocytes, T helpers, T suppressors and natural killer cells. All values returned to normal after 24 h. There were no changes in B cell lymphocytes following exercise (Table 1). Exercise had no effect on serum immunoglobulin's and sub-types of IgG {IgG1, IgG2, IgG3 and IgG4} (Table 2). No differences were observed between gymnasts and untrained girls (46). The changes observed were similar to those found in adults (40).

Our laboratory for leukocyte functions focused within the last 30 years on granulocyte functions and dysfunctions in healthy subjects and in patients suffering from recurrent, severe, opportunistic infections. For the last 15 years, our group focused on neutrophil functions following a single bout of submaximal aerobic exercise (47-50). Neutrophil functions as chemotaxis, oxidative burst, and bactericidal activity were unaffected immediately post-exercise, however neutrophil chemotactic activity was found significantly decreased 24 h after the cessation of the exercise (Table 3) (47).

		Pre exercise		Immediately after exercise		24 h following exercise	
		X	SD	X	SD	X	SD
WBC	gymnasts	5561	596	*7046	1306	*6505	436
	untrained	6340	1043	*8263	1225	*6738	1150
Neutrophils	gymnasts	2710	349	*3554	692	3126	498
	untrained	3570	1000	*4658	1184	3490	805
Lymphocytes	gymnasts	1930	235	*2690	360	*2365	524
	untrained	2106	544	*2671	834	*2464	401
T cell	gymnasts	1590	493	*1860	682	723	340
	untrained	1413	219	*1953	357	1677	458
Th cells	gymnasts	943	251	*1030	248	1003	155
	untrained	792	197	*1059	303	992	334
Ts cells	gymnasts	663	278	* 851	410	776	205
	untrained	550	98	* 784	193	669	173
B cells	gymnasts	306	101	320	96	344	93
	untrained	295	56	329	92	350	103
Natural killer cells	gymnasts	161	132	* 256	119	231	124
	untrained	124	47	* 267	85	139	43
Monocytes	gymnasts	293	61	* 391	127	# 424	72
	untrained	373	82	* 462	125	375	18

* significantly different from pre-exercise value in both groups
# significantly different from pre-exercise value in the gymnasts group only

Table 1. Changes in the cellular components of the immune system. WBC and lymphocyte subpopulations (cells/µl) following exercise in gymnasts and untrained girls (46).

	IgM (mg/dl)		IgA (mg/dl)		IgE (unit/ml)		IgG (mg/dl)		IgG-1 (mg/dl)		IgG-2 (mg/dl)		IgG-3 (mg/dl)		IgG-4 (mg/dl)	
	mean	SD	mean	SD	mean	SD	mean	SD	mean	SD	mean	SD	mean	SD	mean	SD
pre exercise	207.0	83.3	120.6	26.1	81.6	53.2	1194.0	138.2	673.7	108.0	235.3	63.7	69.7	35.5	61.2	24.1
post exercise	199.3	67.6	120.4	21.6	81.1	49.8	1180.7	151.2	705.9	132.6	242.1	66.8	59.1	18.5	63.4	25.1
24 h post exercise	179.4	73.2	116.4	36.4	83.1	56.5	1181.4	147.3	669.9	144.3	232.4	69.0	63.6	22.1	61.4	24.2

Table 2. Immunoglobulin levels pre-exercise, immediately post-exercise among gymnasts (46).

		Pre-exercise (Basal)	Post-exercise	24 h post-exercise
Neutrophils (cells/µl)	trained	2710 ± 349	3554 ± 692	3126 ± 498
	untrained	3570 ± 1000	4658 ± 1184	3490 ± 805
Chemotaxis (cells /field)	trained	58 ± 11	55 ± 13	36 ± 11 *
	untrained	47 ± 7	52 ± 15	42 ± 8 *
Killing (log decrease of colonies) with autologous serum	trained	0.8 ± 0.3 #	0.8 ± 0.2 #	0.8 ± 0.1 #
	untrained	1.1 ± 0.1	1.1 ± 0.1	1.0 ± 0.2
Killing (log decrease of colonies) with homologous serum	trained	0.7 ± 0.2 #	0.8 ± 0.1 #	0.8 ± 0.2
	untrained	1.0 ± 0.1	1.0 ± 0.02	0.9 ± 0.2
Superoxide production (nmol $O_2^-/10^6$ PMNs/min) with PMA stimulation	trained	5.7 ± 0.4	4.4 ± 1.0 *	4.8 ± 1.0 *
	untrained	5.1 ± 0.7	4.7 ± 1.3	4.9 ± 1.2
Superoxide production (nmol $O_2^-/10^6$ PMNs/min) with fMLP stimulation	trained	3.4 ± 1.9	3.2 ± 1.3	2.6 ± 1.3
	untrained	4.1 ± 1.3	3.3 ± 0.5	3.7 ± 0.6

*)<0.05 compared with basal values (before vs. following exercise).
#)<0.05 compared with control group (trained vs. untrained).

Table 3. Effect of exercise on neutrophil count and neutrophil functions (mean+SD), Pre-exercise (basal), immediate post-exercise and 24 h post-exercise (47).

A consistent decrease of neutrophil migration was detected 24 h post-exercise in trained and untrained subjects, children and adults, male and female (47-50). The following studies focused on the recovery time of the impaired neutrophil chemotaxis, using various chemoattractans. We also aimed to learn about the possible mechanisms involved in the post exercise-associated chemotactic defect. We found that the transient impairment shown in the chemotactic activity 24 h post-exercise, returned to normal after 48 h (Figure 1) (49).

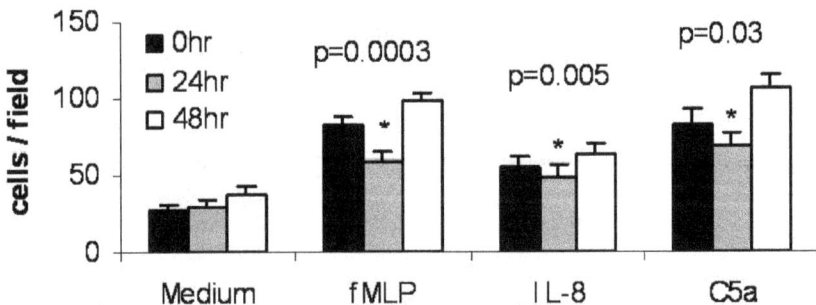

Fig. 1. Kinetics of the neutrophil chemotactic activity in 16 athletes; Pre-exercise, immediately post-exercise and 24 h post-exercise. The chemotaxis was induced by the chemoattractant: fMLP (1 µM), IL-8 (10 nM), or C5a (10 nM). Random migration was conducted in the presence of medium M199. The results were expressed as the number of migrating cells per field (mean±SE) (49).

Looking at the response of the neutrophil specific membrane receptors to the different chemoattractants, we repeatedly found reduction of the chemotaxis following intense exercise, regardless of the chemoattractant used, including Formylated peptides (fMLP), the chemokine IL-8, and the activated complement component(C5a) (49). These chemokines attach to their specific receptors, fMLP-R (N- formyl-Met-Leu-Phe), IL-8-R (CXCR1 and CXCR2), and C5aR, which belong to the seven-transmembrane helix surface receptor family ("serpentine receptors") that transduces signals downstream the cytoskeleton by coupling to heterotrimeric G-proteins (51). Once the signal has been triggered, rapid cytoskeletal rearrangement and chemotaxis take place. "Target" chemoattractants (fMLP, C5a) function primarily through a common signal-transduction pathway by stimulating p38 MAPK, whereas "host" intermediary chemoattractants (IL-8, LTB4) primarily function via the PI3K/Akt pathway (52). The surface density of the chemotactic receptor (C5aR), which serves as a representative model of receptor availability, was not affected 24 h after exercise. Moreover, the integrin CD11b/CD18, which represent one of the main receptors for neutrophil adhesiveness and crucial for normal chemotaxis, was also unaffected by exercise. Therefore, the chemotactic defect is not dependent on the specific receptor of activation, or on its specific pathway of transduction. We could speculate that the chemotactic impairment was related to a common defect at the membrane level, leading to decreased receptor availability or to other factors yet to be elucidated. For achieving appropriate chemotactic responses, an intact cytoskeleton structures are necessary (53,54). Continuous reorganization of the cytoskeleton is required for efficient F-actin polymerization and polarization. Both are important steps in the skeletal rearrangement during migration (55). Consequently, we studied the neutrophil F-actin neutrophil polarization and polymerization (49). Following fMLP stimulation, the cell undergoes sequential morphological changes from round to elongated geometrical forms (figure 2A). These changes reflect the cell activation and the ability to migrate against the chemotactic gradients toward the target (49,53). Using the green phalloidin test we found no correlation between the chemotactic defect and the ability to polymerize F-actin, indicating that the reduction in chemotaxis following exercise was not a result of the F-actin dysfunction. Despite the fact that positive correlation between chemotaxis and F-actin polymerization usually occurs, a lack of correlation in certain conditions has been reported (55).

To elucidate other cell skeletal responses to aerobic exercise, we studied the neutrophil polarization, known to be in tight correlation with the chemotactic activity.

Indeed, the neutrophil polarization was significantly decreased 24 h following aerobic exercise. This change also correlated with the decrease in chemotactic activity ($r= 0.945$; $P= 0.001$) (figure 2B) (49,50).

Since the neutrophil bactericidal activity and the oxidative burst were found to be normal, it seems that the signal transduction pathways are not affected following 30 min of intense aerobic exercise. Rather, it seems that aerobic exercise causes a skeletal impairment, and this eventually could leads to a reduction of the chemotactic activity. Most probably the impaired chemotaxis event, following a short bout of submaximal exercise, occurred at the effectors' machinery level, rather than at the level of the neutrophil membrane receptors. Others found no change in chemotaxis 24 h after a graded exercise to exhaustion (56). Giraldo et. al. reported increased chemotaxis immediately after moderate (45 min of 55% VO2max) and intense (1 hr of 70% VO2max) aerobic exercise that returned to basal values after 24 h (57). These discrepancies are probably related to differences in the type, intensity, and duration of exercise, timing of blood sampling, or use of different laboratory assays.

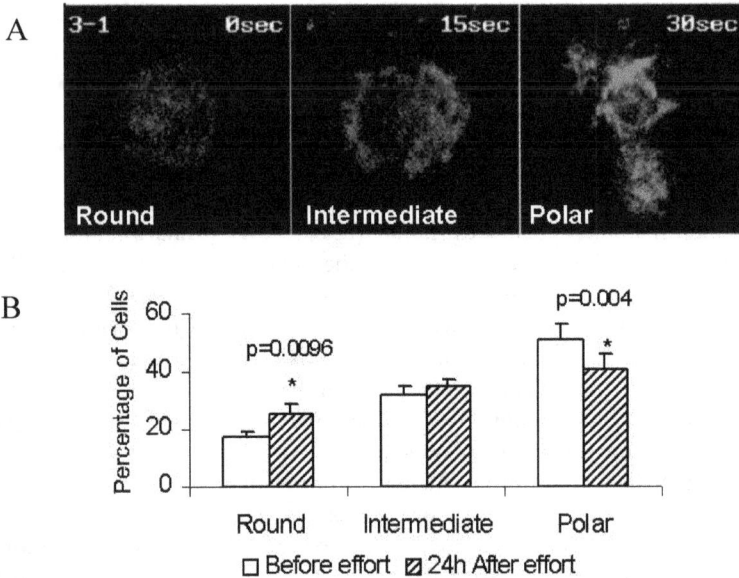

Fig. 2. Neutrophil polarization. A. The cell shape changes that occur following fMLP-stimulation. Three different cell shapes were recorded: non-activated - round cells (R), partially activated - intermediate cells (I), and fully activated - polarized cells (P).
B. Analysis of the cells' morphological changes following fMLP-stimulation, in 11 athletes, before and after effort (mean±SE) (49).

5. Therapeutic approach to exercise-induced immune suppression

Dietary and drug intervention have been reported to boost performance in athletes (58). They could block the transient immune changes, to prevent the oxidative stress and the inflammation induced by prolonged, intense exercise or excessive training. Some supplements as flavonoids were reported to benefit the immune system (59). In endurance events, iron and mineral supplements, together with antioxidant vitamins, help to prevent muscle damage (60). Carbohydrates enhance muscle glycogen stores. Glutamine and aminoacid supplementation did not prove to be beneficial (61).

Vitamin E (VE) and vitamin C, as antioxidants, play an important role in protecting the cells and muscles from damage (62-65). It is well-established that exercise exerts imbalance on the oxidative state by increasing Reactive Oxygen Species (ROS) and decreasing the level of antioxidants (63). As previously shown, intense or prolonged exercise can adversely affect the function of the immune system. It was found that submaximal aerobic activity (1h swim at 75-80% of VO2max) could produce oxidative damage within the neutrophils (64), which lose the appropriate antioxidant defense mechanisms, leading to a defective chemotactic ability (65). This impairment could rise from the increased levels of ROS and lipid peroxidation; both potentially could damage neutrophil function. The enhanced production of ROS, mainly by mitochondria, is associated with excessive oxidation of lipids, proteins, and nucleic acids, causing damage to cell membranes and to the physiological function of proteins and DNA (66-68). To defend themselves from ROS induced damage, cells contain complex antioxidant mechanisms including enzymatic (e.g. superoxide dismutase, glutathione peroxidase, catalase) and non-enzymatic antioxidants (e.g., vitamin E (VE), vitamin C, beta-carotene). VE is the most important lipid-soluble antioxidant due to its abundance in cell and mitochondrial membranes and its ability to act directly on ROS and stop lipid peroxidation. This antioxidant is known to decrease the exercise-induced oxidative stress (69-71) and has been shown to protect against exercise-induced muscle damage (70). Neutrophils play a dual role in exercise-induced oxidative damage. On the one hand, they contribute to ROS formation during intense or prolonged exercise; on the other hand, intense exercise can produce oxidative damage within neutrophils. VE has an important role as anti-oxidant and an important role in maintaining normal neutrophil function. Chemotaxis, adherence, and phagocytic capacities of neutrophils were shown to be reduced in VE deficiency, improving after antioxidant treatment (65,72,73).

Our research focused on the phagocytic immune response to exercise, showing prevention of the impairments by vitamin E supplementation. The results of chemotaxis and polarization are shown in Figure 3, representing the mean +/- SEM of 7 trained men pre- and post-exercise, before and after 28 days of daily VE supplementation (74). We can see that daily supplementation of 800 IU d-alpha tocopheryl succinate, indeed corrected the defective neutrophil chemotaxis and polarization observed 24 hr post-exercise.

A relatively small number of studies have dealt with the effect of VE on neutrophil functions following exercise. To the best of our knowledge, there are no studies addressing the effect of VE on exercise-induced impaired chemotaxis. However, a beneficial effect of VE on chemotaxis was shown in other populations, such as healthy elderly men and women and elderly women with coronary heart disease or major depressive disorder (72,73). Improvement in chemotactic ability after VE supplementation was also found in rats with VE deficiency and in periparturient dairy cows (75,76).

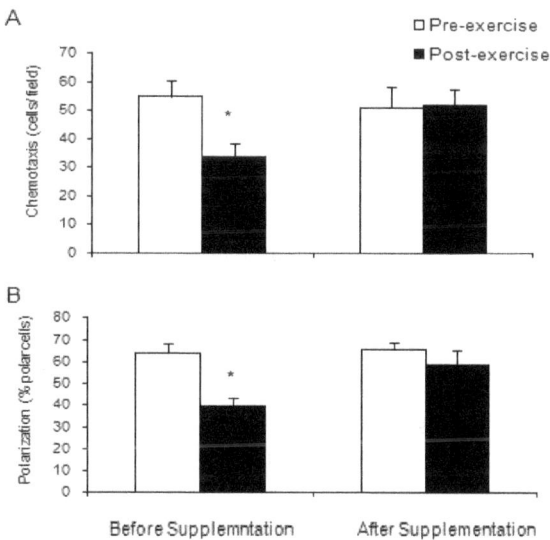

Fig. 3. A. Correction of the defective neutrophil chemotactic activity (observed 24 h post-exercise) by vitamin E supplementation. B. Correction of the defective neutrophil polarization (observed 24 h post-exercise) by vitamin E supplementation (74).

Of note is that recent reports have emphasized that ROS production, through the reversible oxidation of thiol groups, has also important physiological influences on gene transcription and protein synthesis, as part of the adaptive processes that occurs after exercise. High dose antioxidant supplementation may interfere with these processes. Cooper's Group reported gene reorganization after intense exercise (77, 78).

In recent years, it has been reported that regular physical activity can have beneficial role in cancer's prevention and therapy (79,80). There is evidence of a protective effect of physical activity on colon and postmenopausal breast cancer (81). Further, it is also mounting that physical activity reduces risks of lung tumor metastases (82). It has been reported that exercise prevent the loss of muscle mass and functional capacity in chronic deteriorating conditions, beyond the beneficial psychological effects, which certainly improve the quality of life (83-85).

Athletes are not immunocompromised by clinical definition, but could suffer from transitory, persistent immunosuppression, eventually leading to subclinical or clinical diseases. Recovery time is imperative in elite athletes involved in intense training and competitions. The temporary, sometimes multiple, mild impairments of the immune system could change into a chronic more severe immune dysfunction.

The approach should be multidisciplinary, including all care givers as sport medicine physicians, physiologists, immunologists, physiotherapists, nutritionists, psychologists and coaches. To achieve the main goals, an integrated model with programmed activities and clear guidelines for any specific type of sport is imperative. Recommendations should be directed to elite athletes and recreational sports, for sedentary individuals, for moderate and well trained subjects. The target is to maintain the balance of the immune system for the health of the athlete and his optimal performance.

6. References

[1] Larrabee RC, Leukocytosis after violent exercise. J Med Res, 7:76-82, 1902

[2] Cowles WN. Fatigue as a contributory cause of pneumonia. Boston Med Surg J, 179:555, 1918

[3] Baetjer AM. The effect of muscular fatigue upon resistance. Physiol Rev, 12:453-468, 1932

[4] Walsh NP, Gleeson M, Shephard RJ, Gleeson M, Woods JA, Bishop NC, Fleshner M, Green C, Pedersen BK, Hoffman-Goetz L, Rogers CJ, Northoff H, Abbasi A, Simon P. Part one: Immune function and exercise. Exercise Immunol Rev, 17:6-63, 2011

[5] Petersen AM, Pedersen BK. The anti-inflammatory effect of exercise. J Appl Physiol, 98:1154-1162, 2005

[6] Buettner P, Mosig S, Lechtermann A, Funke H, Mooren FC. Exercise affects the gene expression profiles of human white blood cells. J Appl Physiol 102: 26-36, 2007

[7] Nieman DC, Nehlsen-Cannarella SL. The immune response to exercise. Sem Hematol, 31:166-179, 1994

[8] Lamm ME. Current concepts in mucosal immunity. How epithelial transport of IgA antibodies relates to host defense. Am J Physiol, 274:G614-G617, 1998

[9] Gleeson M, Pyne DB. Special feature for the Olympics: effects of exercise in the immune system: exercise effect on mucosal immunity. Immunol Cell Biol, 78:536-544, 2000

[10] Mackinnon LT. Exercise and resistance to infectious diseases. In: Bahrke, Drews, Wentworth (Ed.), Advances in Exercise Immunology. Champaign, IL, pp. 1-26,1999

[11] Wolach B, Baehner RL, Boxer LA. Review: clinical and laboratory approach to the management of neutrophil dysfunction. Isr J Med Sci, 18:897-916, 1982

[12] Boxer LA, Blackwood RA. Leukocyte disorders: quantitative and qualitative disorders of the neutrophil, Part 2. Pediatr Rev, 17:47–50, 1996

[13] Dinauer MC. Disorders of neutrophil function: an overview. Methods Mol Biol, 412:489-504, 2007

[14] Mackinnon LT. Chronic exercise training effects on immune function. Med Sci Sports Exerc, 32(7 Suppl):S369-376, 2000

[15] Friman G, Wesslén L. Special feature for the Olympics: effects of exercise on the immune system: infections and exercise in high-performance athletes. Immunol Cell Biol, 78:510-522, 2000

[16] Peters EM, Bateman ED. Ultramarathon running and URTI. South African Med J, 64:503-584, 1983

[17] Nieman DC. Immune response to heavy exertion. J Appl Physiol, 82:1385-94, 1997

[18] Lehmann M. Foster C, Keul J. Overtraining in endurance athletes: a brief review. Med Sci Sport Exerc, 25:854-862, 1993

[19] Fitzgerald L. Overtraining increases the susceptibility to infection. Int J Sport Med, Suppl 1:S5-8, 1991

[20] Pedersen BK, Ullum H. NK-cell response to physical activity. Possible mechanisms of action. Med Sci Sports Exerc, 26:140-146, 1994

[21] Baron RD, Hutch MH, Kleeman K, Maccromac JN. Aseptic meningitis among members of high school football team. JAMA, 248:1724-1727, 1982

[22] Morse LJ, Bryan JA, Murle JP. The Holly Cross College Football team Hepatitis outbreak. JAJA, 219:706-708, 1972

[23] Nieman DC, Johanssen LM, Lee JW, Arabatzis K. Infectious episodes in runners before and after the Los Angeles Marathon. J Sports Med Phys Fitness, 30:316-328, 1990

[24] Nieman DC. Prolonged aerobic exercise, immune response and risk of infection. In: Exercise and Immune Function, CRC Press, pp.143-161, 1996

[25] Cox AG, Gleeson M, Pyne DB, Callister R, Hopkings WG, Fricker PA. Clinical and laboratory evaluation of upper respiratory symptoms in elite athletes. Clin J Sports Med, 18: 438-445, 2008

[26] Suzuki K, Nakaji S, Yamada M, Totsuka M, Sato K, Sugawara K. Systemic inflammatory response to exhaustive exercise. Cytokine kinetics. Exerc Immunol Rev, 8:6-48, 2002

[27] Cox AJ, Pyne DB, Saunders PU, Callister R, Gleeson M. Cytokine responses to treadmill running in healthy and illness-prone athletes. Med Sci Sports Med, 39:1918-1926, 2007

[28] Bishop NC, Gleeson M. Acute and chronic effects of exercise on markers of mucosal immunity. Front Biosci, 14:4444-4456, 2009

[29] Blanin AK, Robson PJ, Walsh NP, Clark AM, Glennon L, Gleeson M. The effect of exercising to exhaustion at different intensities on saliva immunoglobulin A, protein and electrolyte secretion. Int J Sports Med, 19:547-552, 1998

[30] Allgrove JE, Gomes E, Hough J, Gleeson M. Effects of exercise intensity on saliva antimicrobial proteins and markers of stress in active men. J Sports Sci, 26:653-661, 2008

[31] Sharp JCM. Viruses and the Athlete. Br J Sport Med, 23:47-48, 1989

[32] Eichner ER. Infectious mononucleosis-recognising the condition, 'reactivating' the patient. Physician Sports Med, 24:49-54, 1996

[33] Friman G, Wesslén L, Karjalainen J, Rolf C. Infectious and lymphocytic myocarditis: epidemiology and factors relevant to sports medicine. Scand J Med Sci Sports, 5:269-278, 1995

[34] Russell WR. Poliomyelitis, the paralytic stage and the effect of physical activity on the severity of paralysis. Br Med J, 1:465-471, 1949

[35] Gautmanitan BG, Ghason JL, Lerner AM. Augmentation of the virulence of murine coxsackie virus B3 myocardiopathy by exercise. J Exp Med, 131:1121-1125, 1970

[36] Ortega E. Neuroendocrine mediators in the modulation of phagocytosis by exercise: physiological implications. Exerc Immunol Rev, 9:70-93, 2003

[37] Shephard RJ. Adhesion molecules, catecholamines and leucocyte redistribution during and following exercise. Sports Med, 33:261-284, 2003

[38] Aoi W, Naito Y, Takanami Y, Kawai Y, Sakuma K, Ichikawa H, Yoshida N, Yoshikawa T. Oxidative stress and delayed onset muscle damage after exercise. Free Radic Biol Med, 37:480-487, 2004

[39] Soppi E, Varjo J, Eskola J, Laitinen LA. Effect of strenuous physical stress on circulating lymphocyte number and function before and after training. J Clin Lab Immunol, 8:43-46, 1982

[40] Gabriel H, Schwarz L, Born P, Kindermann W. Differential mobilization of leucocyte and lymphocyte subpopulations into the circulation during endurance exercise. Eur J Appl Physiol, 65:529-534, 1992

[41] Nieman DC, Henson DA, Sampson CS, Herring JL, Stulles J, Conley M, Stone MH, Buttersworth DE, Davis JM. The acute immune response to exhaustive resistance exercise. Int J Sports Med, 16:322-328, 1995

[42] Busse WW, Anderson CL, Hanson PG, Folts JD. The effect of exercise in the granulocyte response to isoproterenol in the trained athlete and unconditioned individual. J Allergy Clin Immunol, 65:358-364, 1980

[43] Hooper S, Mackinnon LT, Howard A, Gordon RD, Bachmann AW. Markers for monitoring overtraining and recovery in elite swimmers. Med Sci Sports Exerc, 27:106-112 1995

[44] Pizza FX, Mitchell JB Davis BH, Starling RD, Holtz RW, Bigelow N . Exercise-induced muscle damage: Effect on circulating leukocyte and lymphocyte subsets. Med Sci Sports Exerc, 27:363-370, 1995

[45] Shinkai S, Shore S, Shek PN, Shephard RJ. Acute exercise and immune function. Relationship between lymphocyte activity and changes in subset counts. Int J Sports Med, 13:452-461, 1992

[46] Eliakim A, Wolach B, Kodesh E, Gavrieli R, Radnay J, Ben-Tovim T, Yarom Y, Falk B. Cellular and humoral immune response to exercise among gymnasts and untrained girls. Int J Sports Med, 18:208-212, 1997

[47] Wolach B, Eliakim A, Gavrieli R, Kodesh E, Yarom Y, Schlesinger M, Falk B Aspects of leukocyte function and the complement system following aerobic exercise in young female gymnasts. Scand J Med Sci Sports, 8:91-97, 1998

[48] Wolach B, Falk B, Gavrieli R, Kodesh E, Eliakim A. Neutrophil function response to aerobic and anaerobic exercise in female judoka and untrained subjects. Br J Sports Med, 34:23-28, 2000

[49] Wolach B, Gavrieli R, Ben-Dror SG, Zigel L, Eliakim A, Falk B. Transient decrease of neutrophil chemotaxis following aerobic exercise. Med Sci Sports Exerc, 37:949-954, 2005

[50] Gavrieli R, Ashlagi-Amiri T, Eliakim A, Nemet D, Zigel L, Berger-Achituv S, Falk B, Wolach B. The effect of aerobic exercise on neutrophil functions. Med Sci Sports Exerc, 40:1623-1628, 2008

[51] Prossnitz ER, Gilbert TL, Chiang S, Campbell JJ, Qin S, Newman W, Sklar LA, Ye RD. Multiple activation steps of the N-formyl- peptide receptor. Biochemistry, 38:2240-2247, 1999

[52] Schraufstatter IU, Chung J, Burger M. IL-8 activates endothelial cell CXCR1 and CXCR2 through Rho and Rac signaling pathways. Am J Physiol Lung Cell Mol Physiol, 280:L1094-L1103, 2001

[53] Chodniewicz D, Zhelev DV. Novel pathways of F-actin polymerization in the human neutrophil. Blood, 102:2251-2258, 2003

[54] Weiner OD, Servant G, M. D. Welch MD, Mitchison TJ, Sedat JW, Bourne HR. Spatial control of actin polymerization during neutrophil chemotaxis. Nature Cell Biol, 1:75-81, 1999

[55] Howard TH, Meyer WH. Chemotactic peptide modulation of actin assembly and locomotion in neutrophils. J Cell Biol, 98:1265-1271, 1984.

[56] Hack V, Strobel G, Rau JP, Weicker H. The effect of maximal exercise on the activity of neutrophil granulocytes in highly trained athletes in a moderate training period. European journal of applied physiology and occupational physiology, 65:520-524, 1992

[57] Giraldo E, Garcia JJ, Hinchado MD, Ortega E. Exercise intensity-dependent changes in the inflammatory response in sedentary women: role of neuroendocrine parameters in the neutrophil phagocytic process and the pro-/anti-inflammatory cytokine balance. Neuroimmunomodulation, 16:237-244, 2009

[58] Walsh NP, Gleeson M, Pyne DB, Nieman DC, Dhabhar FS, Shephard RJ, Oliver SJ, Bermon S, Kajeniene A. Position statement. Part two: Maintaining immune health. Exercise Immunol Rev, 17: 64-103, 2011

[59] Nieman DC. Quercetin's bioactive effects in human athletes. Curr Topic Nutraceut Res, 8:33-44, 2010

[60] Jackson MJ. Redox regulation of adaptive responses in skeletal muscle to contractile activity. Free Radical Biology& Medicine, 47:1267-1275, 2009

[61] Gleeeson M. Dosing and efficacy of glutamine supplementation in human exercise and sport training. J Nutr, 138: 2045S-2049S, 2008

[62] Gomez-Cabrera MC, Domenech E, Romagnoli M, Arduini A, Borras C, Pallardo FV, Sastre J, Viña J. Oral administration of vitamin C decreases muscle mitochondrial biogenesis and hampers training-induced adaptations in endurance performance. American Journal of Clinical Nutrition, 87:142-149, 2008

[63] Finaud J, Scislowski V, Lac G, Durand D, Vidalin H, Robert A, Filaire E. Antioxidant status and oxidative stress in professional rugby players: evolution throughout a season. Int J Sports Med, 27:87-93, 2006

[64] Ferrer, MD, Tauler, P, Sureda, A, Tur, JA and Pons, A. Antioxidant regulatory mechanisms in neutrophils and lymphocytes after intense exercise. J Sports Sci 27: 49-58, 2009

[65] Baehner RL, Boxer LA. Role of membrane vitamin E and cytoplasmic glutathione in the regulation of phagocytic functions of neutrophils and monocytes. American Journal of Pediatric Hematology/Oncology, 1:71-16, 1979

[66] Powers, SK, Lennon SL. Analysis of cellular responses to free radicals: Focus on exercise and skeletal muscle. Proc Nutr Soc, 58:1025-1033, 1999

[67] Sachdev S, Davies KJ. Production, detection and adaptive responses to free radicals in exercise. Free Radic biol Med. 44:215-223, 2008

[68] Finaud J. Lac G, Filaire E. Oxidate stress: relationship with exercise and training Sports Med, 36:327-358, 2006

[69] Silva LA, Pinho CA, Silveira PC, Tuon T, De Souza CT, Dal-Pizzol F, Pinho RA. Vitamin E supplementation decreases muscular and oxidative damage but not inflammatory response induced by eccentric contraction. Journal of Physiological Sciences, 60:51-57, 2010

[70] Bloomer RJ, Goldfarb AH, McKenzie MJ. Oxidative stress response to aerobic exercise: comparison of antioxidant supplements. Medicine & Science in Sports & Exercise, 38:1098-1105, 2006

[71] Williams SL, Strobel NA, Lexis LA, Coombes JS. Antioxidant requirements of endurance athletes: implications for health. Nutrition Reviews, 64:93-108, 2006

[72] De la Fuente M, Ferrández MD, Burgos MS, Soler A, Prieto A, Miquel J. Immune function in aged women is improved by ingestion of vitamins C and E. Canadian Journal of Physiology and Pharmacology, 76:373-380, 1998

[73] De la Fuente M, Hernanz A, Guayerbas N, Victor VM, Arnalich F. Vitamin E ingestion improves several immune functions in elderly men and women. Free Radical Research, 42:272-280, 2008

[74] Gavrieli R, Berger-Achituv S, Ashlagi-Amiri T, Zigel L, Nemet D, Eliakim A, Falk B, and Wolach B. Vitamin E Prevents Neutrophil Impairment after a Single Bout of Intense Aerobic Exercise. Submitted for publication.

[75] Harris RE, Boxer LA, Baehner RL. Consequences of vitamin-E deficiency on the phagocytic and oxidative functions of the rat polymorphonuclear leukocyte. Blood, 55:338-343, 1980

[76] Politis I, Hidiroglou N, White JH, Gilmore JA, Williams SN, Scherf H, Frigg M. Effects of vitamin E on mammary and blood leukocyte function, with emphasis on chemotaxis, in periparturient dairy cows. American Journal of Veterinary Research, 57:468-471, 1996

[77] Cooper DM, Radom-Aizik S, Zaldivar F, Leu SY, Galassetti P. Effects of 30 min of aerobic exercise on gene expression and in human neutrophils. J Appl Physiol, 104:236-243, 2008

[78] Connolly PH, Caiozzo VJ, Zaldivar F, Nemet D, Larson J, Hung S, Heck JD, Hatfield GW, Cooper DM. Effects of exercise on gene expression in human peripheral blood mononuclear cells. J Appl Physiol, 97:1461-1469, 2004

[79] Ben-Eliyahu S, Page GG, Schleifer SJ. Stress, NK cells, and cancer: Still a promissory note. Brain Behav Immun, Review 21:881-887, 2007

[80] Mc Tiernan A. Mechanisms linking physical activity with cancer. Nat Rev Cancer, 8:205-211, 2008

[81] Friedenreitch CM, Gregory J, Kopciuk KA, Mackey JR, Courneya KS. Prospective cohort study of lifetime physical activity and breast cancer survival. Int J Cancer, 124: 1954-1962, 2009

[82] Davis JM, Kohut ML, Jackson DA, Colbert LH, Mayer EP, Ghaffar A. Exercise effects on lung tumor metastases and in vitro alveolar macrophage antitumor cytotoxicity. Am J Physiol, 274:R1454-1459, 1998

[83] Speck RM, Courneya KS, Masse LC, Duval S, Schmitz KH. An update of controlled physical activity trials in cancer survivors: a systematic review and meta-analysis. J Cancer Surviv, 4:87-100, 2010

[84] Hoffman-Goetz L, Husted J. Exercise and Cancer. Do the biology and epidemiology correspond? Exercise Immunology Rev, 1: 81-96, 1995

[85] World Cancer Research Fund. Food, Nutrition, Physical Activity and the prevention of Cancer: a Global Perspective. Washington DC, AICR, 2007

Part 2

Medical Issues in Sports Medicine

Comparison of Seminal Superoxide Dismutase (SOD) Activity Between Elite Athletes, Active and Non Active Men

Bakhtyar Tartibian[1], Behzad Hajizadeh Maleki[1], Asghar Abbasi[2],
Mehdi Eghbali[3], Siamak Asri-Rezaei[3] and Hinnak Northoff[4]
[1]Department of Cellular and Molecular Exercise Physiology,
Faculty of Physical Education and Sport Science, Urmia University, Urmia
[2]Institute of Sport Science, University of Tuebingen
[3]Department of Clinical Science, Faculty of Veterinary Medicine,
Urmia University, Urmia
[4]Institute of Clinical and Experimental Transfusion Medicine (IKET),
University of Tuebingen
[1,3]Iran
[2,4]Germany

1. Introduction

It is increasingly recognized that reactive oxygen species (ROS) originating from the spermatozoa as well as from the leukocytes are of significant pathophysiological importance in the etiology of male infertility (Iwasaki and Gagnon, 1992; Zini et al., 1993; Ochsendorf et al., 1994; Shekarriz et al., 1995; Smith et al., 1996; Agarwal et al., 2006; Tremellen, 2008). ROS, defined as including oxygen ions, free radicals and peroxides, may cause infertility by two principal mechanisms. First, ROS damage the sperm membrane which in turn reduces the sperm's motility and ability to fuse with the oocyte. Secondly, ROS directly damage sperm DNA, compromising the paternal genomic contribution to the embryo (Tremellen, 2008). Due to their high content of polyunsaturated fatty acids and their capacity to generate ROS, human spermatozoa are very sensitive to oxidative stress (Aitken and Clarkson, 1987; Aitken et al., 1989; Smith et al., 1996). To protect spermatozoa from oxidative damage, seminal plasma is endowed with numerous enzymatic antioxidants (AOs) such as superoxide dismutase (SOD), catalase and glutathione peroxidase (Fujii et al., 2003; Garrido et al., 2004; Murawski et al., 2007). It has recently been reported, that superoxide anion (O_2) may be involved in fatty-acid peroxidation (Niess and Simon, 2007). Superoxide dismutase (SOD) and catalase inactivate the superoxide anion (O_2) and peroxide (H_2O_2) radicals by converting them into water and oxygen. SOD as an important element of seminal plasma superoxide anion scavenging capacity plays an essential role in maintaining the balance between ROS generation and degradation. Decrease of its capacity can result in abnormal sperm motility determined as sperm hyperactivation, and hence infertility (De Lamirande and Gagnon, 1993). The addition of SOD to sperm in culture has been confirmed to protect them from oxidative attack (Kobayashi *et al.*, 1991). Although some investigators have shown no association between SOD activity and male fertility (Miesel *et al.*, 1997; Zini *et al.*, 2000; Hsieh *et al.*, 2002), others have reported a reduction in seminal plasma SOD activity in infertile males (Alkan *et al.*, 1997; Sanocka *et al.*, 1997; Siciliano *et al.*, 2001). Recently Murawski et al. (2007) reported a significantly lower semen SOD activity in infertile males, as compared with normospermic men. They showed a positive correlation between SOD activity in seminal plasma and semen quality parameters - sperm concentration and overall motility, which are regarded as most important for normal fertilizing ability of the spermatozoa (Murawski *et al.*, 2007).

Physical exercise has been shown to increase ROS and oxidative stress causing disruptions of homeostasis. Given that generation of oxidative stress is a natural part of physically active people may be susceptible to ROS-induced damage in sperm motility and male infertility, depending on the exercise mode, intensity, and duration as well as antioxidant capacity. Exercise training, on the other hand, has been shown to have modifying effects on oxidative stress, depending on training load, training specificity and the basal level of training. Growing evidence suggests that aerobic exercise training can result in an augmented SOD activity and a reduction in lipid peroxidation (Mena *et al.*, 1991; Ortenblad *et al.*, 1997; Ji, 1998; Suzuki and Ohno, 2000; Niess *et al.*, 2007). It is well documented that due to intensive training programs, trained and athletic people have developed total antioxidant capacity, and in particular high levels of SOD, in several tissues (Banfi *et al.*, 2006; Dekany *et al.*, 2006; Tayler *et al.*, 2006). However, our knowledge about antioxidant capacity in seminal plasma of athletic and trained men is less than meager, and it was up to now unclear if and under which conditions exercise training may influence seminal antioxidant capacity. Nonetheless, the amounts of enzymatic antioxidants in human semen have been well measured in normal and infertile men (Nissen and Kreysel, 1983; Jeuilin *et al.*, 1989; Kobayashi *et al.*, 1991; Alkan *et al.*, 1997; Miesel *et al.*, 1997; Sanocka *et al.*, 1997; Zini *et al.*, 1993).

Taken together, considering the probable positive correlation and beneficial impact of SOD activity on human semen quality parameters and male fertility on the one hand, and the fact that the SOD and antioxidant capacity of various tissues are highly different between individuals with different level of physical fitness on the other hand, we wanted to find an answer to the question if the SOD activity of seminal plasma is different in individuals with different levels of physical activity. Thus, the purpose of this study was to evaluate the SOD activity in elite athletes, recreationally active and non active men.

2. Materials and methods

2.1 Subjects

A total of 40 semen samples were obtained from investigated groups in this study (*Table1*). Of these, 15 samples were obtained from competitive elite athletes (e.g. including wrestlers, runners, football players, and swimmers) who were regularly training 4-5 days per week (Elite group). Thirteen samples were provided by non-obese and physically active males (active group) who participated in educational or recreational physical activities for 4-5 h per week. And 12 samples were obtained from healthy males who had a sedentary lifestyle without practicing in any sport for at least 6 months prior to study (control group). Physical activity of subjects was assessed by a questionnaire and subjects were matched based on training status and training quantity.

To be eligible to participate in the study, subjects were required to meet the following criteria: 1) unmarried men 18–28 year of age; 2) in good health, as determined by a normal physical examination and routine laboratory tests within the previous year; 3) no history of chronic disease, including reproductive disorders; 4) no history of use of medications that could alter the H-P-G axis, such as anabolic steroids; 5) regular eating patterns and no history of depressive illness; 6) normal physical and sexual development; 7) not working in professions where the activity might influence reproductive capacity; 8) no relevance previous surgery (eg, vasectomy reversal or varicocele removal) ; and 9) appropriate history of physical activity for the different groups described above (Lucía et al., 1996; Di Luigi et al., 2001). Informed consent was obtained from each subject. Before the initiation of the study protocol, each of them was introduced to the methods of this investigation. The Human Subject Internal Review Board committee of the Urmia University of IRAN approved the study (approval number 03/686).

Variable	Group	Elite	Active	Control	Sig*
Age (year)		23.1±1.3	23.4±0.9	22.0 ±2.0	0.053
Height (cm)		176.6±6.3	175.8±6.3	175.5±6.3	0.884
Weight (kg)		74.1±12.3	72.1±6.6	75.8±10.9	0.515
BMI (kg/m²)		20.9±2.5	22.1±1.4	24.3±2.6	*0.001
Fat (%)		8.5±3.7	11.2±3.1	15.5±5.1	*0.014

BMI = Body Mass Index.
*: P<0.05, significant difference between groups.

Table 1. Individual physical characteristics of subjects.

All subjects were given clear instructions on how to collect their semen at site. Each subject collected one semen sample by masturbation into a sterile container after at least 3-4 days of abstinence from ejaculations (Chia et al., 1998; Nikoobakht et al., 2005; Kao et al., 2008). The majorities of samples were provided on site or were delivered to the laboratory within 30 min of collection. Each subject also completed a questionnaire concerning the duration (days) of the abstinence before collecting each sample (Jeuilin et al., 1989).

2.2 Seminal SOD activity measurement

Semen analyses were performed according to WHO guidelines (Caballero et al., 1992; Nikoobakht et al., 2005). Semen evaluations were performed on each sample by the same experienced technician throughout the study, for the assessment of SOD activity. All of the semen samples were then cryopreserved using the Test Yolk Buffer with Glycerol as a freezing medium, according to the protocol described in WHO guidelines (4-th edition, 1999).

SOD activity was measured by colorimetric assay (Zini et al., 2000 and 2002). The commercially available colorimetric method was used (Randox Laboratories Ltd, UK). This method employs xanthine and xanthine oxidase to generate superoxide radicals which react with 2-(4-iodophenyl)-3-(4-nitrophenol) - 5-phenyltetrazoliumchloride (I.N.T) to form red formazan dye. The SOD activity is then measured by the degree of inhibition of this reaction. One unit of SOD inhibits reduction of INT by 50% under the conditions of the assay. After thawing, the seminal plasma was diluted 30-fold with 10 mM phosphate buffer, pH 7.0. The assay was performed at 37°C. Phosphate buffer was used as blank. Mixed substrate and xanthine oxidase were added into standards and sample tubes and vortexed well. With spectrophotometer adjusted at a wavelength of 505 nm, the initial absorbance (A1) was read. Final absorbance (A2) was read exactly after 3 minutes, and percentages of inhibition of standards and samples were calculated. The SOD activity was measured using calibration curve of percentage inhibition for each standard against Log10 of standards and SOD activity was expressed as IU/ml.

2.3 Statistical analysis

Data are expressed as means ± SD. Differences among groups were determined by analysis of variance (ANOVA) for continuous variables. If the F-ratio was significant, differences among groups were subsequently identified using a Bonferroni *post-hoc* analysis. The statistical software program SPSS for windows, version 17.0 was used for all data analyses. All statistical tests were performed at a significance level of 0.05.

3. Results

Semen parameters (mean ± SD) were compared between study groups and the results are shown in *Table 2*. No significant differences were observed between groups in semen parameters (P > 0.05) except of normal morphology (P ≤ 0.05). The result of Bonferroni test showed that the observed difference is more pronounced between elite group with active and control groups. However, there was no significant difference between active and control groups.

At this study the seminal SOD activity (IU/ml) of 3 groups was investigated. One-way ANOVA analysis showed that there is a significant difference between three groups (*Table 2*). The result of Bonferroni analysis revealed significantly higher SOD activity in seminal plasma of elite group than those of active and control groups (P ≤ 0.05). However, no statistically significant difference was observed between active and control groups (P > 0.05).

Variable	Group	Elite	Active	Control	Sig*
Total sperm count (*millions*)		89.6±55.1	86.2±52.9	87.4±54.5	0.089
Volume (*ml*)		3.3±1.4	2.7±1.2	2.3±1.3	0.071
Concentration (×10⁶/*ml*)		56.6±2.9	51.7±2.6	53.5±2.8	0.123
Motility (%)		72.8±15.6	66.2±16.1	69.7±14.9	0.068
Viability (%)		80.5±13.5	77.9±12.9	74.7±13.8	0.059
Normal morphology (%)		31.4±10.6	19.1±11.4	23.7±10.1	* 0.034
SOD (*IU/ml*)		34.3±9.4	17.9±5.6	24.2±6.6	* 0.001

*: P<0.05, significant difference between groups.

Table 2. Comparison of Semen parameters and SOD activity between elite athletes, recreationally active and sedentary men.

4. Discussion

The results emerging from this study show that semen from elite athletes have higher SOD content than those of the active and sedentary (control) men. However, no significant difference was observed between samples of active and control groups. Therefore, these results represent that elite athletic men have developed seminal antioxidant capacity at least in the case of SOD, suggesting that spermatozoa from elite athletes may be less susceptible to ROS-induced peroxidative damage, and hence, infertility. ROS have been shown to cause infertility by directly damaging the sperm DNA (Tremellen, 2008). Spermatozoa are susceptible to oxidative damage because their plasma membranes are rich in polyunsaturated fatty acids and have low concentrations of scavenging enzymes. SOD as one of the important elements of seminal plasma superoxide anion scavenging capacity plays an essential role in maintaining the balance between ROS generation and degradation through preventing increases in ROS concentration. Due to the protective effects against peroxidative damage and oxidative stress, seminal SOD has been shown to preserve sperm motility and viability. Sperm motility has been found to associate with men fertility (Jones *et al.*, 1979; Smith *et al.*, 1996; Murawski *et al.*, 2007; Agarwal *et al.*, 2008). The essential role of SOD as antioxidative defense enzyme is inferred from the observation that complete loss of motility of a sperm sample is directly proportional to the SOD activity of that sample (Storey, 1997). In particular, low SOD activity has been shown to be responsible for male infertility (Alkan *et al.*, 1997). Several investigators have reported reductions in SOD activity in semen of infertile men (Alkan *et al.*, 1997; Sanocka *et al.*, 1997; Siciliano *et al.*, 2001), although some have not (Zini *et al.*, 1993; Miesel *et al.*, 1997; Hsieh *et al.*, 2002). Recently Murawski et al. (2007) reported a significantly lower semen SOD activity in infertile men, as compared with normospermic men. They showed a positive correlation between SOD activity in seminal plasma and semen quality parameters - sperm concentration and overall motility, which are regarded as the most important for normal fertilizing ability of the spermatozoa (Murawski *et al.*, 2007).

Although the protective effect of seminal plasma has been well recognized, no study has investigated its antioxidative properties in individuals with different fitness level, in particular in athletic men. To the best of our knowledge, the present study provides the first evidence that elite athletes have an augmented SOD capacity than recreationally active and sedentary control men. Although there is no definitive explanation for this discrepancy, but the notion that high maximal oxygen uptake (VO_{2max}), which is a consequence of systemic endurance training (Tanaka and Swensen, 1998), are correlated to elevated antioxidant enzyme activity in other tissues (Jenkins *et al.*, 1984), can explain some of the disparities in our study. These observations suggest that the fitness level of subject as well as the type and amount of exercise training could be taken into consideration when comparing antioxidant capacity of active people. As the active group in our study were exercising just 4-5h per week, it seems possible that this amount of exercise is not enough to enhance antioxidant capacity. Dekany et al. (2006) have also referred to fitness level of athletes and type of exercise as important factors determining the blood level of antioxidant enzymes (Dekany *et al.*, 2006). In the review by Clarkson (1995) it has been documented that the ``weekend athlete`` may not have the augmented antioxidant defense system produced through continued training (Clarkson, 1995). This may make them more susceptible to oxidative stress.

The fact that rigorous exercise training programs may be required to promote antioxidant enzyme activity in skeletal muscle (Powers and Leeuwenburgh, 1999), can support our results. Intensive endurance training has been postulated as a potential muscle`s antioxidant defense system up-regulator (Fatouros *et al.*, 2004). Powers et al. (1994) experimentally analyzed the relationship between the magnitude of the training stimulus (i.e., exercise intensity and daily duration) and the activity of SOD in locomotor skeletal muscles. Nine groups of rats ran at three different daily durations (i.e., 30, 60, 90 min.d) and three different exercise intensities (i.e., 55, 65, and 75% of VO_{2max}) (**Powers** *et al.*, 1994). Furthermore, previous studies have reported that high-intensity running training can elevate antioxidant enzyme activities in erythrocytes and decrease neutrophil superoxide anion production both at rest and in response to exhaustive acute exercise (Miyazaki et al., 2001). These data clearly show that high intensity long-term exercise training is superior to recreationally exercise in the up-regulation of seminal plasma SOD activity, representing adaptation to regular training. In fact, the training-stressed cells provide high antioxidant enzyme content. It has been generally believed that training induction of antioxidant enzymes is a cellular adaptation to oxidative stress caused by free radical generation during heavy exercises (Jenkins, 1988; Ji, 1998).

Prior to this work, numerous studies have been published focusing on the adaptation of different tissue's antioxidant capacity to exercise training (Mena et al., 1991; Ortenblad et al., 1997; Ji, 1998; Suzuki et al., 2000; Banfi et al., 2006; Dekany et al., 2006; Tayler et al., 2006; Garcia-Lopez et al., 2007; Niess et al., 2007). Recently Garcia Lopez et al. (2007) showed an increase in MnSOD mRNA levels of peripheral mononuclear cell (PBMC) in response to endurance training in middle-aged men (Garcia-Lopez et al., 2007). Tauler et al. (2006) reported an increase in erythrocyte superoxide dismutase activity after the training/competition period for amateur trained male athletes (Tayler et al., 2006). Banfi et al. (2006) showed a significantly higher plasma Glutathione reductase (GR) activity in trained elite soccer players, as compared with sedentary controls (Banfi et al., 2006). Investigating antioxidant status of interval-trained athletes, Dekany et al. (2006) reported high level of blood enzymatic antioxidants in highly trained athletes (Dekany et al., 2006). Ravi et al. (2004) showed a significantly increase in myocardium superoxide dismutase after 4 weeks low-intensity swim training in rats (Ravi et al., 2004). Also, Yamamoto et al. (2002) reported higher superoxide dismutase activity and antioxidant capacity for physically active rats in compared to sedentary rats (Yamamoto et al., 2002). However, both in treadmill-trained rats (Leeuwenburgh et al., 1994) and running trained humans (Tiidus et al., 1996) endurance training did not affect antioxidant defense.

Some limitations of the present study should be taken into consideration. First, we measured the SOD activity just in seminal plasma and did not measure in spermatozoa. Secondly, five subjects (active group n=2, and control group n=3) could not provide the semen sample in time and were excluded from the study. This might influence the compared results. Thirdly, this study comprised a relatively small sample thus limiting statistical power to detect differential effects. However, this is, to our knowledge, the first study analyzed the seminal antioxidant activity in individuals with different level of physical fitness.

In conclusion, the results of present study demonstrate that in compared to recreationally active and sedentary men, the elite athletes have developed SOD capacity. The mechanisms responsible for this increase are unknown and remain an active area of research. However, this raises the question that does the training-induced increase in seminal plasma SOD capacity provide increased protection against ROS-induced sperm dysfunction and infertility in high level athletes? If it does, we are able to provide novel insights into athletic health and male fertility. Further studies are warranted to deal the antioxidant capacity of seminal plasma and spermatozoa of individuals with different level of physical fitness as well as the effect of various exercise programs on seminal antioxidant capacity.

5. Acknowledgment

We would like to thank the subjects for their participation and effort. This research did not receive any specific grant from any funding agency in the public, commercial or not-for-profit sector.

6. References

Agarwal, A. Prabakaran, S. & Allamaneni, S. (2006). What an andrologist/urologist should know about free radicals and why? *Journal of Urology*, 67 (1): 2-8, ISSN 00904295.

Agarwal, A. Kartikeya, M. & Sharma, R. (2008). Clinical relevance of oxidative stress in male factor infertility: an update. *American Journal of Reproductive Immunology*, 59 (1): 2-11, ISSN 1677-5538.

Aitken, RJ. & Clarkson, JS. (1987). Cellular basis of defective sperm function and its association with the genesis of reactive oxygen species by human spermatozoa. *Journal of Reproduction and Fertility*, 81 (2): 459-469, ISSN 0022-4251.

Aitken, RJ. Irvine, MD. & Wu, FC. (1989). Prospective analysis of sperm-oocyte fusion and reactive oxygen species generation as criteria for the diagnosis of infertility. *American Journal of Obstetrics and Gynecology*, 164 (2): 542-551, ISSN 0002-9378.

Alkan, I. Simsek, F. Haklar, G. Kervancioglu, E. Ozveri, H. Yalcin, S. & Akdas, A. (1997). Reactive oxygen species production by the spermatozoa of patients with idiopathic infertility: relationship to seminal plasma antioxidants. *Journal of Urology*, 157 (1): 140-143, ISSN 00904295.

Banfi, G. Malavazos, A. Iorio, E. Dolci, A. Doneda, L. Verna, R. & Corsi, MM. (2006). Plasma oxidative stress biomarkers, nitric oxide and heat shock protein 70 in trained elite soccer players. *European Journal of Applied Physiology*, 96(5): 483-486, ISSN 1439-6319.

Caballero, MJ. Mena, P. & Maynar, M. (1992). Changes in sex hormone binding globulin, high density lipoprotein cholesterol and plasma lipids in male cyclists during training and competition. *European Journal of Applied Physiology and Occupational Physiology*, 64 (1): 9-13, ISSN 1432-1025.

Chia, SE. Tay, SK. & Lim, ST. (1998). What constitutes a normal seminal analysis? Semen parameters of 243 fertile men. *Human Reproduction*, 13 (12): 3394-3398, ISSN 0268-1161.

Clarkson, PM. (1995). Antioxidants and physical performance. *Critical Review in Food Science and Nutrition*, 35(1-2): 131-141, ISSN 1040-8398.

Dekany, M. Nemeskeri, V. Györe, I. Harbula, I. Malomski, J. & Pucsok, J. (2006). Antioxidant status of interval-trained athletes in various sports. *International Journal of Sports Medicine*, 27(2): 112-116, ISSN 0172-4622.

De Lamirande, E. & Gagnon, C. (1993). Human sperm hyperactivation in whole semen and its association with low superoxide scavenging capacity in seminal plasma. *Fertility and Sterility*, 59 (6): 1291-1295, ISSN 1556-5653.

Di Luigi, L. Gentile, V. Pigozzi, F. Parisi, A. Giannetti, D. & Romanelli, F. (2001). Physical activity as a possible aggravating factor for athletes with caricocele: impact on the semen profile. *Human Reproduction*, 16 (6): 1180–1184, ISSN 0268-1161.

Fatouros, IG. Jamurtas, AZ. Villiotou, V. Pouliopoulou, S. Fotinakis, P. Taxildaris, K. & Deliconstantinos, G. (2004). Oxidative stress responses in older men during endurance training and detraining. *Medicine and Science in Sports and Exercise*, 36 (12): 2065–2072, ISSN 1530-0315.

Fujii, J. Iuchi, Y. Matsuki, S. & Ishii, T. (2003). Cooperative function of antioxidant and redox systems against oxidative stress in male reproductive tissues. *Asian Journal of Andrology*, 5 (3): 231–242, ISSN 1008-682X.

Garcia-Lopez, D. Häkkinen, K. Cuevas, MJ. Lima, E. Kauhanen, A. Mattila, M. Sillanpää, E. Ahtiainen, JP. Karavirta, L. Almar, M. & González-Gallego, J. (2007). Effects of strength and endurance training on antioxidant enzyme gene expression and activity in middle-aged men. *Scandinavian Journal of Medicine and Science in Sports*, 17 (5): 595-604, ISSN 0905-7188.

Garrido N, Meseguer M, Simon C, Pellicer A & Remohi J. (2004). Pro-oxidative and anti-oxidative imbalance in human semen and its relation with male fertility. *Asian Journal of Andrology*, 6 (1): 59–65, ISSN 1008-682X.

Hsieh, YY. Sun, YL. Chang, CC. Lee, YS. Tsai, HD. & Lin, CS. (2002). Superoxide dismutase activities of spermatozoa and seminal plasma are not correlated with male infertility. *Journal of Clinical and Laboratory Analysis*, 16 (3): 127–131, ISSN 1098-2825.

Iwasaki, A. & Gagnon, C. (1992). Formation of reactive oxygen species in spermatozoa of infertile patients. *Fertility and Sterility*, 57 (2): 409–416, ISSN 1556-5653.

Jenkins, RR. Friedland, R. & Howald, H. (1984). The relationship of oxygen consumption to superoxide dismutase and catalase activity in human skeletal muscle. *International Journal of Sports Medicine*, 5 (1): 11–14, ISSN 0172-4622.

Jenkins, R. (1988). Free radical chemistry: relationship to exercise. *Sports Medicine*, 5 (3): 156-170, ISSN 0112-1642.

Jeuilin, C. Soufir, JC. & Weber, P. (1989). Catalase activity in human spermatozoa and seminal plasma. *Gamete Research*, 24 (2): 185-191, ISSN 0148-7280.

Ji, LL. (1998). Antioxidant enzyme response to exercise and training in the skeletal muscle. In: Oxidative Stress in skeletal muscle, ed. A.Z. Reznik. L. Packer, C.K. Sen, J.O. Holloszy & M.J.Jackson, 103-125. Basel: Bikhaeuser Verlag.

Jones, R. Mann, T. & Shenns, R. (1979). Peroxidative breakdown of phosphohpids in human spermatozoa, spermicidal properties of fatty acid peroxides, and protective action of seminal plasma. *Fertility and Sterility*, 31 (5): 531-537, ISSN 1556-5653.

Kao, SH. Chao, HT. Chen, HW. Hwang, TI. Liao, TL. & Wei, YH. (2008). Increase of oxidative stress in human sperm with lower motility. *Fertility and Sterility*, 89(5): 1183-1190, ISSN 1556-5653.

Kobayashi, T. Miyazaki, T. Natori, M. & Nozawa, S. (1991). Protective role of superoxide dismutase in human sperm motility: superoxide dismutase activity and lipid peroxide in human seminal plasma and spermatozoa. *Human Reproduction*, 6 (7): 987–991, ISSN 0268-1161.

Leeuwenburgh, C. Fiebig, R. Chandwaney, R. & Ji, LL. (1994). Aging and exercise training in skeletal muscle: responses of glutathione and antioxidant enzyme systems. *American Journal of Physiology*, 267 (2): 439–445, ISSN 0363-6143.

Lucía, A. José, L. Chicharro, A. Pérez, M. Serratosa, L. Bandrés, F. & Legido, JC. (1996). Reproductive function in male endurance athletes: sperm analysis and hormonal profile. *Journal of Applied Physiology*, 81 (6): 2627-2636, ISSN 8750-7587.

Mena, P. Maynar, M. Gutierrez, JM. Maynar, J. Timon, J. & Campillo, JE. (1991). Erythrocyte free radical scavenger enzymes in bicycle professional racers, adaptation to training. *International Journal of Sports Medicine*, 12 (6):563-566, ISSN 0172-4622.

Miesel, R. Jedrzejczak, P. Sanocka, D. & Kurpisz, MK. (1997). Severe antioxidase deficiency in human semen samples with pathological spermiogram parameters. *Andrologia*, 29 (2): 77–83, ISSN 0303-4569.

Miyazaki, H. Oh-ishi, S. Ookawara, T. Kizaki, T. Toshinai, K. Ha, S. Haga, S. Ji, LL. & Ohno, H. (2001). Strenuous endurance training in humans reduces oxidative stress following exhausting exercise. *Journal of Applied Physiology*, 84 (1-2): 1-6, ISSN 8750-7587.

Murawski, M. Saczko, J. Marcinkowska, A. Chwikowska, A. Grybooe, M. & Banaoe, T. (2007). Evaluation of superoxide dismutase activity and its impact on semen quality parameters of infertile men. *folia histochemica et cytobiologica*, 45 (1): 123-126, ISSN 02398508.

Niess, AM. & Simon, P. (2007). Response and adaptation of skeletal muscle to exercise: the role of reactive oxygen species. *Frontiers in Bioscience*, 1 (12): 4826-4838, ISSN 1093-9946,

Nikoobakht, M. Aloosh, M. & Hasani, M. (2005). Seminal Plasma Magnesium and Premature Ejaculation: a Case-Control Study. *Journal of Urology*, 2 (2): 102-105, ISSN 00904295.

Nissen, HP. & Kreysel, HWA. (1983). Superoxide dismutase in human semen. *Klin Wochenschr*, 61 (1): 63-65, ISSN 0023-2173.

Ochsendorf, FR. Thiele, J. Fuchs, J. Schuttau, H. Freisleben, HJ. Buslau, M. & Milbradt, R. (1994). Chemiluminescence in semen of infertile men. *Andrologia*, 26 (5): 289-293, ISSN 0303-4569.

Ortenblad, N. Madsen, K. & Djurhuus, MS. (1997). Antioxidant status and lipid peroxidation after short term maximal exercise in trained and untrained humans. *American Journal of physiology*, 272 (2): 1258-1263, ISSN 0363-6143.

Powers, SK. Criswell, D. Lawler, J. Ji, LL. Martin, D. Herb, RA. & Dudley, G. (1994). Influence of exercise and fiber type on antioxidant enzyme activity in rat skeletal muscle. *American Journal of physiology*. 266 (2): 375-380, ISSN 0363-6143.

Powers, SK. & Leeuwenburgh, C. (1999). Exercise training-induced alterations in skeletal muscle antioxidant capacity: a brief review. *Medicine and Science in Sport and Exercise*, 31 (7): 987-997, ISSN 1530-0315.

Ravi, KT. Subramanyam, MV. & Asha, DS. (2004). Swim exercise training and adaptation in the antioxidant defense system of myocardium of old rats: relationship to swim intensity and duration. *Comparative Biochemistry and Physiology Part B: Biochemistry and Molecular Biology*, 137 (2): 187-196, ISSN 1095-6433.

Sanocka, D. Miesel, R. Jedrzejczak, P. Chelmonska-Soyta, AC. & Kurpisz, M. (1997). Effect of reactive oxygen species and the activity of antioxidant systems on human semen; association with male infertility. *International Journal of Andrology*, 20 (5): 255-264, ISSN 1365-2605.

Shekarriz, M. Thomas, AJ. & Agarwal, A. (1995). Incidence and level of seminal reactive oxygen species in normal men. *Journal of Urology* 45 (1): 103-107, ISSN 00904295.

Siciliano, L. Tarantino, P. Longobardi, F. Rago, V. De Stefano, C. & Carpino, A. (2001). Impaired seminal antioxidant capacity in human semen with hyperviscosity or oligoasthenozoospermia. *Journal of Andrology*, 22 (5): 798-803, ISSN 0196-3635.

Smith, R. Vantman, J. Ponce, J. Escobar, A. & Lissi, E. (1996). Total antioxidant capacity of human seminal plasma. *Human Reproduction*, 11 (8): 1655-1660, ISSN 0268-1161.

Storey, BT. (1997). Biochemistry of the induction and prevention of lipoperoxidative damage in human spermatozoa. *Molecular Human Reproduction*, 3 (3): 203-213, ISSN 1360-9947.

Suzuki K, Ohno H, Oh-ishi S, Kizaki T, Ookawara T, Fujii J, Radák Z, and Taniguchi N. Superoxide dismutases in exercise and disease. In: *Handbook of Oxidants and Antioxidants in Exercise*, edited by Sen CK, Packer L, and Hänninen O. Amsterdam: Elsevier, 2000, p. 243–295.

Tanaka, H. & Swensen, T. (1998). Impact of resistance training on endurance performance. A new form of cross-training. *Sports Medicine*, 25 (3): 191-200, ISSN 0112-1642.

Tayler, P. Aquilo, A. Gimeno, I. Fuentespina, E. Tur, JA. & Pons, A. (2006). Response of blood cell antioxidant enzyme defence to antioxidant diet supplementation and to intense exercise. *European Journal of Nutrition*, 45 (4): 187-195, ISSN 1436-6215.

Tiidus, PM. Pushkarenko, J. & Houston, ME. (1996). Lack of antioxidant adaptation to short-term aerobic training in human muscle. *American Journal of Physiology*. 271 (4): 832–836, ISSN 0363-6143.

Tremellen, K. (2008). Oxidative stress and male infertility-a clinical perspective. *Human Reproduction Update,* 14 (3): 243–258, ISSN 1355-4786.

Yamamoto, T. Ohkuwa, T. Itoh, H. Sato, Y. & Naoi, M. (2002). Effect of gender differences and voluntary exercise on antioxidant capacity in rats. *Comparative Biochemistry and Physiology Part C: Toxicology and Pharmacology*, 132 (4): 437-444, ISSN 1532-0456.

Zini, A. de Lamirande, E. & Gagnon, C. (1993). Reactive oxygen species in semen of infertile patients: levels of superoxide dismutase- and catalase-like activities in seminal plasma and spermatozoa. *International Journal of Andrology*, 16 (3): 183–188, ISSN 1365-2605.

Zini, A. Garrels, K. & Phang, D. (2000). Antioxidant activity in the semen of fertile and infertile men. *Urology*, 55 (6): 922-926, ISSN 00904295.

11

Effects of Exercise on the Airways

Maria R. Bonsignore[1,4], Nicola Scichilone[1], Laura Chimenti[1],
Roberta Santagata[1], Daniele Zangla[2] and Giuseppe Morici[3,4]

[1]*Biomedical Department of Internal and
Specialistic Medicine (DiBiMIS), Section of Pneumology,
[2]Department of Motor Sciences (DISMOT),
[3]Department of Experiental Biomedicine and
Clinical Neurosciences (BIONEC), University of Palermo,
[4]Institute of Biomedicine and Molecular Immunology (IBIM),
National Research Council, Palermo
Italy*

1. Introduction

In the last ten years, the effects of exercise on bronchial epithelial cells and inflammatory cells in the airways have been studied in detail, and such new information has been combined with previous knowledge on bronchial reactivity and asthma evoked by exercise in asthmatic patients and athletes. The resulting picture is very complex, and the potential clinical consequences are often contradictory, suggesting the opportunity to define different phenotypes of exercise-associated airway changes (Lee & Anderson, 1985; Haahtela et al., 2008; Moreira et al., 2011a).

Studies in asthmatic athletes in the 90' had began to explore the possibility that airway inflammation might be involved in exercise-associated respiratory symptoms. However, studies in non-asthmatic athletes also found increased number of inflammatory cells not only at rest, but also after strenuous endurance exercise (Bonsignore et al., 2001). It was therefore hypothesized that endurance exercise may physiologically cause influx of inflammatory cells into the airways, associated with low or absent inflammatory activation (Bonsignore et al., 2003a). Subsequent studies in athletes and animal models have extended these finding, but the mechanisms of inflammatory cell recruitment into the airways and the tight control of inflammatory activation physiologically associated with exercise remain poorly understood.

Exercise is a known cause of bronchoconstriction in asthmatic patients (Cabral et al., 1999) and athletes (Parsons & Mastronarde, 2005). A large number of asthmatic elite athletes participate to international top-level competitions, and guidelines regarding management of asthmatic athletes (Fitch et al., 2008) and rules on the use of anti-asthmatic drugs have been issued (World Anti-Doping Agency, WADA, Oct. 18 2010 report). However, exercise is a powerful physiologic stimulus for bronchodilatation, and some reports underlined that exercise training may actually downmodulate bronchial reactivity in normal subjects (Scichilone et al., 2005, 2010), asthmatic children (Bonsignore et al., 2008) and animal models of asthma (Hewitt et al., 2010).

This chapter will summarize the changes induced by acute exercise and training in bronchial reactivity and airway cells in both humans and animal models. It will also discuss the changing paradigm regarding the impact of physical activity in patients with bronchial asthma, and the new perspectives of exercise-based rehabilitation in patients with respiratory diseases such as chronic obstructive pulmonary disease (COPD).

2. Exercise-induced bronchoconstriction

In patients with bronchial asthma, occurrence of bronchoconstriction and symptoms after exercise is common and has been known for a long time (Lee & Anderson, 1985; Cabral et al., 1999). Exercise-induced bronchoconstriction (EIB) is characterized by respiratory symptoms, such as wheezing and chest tightness, secondary to an acute, transient airway narrowing that typically occurs in the first 15-20 min after cessation of exercise. In some instances, a late-phase response also occurs 3 to 13 h after completing exercise (Freed, 1995; Speelberg et al., 1989). In asthmatic patients, exercise-induced symptoms are considered as clinically important indicators of insufficient asthma control, and suggest the opportunity to increase or change the medication regimen.

In the laboratory, EIB is defined as a decrease in forced expiratory volume of 1s (FEV_1) $\geq$ 10% from the baseline value after appropriate exercise provocation (Kyle et al., 1992). Exercise is the most common trigger of bronchospasm in those who are known to be asthmatic, and 50% to 90% of asthmatic individuals have airways that are hyperreactive to exercise (Rundell et al., 2002).

EIB also occurs in up to 10% of subjects who are not known to be atopic or asthmatic (Gotshall et al., 2002). Prevalence of EIB or exercise-induced symptoms in elite athletes is high (Parsons & Mastronarde, 2005; Turcotte et al., 2003), and asthma in athletes may develop according to different phenotypes, likely influenced by environmental exposures during exercise (Haahtela et al., 2008). Prevalence of asthma is high in athletes of winter sports and endurance sports such as swimming or running (Helenius & Haahtela, 2000; Karjalainen et al., 2000; Lumme et al., 2003; Langdeau et al., 2004; Durand et al., 2005; Vergès et al., 2005, Lund et al., 2009), even in subjects who do not report symptoms during childhood, atopy or a family history of asthma (Langdeau et al., 2004). On the other hand, exercise-induced symptoms are poor predictors of EIB (Parsons, 2009) since they are variably associated with objectively documented bronchial hyperreactivity to exercise (Sue-Chu et al., 1996; Rundell et al., 2001; Langdeau et al., 2000, 2004; Bougault et al., 2010). Finally, a gender effect has been recently underlined, with female athletes reporting more exercise-associated symptoms and showing a higher prevalence of bronchial hyperreactivity at rest compared to male athletes (Langdeau et al., 2009). Unfortunately, data on prevalence of EIB according to gender are not available, and more studies are necessary to ascertain whether exercise-associated bronchoconstriction is more common in women than in men, and the mechanism(s) responsible for such an effect.

2.1 Pathophysiology of EIB: Main theories

While bronchial asthma is known to be associated with a complex inflammatory picture at the airway level usually triggered by exposure to allergens or exercise, EIB in otherwise healthy subjects is difficult to explain. To this aim, two theories have been proposed, based on the possibility of post-exercise engorgement of bronchial vessels with decreased bronchial luminal area (the vasomotor hypothesis) and the hypothesis of insufficient conditioning of inspired air (the hyperosmolar theory).

The vasomotor hypothesis proposed that cooling of the airways followed by rapid re-warming may cause vasocostriction followed by reactive hyperemia of the bronchial microcirculation, together with edema of the airway wall (McFadden, 1990). Nevertheless, neither airway cooling or re-warming appear necessary for EIB to occur (Lee & Anderson, 1985; Anderson & Daviskas, 1992; Anderson & Daviskas, 2000; Anderson & Kippelen, 2008). The main theory on EIB pathophysiology is that exercise hyperventilation causes drying of the airways, thus increasing osmolarity of the airway surface lining fluid (Anderson et al., 1989; Boulet & Turcotte, 1991; Anderson & Daviskas, 1992, 2000; Freed, 1995; Anderson & Kippelen, 2008). As water evaporates, the airway surface liquid becomes hyperosmolar and provides an osmotic stimulus for water to move from any cell nearby, resulting in cell volume loss. Therefore, the change in regulatory volume after cell shrinkage is believed to be the key event, which results in release of inflammatory mediators that cause airway smooth muscle to contract and the airways to narrow (Anderson & Daviskas, 2000). It has been calculated that severe hyperosmolarity can occur in the airways during intense exercise (Anderson & Daviskas, 1992), and clinical tests based on hyperosmolar stimulation, such as eucapnic voluntary hyperventilation (EVH) (Anderson et al., 2001) or mannitol inhalation (Holzer et al., 2003; Anderson et al., 2009), are widely used, instead of exercise provocation tests, to assess the predisposition to develop EIB in the laboratory.

Both hyperosmolarity and vasomotor changes might be involved in the pathogenesis of EIB in asthmatic patients (Kanazawa et al., 2002). Bronchial epithelial cells *in vitro* release IL-8 upon stimulation with either hyperosmolar solutions or cooling-rewarming, indicating that the proposed mechanisms are capable of activating the bronchial epithelium (Hashimoto et al., 1999). In addition, corticosteroids have been shown to inhibit the activation of bronchial epithelial cells caused by hyperosmolar exposure (Hashimoto et al., 2000).

2.2 EIB in athletes of different sports

In athletes involved in winter sports, EIB is especially frequent (Durand et al, 1995; Provost-Craig et al., 1996, Lumme et al., 2003) and a specific clinical picture has been described in cross-country skiers ("ski asthma"). Similar to other athletes, elite cross-country skiers show a high prevalence of exercise-induced respiratory symptoms, which however resulted poorly correlated with the degree of bronchial hyperresponsiveness (Durand et al., 2005; Stenfors, 2010). Ski asthma shows some peculiar features, such as evidence of airway remodelling and inflammation (Sue-Chu et al., 1999; Karjalainen et al, 2000), lymphoid aggregates in endobronchial biopsies (Sue-Chu et al., 1998), and lack of clinically significant response to corticosteroids (Sue-Chu et al., 2000).

Summer sports can also be associated with asthma and EIB, possibly because of increased allergen exposure during outdoor activities (Helenius & Haahtela, 2000). Asthma and EIB show the highest frequency among adult elite swimmers, possibly due to the prolonged exposure to the irritant effects of chlorine in indoor swimming pools (Helenius et al, 1998a; Langdeau et al, 2000). A role of swimming on bronchial reactivity and airway inflammation is confirmed by reversibility of such changes upon cessation of intense training in adult athletes (Helenius et al., 2002; Bougault et al., 2011). In young swimmers, the relevance of exposure to chlorine-derived products in causing pathological airway changes has been recently questioned (Pedersen et al., 2008; Font-Ribera et al., 2011; Piacentini et al., 2011). Nevertheless, the increasing popularity of swimming suggests the opportunity to further assess the potential detrimental effect of exposure to chlorine associated with swimming, especially at young age (Bernard et al., 2008, 2009, 2011; Voisin et al., 2010).

2.3 Do acute exercise and training decrease bronchial reactivity?

Exercise is a very powerful bronchodilator stimulus, in both normal subjects and asthmatic patients. Even symptomatic patients with insufficiently controlled mild or moderate asthma showed bronchodilatation during acute incremental exercise, with preserved maximal ventilation and oxygen consumption (Crimi et al., 2002). The effects of acute incremental exercise were about 60% of the maximal bronchodilatation obtained after inhalation of albuterol (Milanese et al., 2009). The response to bronchoconstrictor agents in asthmatic patients was also lower during submaximal exercise compared to resting conditions (Stirling et al., 1983; Inman et al., 1990). The effects of constant-load submaximal exercise are somewhat controversial, since some studies reported persistent bronchodilatation in asthmatics (Mansfield et al., 1979; Inman et al, 1990), while others found that initial bronchodilation was followed by progressive bronchoconstriction during exercise in adult asthmatic patients (Milanese et al., 2009). Finally, eucapnic voluntary hyperventilation, mimicking the ventilation profile observed during exercise in asthmatic patients, was associated with bronchodilatation (Stirling et al., 1983; Gelb et al., 1985), while sympathoadrenal activation did not appear to play a major role (Gilbert et al., 1988; Hulks et al, 1991). Therefore, during acute exercise, the behaviour of airways appears quite similar in asthmatic patients and normal subjects.

Recent data indicate that intensive physical training may profoundly affect the airways and could decrease airways responsiveness (Scichilone et al., 2005). The intricate mechanisms underlying the pathophysiology of increased airway responses to inhaled broncoconstrictors, and the impact of physical activity on the occurrence and/or worsening of bronchial hyperreactivity, imply that research should first focus on interventions in healthy, non-asthmatic subjects. Therefore, we tested whether bronchial reactivity at rest differed between trained non-asthmatic amateur athletes and sedentary non-asthmatic controls, and found that the airway response to a spasmogen was lower in amateur runners than in sedentary individuals (Scichilone et al., 2005). Moreover, the "airway hyporesponsiveness" state of the athletes became more pronounced immediately after a competitive marathon.

This phenomenon can be explained by airway smooth muscle alterations induced by habitual heavy exercise. We speculated that the increased frequency of airway stretch that occurs with exercise hyperpnea could change the plasticity of airway smooth muscle cytoskeleton (Gunst & Tang, 2000; Gunst & Wu, 2001) or the myosin-actin interactions (Fredberg et al., 1996; Fredberg et al., 1997), enabling the smooth muscle fibers to become more resistant to spasmogens. Reorganization of the contractile apparatus of the airway smooth muscle may take place with habitual endurance exercise, thus enabling the smooth muscle fibers to adapt to changes in cell shape. Although we favour the mechanical explanation, other mechanisms, such as changes in the neural and/or biochemical control of the airways induced by physical training, may also contribute (Moreira et al., 2011a).

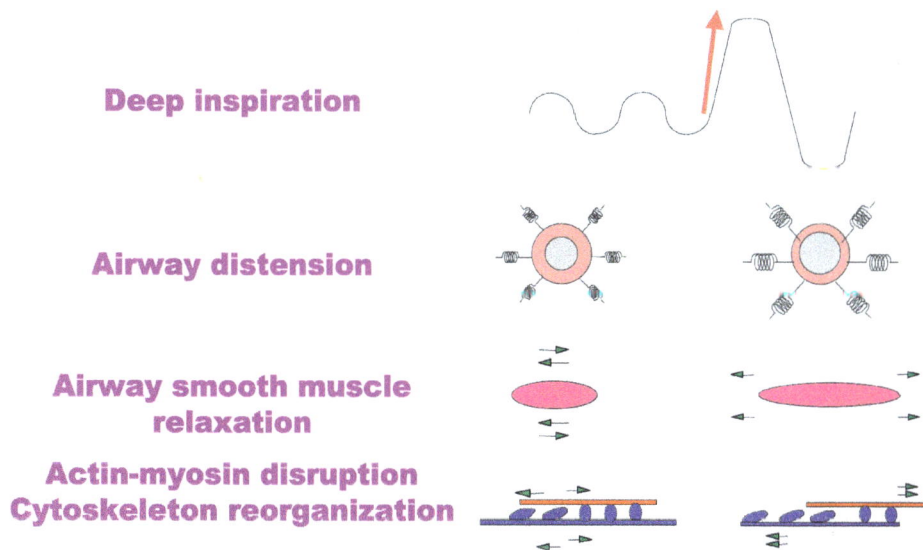

Deep inspiration

Airway distension

Airway smooth muscle relaxation

Actin-myosin disruption Cytoskeleton reorganization

Fig. 1. Cascade of events that likely contribute to reduce airway smooth muscle contractility during lung inflation

In this scenario, development of asthma in atopic individuals could be in part secondary to lack of exercise and a sedentary lifestyle. In the European Community Respiratory Health Survey (ECRHS) II study, both frequency and duration of physical activity, as assessed by questionnaires, were inversely related to bronchial reactivity in a large population cohort independent of other variables (Shaaban et al., 2007). In a cohort of 411 Danish children born to mothers with asthma and closely monitored for occurrence of symptoms suggestive of asthma, the amount of habitual physical activity correlated inversely with occurrence of bronchial reactivity (Brasholt et al., 2010). These epidemiological data suggest that increased prevalence of asthma could be a consequence of changes in lifestyle related to physical activity and dietary habits, as confirmed by the increased prevalence of obesity worldwide, also at young age. In addition, a large longitudinal study recently found a decreased risk of asthma exacerbations associated with regular physical activity in older women (Garcia-Aymerich et al., 2009), suggesting that exercise may positively affect asthma control.

2.3.1 Results of methacholine tests in the absence of deep breaths in sedentary subjects and nonasthmatic athletes

Altered airway responsiveness in asthmatics has been primarily attributed to enhanced shortening ability of the airway smooth muscle. However, a wealth of evidence has accumulated to support the concept that factors other than smooth muscle reactivity are implicated in the overall response to a spasmogen. Indeed, changes in breathing pattern can modulate the response to bronchoconstrictor stimulation in healthy subjects, since the response to methacholine becomes almost indistinguishable from that of asthmatics when only shallow breaths are allowed (Skloot et al., 1995). Thus, excessive airway narrowing likely results from an imbalance of opposing factors: on one hand, the forces generated by airway smooth muscle contraction; on the other hand, the effects of increased lung volumes, which may mechanically counteract smooth muscle shortening (Macklem, 1989).

Deep inspirations have been demonstrated to play a central role in opposing to airway narrowing, in that they are able to prevent bronchoconstriction in nonasthmatic subjects (Kapsali et al., 2000). Interestingly, such physiological function of lung inflation fails to occur in subjects who have airways hyperresponsiveness. In addition, deep inspirations can also reverse bronchoconstriction in both healthy subjects and patients with mild asthma (Scichilone et al., 2001); this phenomenon tends to decrease with increasing severity of asthma (Scichilone et al., 2007). Taken together, these observations imply that at least three factors are involved in the hyperreactive phenotype: the smooth muscle contractile properties and the bronchoprotective and bronchodilatory effects of deep inspirations.

We reasoned that by avoiding any effect of deep inspiratory maneuver thoroughout a bronchoprovocation protocol, the "true" smooth muscle reactivity could be assessed. Our group applied a single dose methacholine bronchoprovocation test to specifically study the response to spasmogen in the absence of large lung inflations (Scichilone et al., 2001). This modified bronchoprovocation challenge is more sensitive than the conventional challenge with incremental methacholine doses, as it causes substantial bronchoconstriction even in healthy individuals. In such protocol, the response to methacholine can be evaluated based on the dose of spasmogen inhaled, and the degree of bronchoconstriction obtained.

Nonasthmatic amateur runners responded less to methacholine in the absence of deep inspirations (higher amount of methacholine and lower degree of bronchial obstruction) than age-matched sedentary subjects (Scichilone et al., 2005). These findings suggest that smooth muscle of the athletes underwent exercise-induced structural changes, thus becoming more resistant to the effect of a bronchial spasmogen (bronchoprotective effect). The decreased reactivity in the athletes did not appear to depend on higher lung volumes at baseline compared to sedentary subjects (Scichilone et al., 2005). Deep inspiration may also exert a stronger bronchodilatory effect in athletes compared to the sedentary controls, but this hypothesis has not been tested yet.

Following this cross-sectional study, we longitudinally tested the effects of training in a group of healthy sedentary subjects undergoing intensive rowing training for 3 months. A significant reduction in the degree of bronchial reactivity in the absence of deep breaths was recorded during and at the end of the study (Scichilone et al., 2010). This observation shed new light in the field of bronchial hyperreactivity, since it indicates a significant effect of regular intensive exercise. Interestingly, Hewitt and colleagues recently reported that repeated bouts of moderate-intensity aerobic exercise (Hewitt et al., 2010), but not acute exercise (Hewitt et al., 2009), improved bronchial reactivity in OVA-treated mice. In amateur endurance athletes training in the Mediterranean area, no evidence was found for increased prevalence of EIB, suggesting that moderate intensity training does not worsen respiratory health (Kippelen et al., 2004). Therefore, moderate physical training could become a new, still relatively unexplored, management tool in asthma. In addition, given the potential to affect the progression of asymptomatic bronchial reactivity to asthma, we could conclude as stated in the editorial from Chapman and colleagues in 2010: "*the next time a physician hands an asthmatic patient a prescription and exclaims "take two at a time", the response may be – "do you mean pills or stairs?"* (Chapman et al., 2010).

2.3.2 Experimental data on the effects of deep inspirations on airway smooth muscle

Airway smooth muscle is subjected to mechanical strain associated with tidal breathing, and more so when deep inspirations take place. In 1995, it was shown that the active force generated by the airway smooth muscle decreases with increasing the amplitude of stretch (Pratusevich et al., 1995). In another *in vitro* study (Gump et al., 2001), a 3% increase of muscle length reduced force generation by 50%, which was comparable to the effect of isoproterenol treatment. *In vitro* experiments also showed that the magnitude of force generation of the airway smooth muscle decreases in parallel with increasing amplitude and duration of length oscillations applied to the relaxed muscle.

After a deep inspiration, the smooth muscle is believed to increase its length by 12% from its baseline value, and greater values can be reached during exercise (Fredberg et al., 1997). Bridge dynamic disruption (Fredberg et al., 1996, Fredberg et al., 1997) and plastic reorganization of the cytoskeleton (Gunst & Wu, 2001) both of which can lead to a state of lower airway smooth muscle contractility, have been advocated to explain the effect of lung inflation on airways. Kuo and colleagues showed that the density of thick myosin filaments decreases with varying the length of the airway smooth muscle (Kuo et al., 2001).

Prolonged changes in the contractile function of airway smooth muscle have been shown after long-term alterations in smooth muscle resting length. Chest strapping to maintain low end-expiratory lung volume in sheep increased airway smooth muscle contractility (McClean et al., 2003), while prolonged application of continuous positive airway pressure, which increased end-expiratory volume, decreased airway smooth muscle contractility in ferrets (Xue et al., 2008).

In summary, there is growing evidence indicating a major effect of deep inspiration in modulating airway smooth muscle cell reactivity. Habitual exercise training, with repeated intense hyperpnea, may be an important factor in regulation of bronchial reactivity in healthy and asthmatic subjects. More studies, however, are needed to extend the available results and identify optimal frequency and intensity of training to evoke positive changes in bronchial reactivity in humans.

3. Exercise-induced changes in airway cells

Exercise–induced changes in airways cells were initially studied in relation to occurrence of EIB. It was hypothesized that, similar to bronchial asthma, subjects developing EIB after intense exercise might also show a background of inflammatory activation in their airways.

In asthmatic patients, occurrence of EIB was found to be associated with intense eosinophilic inflammation (Yoshikawa et al., 1998). Asthmatic patients with EIB showed increased bronchial epithelial cells and eosinophil counts, as well as increased histamine, cysteinyl-leukotrienes and tryptase, and decreased prostaglandin E2 (PGE2) and thromboxane B2 in induced sputum after exercise challenge (Hallstrand et al., 2005a, 2005b). Leukotrienes are believed to be major players in EIB and asthma (Hallstrand et al., 2010), and increased leukotriene concentrations have been reported in exhaled breath condensate in asthmatic children with EIB (Carraro et al., 2005). A role for oxidative stress was also suggested by increased 8-isoprostane levels in exhaled breath condensate collected in asthmatic children developing EIB (Barreto et al., 2009). For further information, the reader is referred to a comprehensive review on EIB in asthmatic patients (Brannan & Turton, 2010). Finally, recent data suggest a relationship between neutrophilic inflammation and airway dehydration in asthmatics (Loughlin et al., 2010), indicating that asthma and EIB may share the common pathophysiological mechanism of airway drying and hyperosmolarity. However, more studies are needed to confirm this hypothesis.

Studies in athletes found that changes in airways cells are common and occur independent of exercise-associated symptoms or spirometric changes. Increasing evidence suggest that habitual training is associated with airway inflammation in athletes of different endurance sports performed in cold or temperate environments (Bonsignore et al 2001, 2003b; Karjalainen et al., 2000; Sue-Chu et al., 1999; Lumme et al. 2003; Morici et al., 2004). However, the degree and type of airway inflammation under resting conditions is variable in athletes who perform different sports, and the role of inflammatory cells in the airways is currently unclear. Furthermore, airway inflammation in endurance athletes shows some peculiarities, since it may not be associated with bronchial hyperreactivity, post-exercise respiratory symptoms (Karjalainen et al., 2000; Bonsignore et al., 2001) or clear evidence of cell activation after acute exercise in humans or mice (Bonsignore 2001, 2003b; Morici et al., 2004; Hewitt et al., 2008) or after training in animal models (Chimenti et al. 2007, 2009; Silva et al., 2010; Vieira et al., 2007, 2011).

3.1 Studies in human athletes

Airway inflammation has been well characterized in athletes who exercise in a very cold environment (e.g skaters, ice hockey players, cross-country skiers) (Provost-Craig et al., 1996 ; Karjalainen et al., 2000, Lumme et al., 2003; Bougault et al., 2009). In cross-country skiers studied at rest, lymphocytes were increased in bronchoalveolar lavage fluid (Karjalainen et al., 2000), and endobronchial biopsies of proximal airways showed increased lymphocytes, but also neutrophils and eosinophils and evidence of airway remodelling, i.e. increased tenascin expression in the basement membrane (Sue-Chu et al., 1999). Skiers showed neutrophil infiltration, and relatively mild infiltration with eosinophils, mast cells, and macrophages. These results suggested that the inflammatory process in these athletes is different from classic asthma. Moreover, bronchial biopsy findings did not correlate with bronchial reactivity, atopy, or symptoms of asthma (Sue-Chu et al., 1999). Ice hockey players also showed increased neutrophil and eosinophil counts in induced sputum (Lumme et al., 2003). All these data were obtained in athletes under resting conditions, and the effects of acute exercise on airway cells in skiers have not been assessed, at least in part because of the objective environmental difficulties in collecting samples in these athletes.

Airway inflammation has been found in endurance athletes who perform sports in a temperate climate. In non-asthmatic amateur runners, neutrophil counts in induced sputum were increased after a marathon race compared to baseline level (Bonsignore et al, 2001); under resting conditions, the percentage of neutrophils in induced sputum of runners was higher than in sedentary controls, suggesting a chronic increase in neutrophils in the airways possibly related to habitual training (Bonsignore et al, 2001; Kippelen et al., 2004; Denguezli et al., 2008; Bougault et al., 2009). More recently, increased bronchial epithelial cell counts and interleukin-8 concentration, and apoptosis of bronchial epithelial cells, were found in induced sputum collected in nonasthmatic runners shortly after a half-marathon race, while neutrophil absolute counts were unchanged (Chimenti et al., 2010). Induced sputum samples collected the morning after a half-marathon race showed a slight increase in neutrophils compared to resting conditions (Chimenti et al., 2009). Increased bronchial epithelial cell counts were also reported in induced sputum of elite swimmers collected at rest (Bougault et al. 2009).

These data suggest that neutrophil influx into the airways might be secondary to mild bronchial epithelial damage caused by intense exercise, but requires some time to occur. Similar to runners, well-trained young competitive rowers with normal bronchial reactivity to methacholine showed predominance of neutrophils in induced sputum both at rest and after exercise, and increased bronchial epithelial cell counts in induced sputum collected after a short bout of very intense exercise (Morici et al., 2004; Bonsignore et al, unpublished observations). Therefore, studies on the effects of exercise should take into account both the duration and the intensity of exercise; in addition, the time course of airway cell changes is likely to be complex, explaining some discrepancies between results of different studies.

The inflammatory pattern found in swimmers is very complex, as recently underlined (Haahtela et al., 2008), and different phenotypes of asthma in swimmers likely exist. On one hand, swimming is traditionally considered as a good type of physical activity for asthmatic patients, since it is associated with low allergen exposure. On the other hand, data in elite swimmers do suggest an important pro-inflammatory role played by environmental exposure to chlorine-derived compounds. Some time, however, might be required for airway cell changes to develop, as suggested by the negative results recently found in adolescent elite swimmers (Pedersen et al., 2008). Adult elite swimmers at rest, about half of them hyperreactive to methacholine, showed more eosinophils and neutrophils in induced sputum than sedentary subjects, with some evidence of inflammatory activation (Helenius et al., 1998a). Airway inflammation increased at 5-year follow-up in swimmers who continued training, but decreased in swimmers who had stopped competitive activity (Helenius et al., 2002). In adult non-asthmatic swimmers habitually training in an outdoor pool, airway neutrophil differential counts at baseline were higher than in sedentary controls but cell counts did not change significantly after a 5-km trial (Bonsignore et al., 2003b). After a 5-km competition in the sea, a condition of potential hypertonic airway exposure during exercise, the same swimmers showed slightly increased eosinophil and lymphocyte differential counts in induced sputum (Bonsignore et al., 2003b). These results suggested that the effects of chlorine exposure might be limited in athletes training in outdoor swimming pools; however, a study in adolescents swimmers attending outdoor pools confirmed an elevated risk of asthma also in this population (Bernard et al., 2008). More recently, asthmatic and nonasthmatic swimmers showed increased neutrophil counts in induced sputum, which correlated with increased airway vascular permeability assessed as the ratio of albumin in sputum and serum (Moreira et al., 2011b). Conversely, other studies found increased airway neutrophils only in swimmers who were hyperreactive to methacholine (Boulet et al., 2005; Belda et al., 2008, Bougault et al., 2009). Finally, a mixed type of inflammation, with increased eosinophil and neutrophil counts in induced sputum at rest, was reported in elite swimmers who showed hyperreactivity to methacholine (Moreira et al., 2008).

To our knowledge, only one study assessed airway cells in non-asthmatic athletes experiencing EIB (Parsons et al., 2008). The study shows some methodological limitations, such as EIB assessment only as response to eucapnic voluntary hyperventilation, and lack of baseline induced sputum samples. This study reported increased inflammatory mediators in

EIB+ athletes. However, airway cell counts were similar in EIB+ and EIB- athletes and did not correlate with concentration of mediators in sputum supernatants (Parsons et al., 2008). Our study on the effects of training in non-asthmatic subjects found that changes in airway cells and in the response to methacholine in the absence of deep inhalations showed different time courses (Scichilone et al., 2010). The picture can be further complicated by interactions between airway epithelial cells and smooth muscle cells, as suggested by a study showing that hyperosmotic stimuli induce epithelial dependent relaxation in the guinea pig trachea *in vitro* (Munakata et al., 1988). Therefore, further studies are needed to better characterize the role of airway epithelium in airway inflammation and its relationship with occurrence of EIB.

3.2 Studies in animal models and cultured bronchial epithelial cells

The functional and cellular events triggered by exercise hyperventilation have been studied in animal models, confirming that bronchial epithelial cells likely play an important role in exercise-induced airway changes. Besides functioning as a barrier against environmental toxins and injury, bronchial epithelial cells may modulate the immune response. In addition, in the long term, epithelial damage may favour sensitization to allergens, at least partly explaining the high prevalence of asthma in elite athletes (Helenius et al, 1998b).

In anesthetized dogs challenged with high flows of air into a lung segment during bronchoscopy, hyperventilation with dry air caused hyperosmolarity of airway surface lining (Freed & Davis, 1999) and bronchoconstriction (Freed et al., 1985). Repeated dry air challenges (DACs) in the same model, mimicking chronic exposure such as during training, caused epithelial damage with eosinophil and neutrophil influx, and increased peptidoleukotriene concentrations in bronchoalveolar lavage fluid (BALF) (Davis et al., 2001). Bronchial epithelial damage also occurred in horses after exercise while breathing cold air (Davis et al., 2002). In cultured human bronchial epithelial cells, exposure to a hyperosmolar medium or cooling-rewarming increased the expression of IL-8 and RANTES partly through the activation of p38 MAP Kinase (Hashimoto et al., 1999, 2000). Therefore, both hyperventilation and airway hyperosmolarity appear capable to cause bronchoconstriction and inflammatory response.

Data obtained in a normal mouse model of endurance training support the interpretation that exercise causes limited inflammation in small airways but may damage bronchial epithelium. Increased leukocyte infiltrate was observed in bronchiolar walls and lumen of endurance-trained mice undergoing mild-intensity training for 45 days (Chimenti et al., 2007). Bronchiolar epithelium showed progressive changes during training. In mice trained for 45 days, the number of ciliated epithelial cells was significantly lower compared to sedentary mice, and apoptosis of bronchiolar epithelial cells increased. Epithelial thickness was increased in trained compared to sedentary mice. Bronchiolar epithelium of trained mice showed an increased number of proliferating cells, suggesting that habitual exercise may increase epithelial turnover in the airways (Chimenti et al., 2007).

Bronchial epithelial cells play a crucial role in the asthma pathophysiology. A number of studies have demonstrated the beneficial effects of aerobic exercise in chronic allergic airway inflammation (Table 1).

Author, yr	Animal model	Aerobic training intensity	Aerobic training duration	Airway inflammation	BHR	Other post-training data
Pastva et al., 2004	OVA-sensitized mice	Moderate	4 wk	Trained mice showed ↓ inflammation when OVA-tested	Not tested	↓ NFkB expression
Davis et al., 2003	Sled dogs	High	2-4 mo	Not tested	=, but increased pre-training compared to control dogs	-
Chimenti et al., 2007	Normal mice	Low-moderate	45 d	↑inflammatory cells, ↓ NFkB expression in small airways	Not tested	-
Vieira et al, 2007	OVA-sensitized mice	Low-moderate	30 d	Trained OVA+ mice showed ↓ inflammation	Not tested	↓ remodeling
Vieira et al, 2008	OVA-sensitized mice	Low-moderate	30 d	Trained OVA+ mice showed ↓ vascular and parenchymal inflammation	Not tested	
Hewitt et al, 2009	OVA-sensitized mice	Moderate	4 wk	Not tested	↓	B2AR involved in BHR response
Silva et al., 2010	OVA-sensitized mice	Moderate	4 wk	Trained OVA+ mice showed ↓ inflammation		↓ remodeling
Lowder et al., 2010	OVA-sensitized mice	Moderate	4 wk	trained OVA+ mice showed ↓ inflammation associated with ↑ Treg cell response	Not tested	-
Vieira et al., 2011	OVA-sensitized mice	Moderate	4 wk	Trained OVA+ mice showed ↓ inflammation	Not tested	↓ remodeling; ↑ IL-10 in bronchial epithelium in OVA+ and OVA- trained mice

Table 1. Effects of training on airway inflammation and bronchial reactivity in animal models. Abbreviations: BHR: bronchial hyperreactivity; OVA: ovalbumin; B2AR: beta2-adrenergic receptor; NFkB: nuclear factor k B; = unchanged; ↑: increased; ↓ decreased; IL-10: interleukin-10

Regular aerobic exercise performed at low or moderate intensity decreased eosinophilic and lymphocytic inflammation and Th-2 immune response in a murine model of allergic asthma (Pastva et al., 2004; Vieira et al., 2007, 2008, 2011; Hewitt et al., 2009, 2010; Lowder et al., 2010). These studies showed that the effects of exercise training were mediated by reduced activation and expression of NF-kB, insulin like growth factor 1 (IGF-1), RANTES (CCL2) and glucocorticoid receptors. Exercise training increased the expression of interleukin 10 (IL-10) and of the receptor antagonist of IL-1 (IL-1ra) suggesting an immune-regulatory role of habitual exercise on airway epithelium.

3.2.1 Markers of airway inflammation

To assess whether the increased inflammatory cells in the airways were activated, markers of inflammation were analysed in endurance athletes or animal models. According to some studies, the increased number of airway inflammatory cells was not associated with major signs of inflammatory activation in BALF or induced sputum in cross-country skiers at rest (Sue-Chu et al., 2000), or in induced sputum of runners studied at rest and after a marathon race (Bonsignore at al., 2001). In amateur swimmers who trained outdoor throughout the year, there was no evidence of inflammatory cell activation at rest or after exercise in outdoor pool or sea as suggested by low levels of neutrophil elastase and decreased expression of L-selectin by airway cells (Bonsignore et al., 2003b). However, in runners IL-8 concentration in induced sputum supernatants doubled after a half-marathon and was positively correlated with absolute bronchial epithelial cell counts (Chimenti et al., 2010). We speculate that the increase in neutrophils found in large airways of athletes after prolonged exercise (Bonsignore et al., 2001) or the morning post-race (Chimenti et al., 2009) might be at least partly secondary to release of chemotactic factors, such as IL-8, by bronchial epithelial cells during exercise. On the other hand, IL-8 concentration in sputum supernatants collected on the morning after a half-marathon race was low (Chimenti et al., 2009), suggesting that exercise-induced inflammatory activation is transient. In runners, increased IL-8 in induced sputum at rest was found during a competitive period, but did not correlate with sputum cells counts (Denguezli et al., 2008).

Data on lung-derived proteins measured in serum or urine, suggest that pulmonary epithelial permeability may increase after intense exercise (Hermans et al., 1999; Chimenti et al., 2010, Romberg et al., 2011) or after eucapnic hyperventilation, independent of training status or occurrence of EIB (Bolger et al., 2011). In amateur runners, CC-16 levels did not correlate with air pollutants levels, and were normal in samples collected the morning after a half-marathon race (Chimenti et al., 2009). Thus, intense exercise appears to transiently increase epithelial permeability.

Data obtained in a murine model of allergic asthma suggest that inflammatory activation in the airways may actually be inhibited by exercise training (Table 1). In ovalbumin-sensitized mice, nuclear translocation of nuclear-factor-κB (NF-κB) in airway cells was lower in trained compared to sedentary animals (Pastva et al., 2004). More recently, exercise training in ovalbumin-sensitized mice decreased epithelial expression of IL-4, IL-5, IL-13, CCL11, CCL5, adhesion molecules ICAM-1 and VCAM-1, iNOS and NF-kB, while the expression of the anti-inflammatory cytokine IL-10 increased, suggesting a positive effect of training on control of inflammation in asthmatic airways (Vieira et al., 2011). In small airways of endurance-trained nonasthmatic mice, NF-κB translocation and inhibitor-alpha of NF-κB (IκBα) phosphorylation were not affected, and goblet cells in bronchioles were negative at

Alcian-PAS staining, indicating that training did not cause excess mucus production (Chimenti et al., 2007).

Other studies found increased airway inflammatory markers in athletes. Increased concentrations of eosinophil peroxidase and neutrophil lipocalin in induced sputum were observed in elite swimmers of the Finnish National team (Helenius et al., 1998). In young athletes, concentration of cysteinil-leukotrienes, prostaglandin E2 (PGE-2), histamine, thromboxane B2 (TXB2), and leukotriene B4 (LTB4) in induced sputum after a eucapnic voluntary hyperventilation challenge were higher in subjects with than without EIB (Parsons et al., 2008).

In summary, data from athletes or animal models are somewhat controversial, as some studies did not show any clear evidence of significant inflammatory activation in the airways, while others reported increased inflammatory mediators. These studies did not assess exercise-induced changes but only examined airway cells and mediators under resting conditions. The few data available on the effects of acute exercise suggest that changes in inflammatory markers, if any, might be transient. The relationship between EIB and inflammation is still unclear, and its assessment is often complicated by the concomitant occurrence of asthma and bronchial hyperreactivity in athletes.

4. Could exercise training be useful in patients with respiratory disease?

The possibility that habitual exercise may affect inflammatory processes in the airways opens the way to a new perspective regarding exercise-based rehabilitation. Until recently, exercise training in patients with respiratory diseases, such as asthma or chronic obstructive pulmonary disease (COPD), was based on the assumption that the main effect of rehabilitation was to improve muscle function and decrease ventilatory requirements. While this holds true, especially in physically deconditioned patients, the possibility that exercise training may also modulate airway cell biology is being increasingly considered. The following paragraphs report a summary of recent findings suggesting that this could well be the case in patients with asthma or COPD, respectively.

4.1 Asthma

In subjects with asthma, the level of activity is restricted mainly because bronchoconstriction occurs after exercise. On the other hand, physical training increases the capacity for physical work (Freedman, 1992; Arborelius & Svenonius, 1984), and the anaerobic threshold (i.e., the level at which lactic acid production, and the associated increase in ventilation, occur). Consequently, hyperpnea, one of the major stimuli for EIB, is delayed and exercise tolerance improves after aerobic training. Ventilatory muscle training might also improve the capacity for sustaining physical activity, or, at least, minimize muscle fatigue (Leith & Bradley, 1976).

In asthmatic patients, an exercise-based training program improved asthma symptoms (Arborelius & Svenonius, 1984; Haas et al., 1987), even though baseline lung function remained unchanged. None of these studies tested whether airway responsiveness was affected by exercise training.

Table 2 summarizes the studies on the effects of physical training in normal subjects and patients with asthma. Some studies examined the effects of training on inflammation, other studies tested bronchial reactivity before and after training, and some did analyze other aspects such as quality of life and asthma control.

Author, yr	n	Training type	Training duration	Airway inflammation	BHR	Other post-training data
Matsumoto et al., 1999	8 children with mild-moderate asthma	swimming	6 wk	Not tested	=	Lac Thr ↑
Neder et al., 1999	42 children with mild-moderate asthma	aerobic	2 mo	Not tested	=	↓ use of B2A
Hallstrand et al., 2000	5 pts with mild asthma, 5 controls	aerobic	10 wk	Not tested	Not tested	Less HV during exercise
Kippelen et al., 2005	13 healthy subjects	aerobic	1 yr	Not tested	Not tested	Lung function=
Fanelli et al, 2007	Moderate-severe persistent asthma (21 T, 17 C children)	mixed	16 wk	Not tested	↓ EIB in trained group	↑ QoL
Bonsignore et al., 2008	Mild asthma (25 placebo, 25 montelukast, M, children)	aerobic	12 wk	=	↓ Mch PC20 in both groups	↓ FEV1 slope and exacerbations in M group
Moreira et al., 2008	34 asthmatic children (17 T, 17 C)	aerobic	12 wk	Not worsened by training, possible ↓ in IgE	Not tested	-
Dengzueli et al., 2008	10 endurance runners	aerobic	1 yr	↑ in precompetitive period	Not tested	Lung function =
Mendes et al., 2010	Moderate-severe persistent asthma (51 C, 50 T)	aerobic	3 mo	Not tested	Not tested	↑ asthma control and QoL
Scichilone et al., 2010	10 sedentary healthy subjects	rowing	10 wk	↑IL-8 in induced sputum supernatants at 10 wk	↓ response to Mch in the absence of deep inspiration at wk 5 and 10	-
Dogra et al., 2011	Incompletely controlled asthma (15 C, 21 T adults)	Mostly aerobic	24 wks	Not tested	Not tested	↑ asthma control and QoL
Mendes et al., 2011	Moderate-severe persistent asthma (24 C, 27 T adults)	Aerobic	3 mo	↓ only in trained group	Not tested	↑ asthma control

Table 2. Effects of training on airway inflammation and reactivity in normal and asthmatic subjects. Abbreviations: BHR: bronchial hyperreactivity; Lac Thr: lactate threshold; T: trained; C: control; B2A: beta2-agonist; FEV1: forced expiratory volume in 1 second; HV: hyperventilation; Mch: methacholine; PC20: provocative concentration causing 20% fall in FEV1; QoL: quality of life; NFkB: nuclear factor k B; = unchanged; ↑: increased; ↓ decreased; IL-8: interleukin-8.

Overall, the data in humans show no worsening or improvement of asthma after exercise training. The studies in animal models (Table 1) are much more refined in term of assessment of mediators and potential mechanisms involved. Therefore, additional work is required to improve our understanding of the effects of exercise training in human patients with asthma. The asthmatic athlete, on the other hand, might be considered a "special case", given the high intensity/frequency of training and the role of environmental exposures.

4.2 Chronic obstructive pulmonary disease

The literature on the physiological effects of pulmonary rehabilitation in COPD is large, but the majority of studies have examined the effects of training on skeletal muscles and markers of systemic inflammation, while changes in airway cells occurring during exercise or physical training in COPD patients remain largely unknown. The most recent studies have focused their attention on the amount, intensity, and pattern of daily physical activity in COPD patients, rather than the degree of physical fitness examined by traditional exercise stress tests, since the former is a better indicator of the impact of the disease on the quality of life of the patients. These studies are made easier today by the availability of accelerometers, which are very useful tools to objectively assess daily physical activity in and elderly population such as COPD patients. At least two meta-analyses have shown that daily physical activity in COPD patients is lower than in controls (Bossenbrock et al., 2011; Vorrink et al., 2011), but the involved mechanism are far from being clarified.

Interestingly, similar to studies on asthmatic patients, some epidemiological studies highlighted the prognostic importance of maintaining a good level of daily physical activity in COPD. Patients maintaining a regular level of physical activity underwent less hospital admission for COPD exacerbations (Garcia-Aymerich et al., 2006; Benzo et al. 2010). Moreover, in a population-based cohort the decline in lung function and the risk to develop COPD were found to be lower in smokers with an active lifestyle compared to smokers with a sedentary lifestyle (Garcia-Aymerich et al., 2007). Finally, an active lifestyle was associated with a more favorable clinical and functional status in a large sample of COPD patients (Garcia-Aymerich et al., 2009). An inverse association between life-long physical activity and the risk of COPD has also been recently reported by a case-control study conducted in Japan (Hirayama et al., 2010). Therefore, increasing evidence suggests a protective effect of an active life against the development of COPD and disease severity.

No study is available yet in humans on training-associated changes in airway responses in COPD patients. In a mouse model of COPD, favourable effects of 24-week exercise training in animals chronically exposed to cigarette smoke compared to the sedentary group have been reported (Toledo et al., 2011). Regular aerobic physical training of moderate intensity reduced oxidative stress and the development of emphysema in mice (Toledo et al., 2011). Therefore, it can be expected that studies in the near future will increasingly examine the protective effects of exercise training in the lung of COPD patients.

5. Conclusions

The effects of acute exercise and training on bronchial reactivity and airway inflammation are still a puzzle with many missing elements, but the general picture is appearing with an increasing number of details. In elite athletes, the combination of high exercise intensity, environmental exposure and genetic background is likely responsible for the varying airway involvement described for different sports. However, it is likely that the levels of exercise commonly observed in the active population are associated with positive effects on bronchial reactivity and tight control of airway inflammation.

The majority of studies in patients with asthma similarly suggest a beneficial effect of training on the control of airway inflammation, although little evidence is currently available on the potentially beneficial effects of habitual exercise on bronchial reactivity. Instead, the only evidence in favour of physical activity in COPD patients comes from epidemiological observations and limited experimental results. A better understanding of the pathophysiology of exercise training in patients with asthma and COPD will be the first step towards a rational, evidence-based development of specific recommendations targeted to improve the quality of life and possibly the prognosis of these patients.

6. Acknowledgments

This work has been funded by University of Palermo, Italy and the Institute of Biomedicine and Molecular Immunology (IBIM) of National Research Council of Italy (CNR). Publication costs were covered by institutional funding of DISMOT, University of Palermo, Italy.

7. References

Anderson, S.D., Daviskas, E., & Smith, C.M. (1989). Exercise-induced asthma: a difference in opinion regarding the stimulus. *Allergy Proc*, Vol. 10, No. 3, (May-Jun 1989), pp. 215-226, ISSN 1046-9354

Anderson, S.D., & Daviskas, E. (1992). The airway microvasculature and exercise induced asthma. *Thorax*, Vol. 47, No. 9, (September 1992), pp. 748-752, ISSN 0040-6376

Anderson, S.D. & Daviskas, E. (2000). The mechanism of exercise-induced asthma is.... *J Allergy Clin Immunol*, Vol. 106, No. 3, (March 2000), pp. 453-459, ISSN 0091-6749

Anderson, S.D., Argyros, G.J., Magnussen, H. & Holzer, K. (2001). Provocation by eucapnic voluntary hyperpnoea to identify exercise induced bronchoconstriction. *Br J Sports Med*, Vol.35, No. 5, (October 2001), pp. 344–347, ISSN 0306-3674

Anderson, S.D. & Kippelen, P. (2008). Airway injury as a mechanism for exercise-induced bronchoconstriction in elite athletes. *J Allergy Clin Immunol*, Vol. 122, No. 2,(August 2008), pp. 225-235, ISSN 0091-6749

Anderson, S.D., Charlton, B., Weiler, J.M., Nichols, S., Spector, S.L., Pearlman, D.S.; & A305 Study Group. (2009). Comparison of mannitol and methacholine to predict exercise-induced bronchoconstriction and a clinical diagnosis of asthma. *Respir Res*, Vol. 10, (23 January 2009), pp. 4, ISSN 1465-993X

Arborelius, J.M., & Svenonius, E. (1984). Decrease of exercise-induced asthma after physical training. *Eur J Resp Dis Suppl*, Vol. 136, pp. 25-31, ISSN 0106-4347

Barreto, M., Villa, M.P., Olita, C., Martella, S., Ciabattoni, G., & Montuschi, P. (2009). 8-isoprostane in exhaled breath condensate and exercise-induced bronchoconstriction in asthmatic children and adolescents. *Chest*, Vol. 135, No. 1, (January 2009), pp. 66-73, ISSN 0012-3692

Belda, J., Ricart, S., Casan, P., Giner, J., Bellido-Casado, J., Torrejon, M., Margarit, G. & Drobnic, F. (2008). Airway inflammation in the elite athlete and type of sport. *Br J Sports Med*, Vol. 42, No. 4, (April 2008), pp. 244-248, ISSN 0306-3674

Benzo, R.P., Chang, C.C., Farrell, M.H., Kaplan, R., Ries, A., Martinez, F.J., Wise, R., Make, B., Sciurba, F., & NETT Research Group. (2010). Physical activity, health status and risk of hospitalization in patients with severe chronic obstructive pulmonary disease. *Respiration*, Vol. 80, No. 1, (June 2010), pp. 10-18, ISSN 0025-7931

Bernard, A., Nickmilder, M., & Voisin, C. (2008). Outdoor swimming pools and the risks of asthma and allergies during adolescence. *Eur Respir J*, Vol. 32, No. 4, (October 2008), pp. 979-988, ISSN 0903-1936

Bernard, A., Nickmilder, M., Voisin, C., & Sardella, A. (2009). Impact of chlorinated swimming pool attendance on the respiratory health of adolescents. *Pediatrics*, Vol. 124, No. 4, (October 2009), pp. 1110-1118, ISSN 0031-4005

Bernard, A., Voisin, C., & Sardella, A. (2011). Corr. Respiratory risks associated with chlorinated swimming pools. A complex pattern of exposure and effects. *Am J Respir Crit Care Med*, Vol. 183, No. 5, (1 March 2011), pp. 570-573, ISSN 1073-449X

Bolger, C., Tufvesson, E., Sue-Chu, M., Devereux, G., Ayres, J.G., Bjermer, L., & Kippelen, P. (2011). Hyperpnea-induced bronchoconstriction and urinary CC16 levels in athletes. *Med Sci Sports Exerc*, Vol. 43, No. 7, (July 2011), pp. 1207-1213, ISSN 0195-9131

Bonsignore, M.R., Morici, G., Riccobono, L., Insalaco, G., Bonanno, A., Profita, M., Paternò, A., Mirabella, A., Vassalle, C. & Vignola, A.M. (2001). Airway inflammation in nonasthmatic amateur runners. *Am J Physiol Lung Cell Mol Physiol*, Vol. 281, No. 3, (September 2001), pp. L668-L676, ISSN 1040-0605

Bonsignore, M.R., Morici, G., Vignola, A.M., Riccobono, L., Bonanno, A., Profita, M., Abate, P., Scichilone, N., Amato, G., Bellia, V. & Bonsignore, G. (2003a). Increased airway inflammatory cells in athletes: what do they mean?. *Clin Exper Allergy*, Vol. 33, No. 1, (January 2003), pp. 14-21, ISSN 0954-7894

Bonsignore, M.R., Morici, G., Riccobono, L., Profita, M., Bonanno, A., Paternò, A., Di Giorgi, R., Chimenti, L., Insalaco, G., Cuttitta, G., Abate, P., Mirabella, F., Vignola, A.M. & Bonsignore, G. (2003b). Airway cells after swimming outdoors or in the sea in nonasthmatic athletes. *Med Sci Sports Exerc*, Vol. 35, No. 7, (July 2003), pp. 1146-1152, ISSN 0195-9131

Bonsignore, M.R., La Grutta, S., Cibella, F., Scichilone, N., Cuttitta, G., Interrante, A., Marchese, M., Veca, M., Virzì, M., Bonanno, A., Profita, M. & Morici, G. (2008). Effects of exercise training and montelukast in children with mild asthma. *Med Sci Sports Exerc.*, Vol. 40, No. 3, (March 2008), pp. 405-412, ISSN 0195-9131

Bossenbroek, L., de Greef, M.H., Wempe, J.B., Krijnen, W.P., & Ten Hacken, N.H. (2011). Daily physical activity in patients with chronic obstructive pulmonary disease: A systematic review. *COPD*, (5 July 2011), Epub ahead of print, ISSN 1541-2555

Bougault, V., Turmel, J., St-Laurent, J., Bertrand, M. & Boulet, L.P. (2009). Asthma, airway inflammation and epithelial damage in swimmers and cold-air athletes. *Eur Respir J*, Vol. 33, No. 4, (April 2009), pp. 740-746, ISSN 0903-1936

Bougault, V., Turmel, J., & Boulet, L.P. (2010). Bronchial challenges and respiratory symptoms in elite swimmers and winter sport athletes: Airway hyperresponsiveness in asthma: its measurement and clinical significance. *Chest* Vol. 138, No. 2 Suppl, (August 2010), pp. 31S-37S, ISSN 0012-3692

Bougault, V., Turmel, J., & Boulet, L.P. (2011). Airway hyperresponsiveness in elite swimmers: Is it a transient phenomenon? *J Allergy Clin Immunol*,.Vol. 127, No. 4, (April 2011), pp. 892-898, ISSN 0091-6749

Boulet, L.P., & Turcotte, H. (1991). Influence of water content of inspired air during and after exercise on induced bronchoconstriction. *Eur Respir J*, Vol. 4, No. 8, (September 1991), pp. 979-984, ISSN 0903-1936

Boulet, L.P., Turcotte, H., Langdeau, J.B. & Bernier, M.C. (2005). Lower airway inflammatory responses to high-intensity training in athletes. *Clin Invest Med*, Vol. 28, No. 1, (February 2005), pp. 15-22, ISSN 0147-958X

Brannan, J.D., & Turton, J,A. (2010). The inflammatory basis of exercise-induced bronchoconstriction. *Phys Sportsmed*, Vol. 38, No. 4, (December 2010), pp. 67-73, ISSN 0091-3847

Brasholt, M., Baty, F., & Bisgaard, H. (2010). Physical activity in young children is reduced with increasing bronchial responsiveness. *J Allergy Clin Immunol*, Vol. 125, No. 5, (May 2010), pp. 1007-1012, ISSN 0091-6749

Cabral, A.L., Conceição, G.M., Fonseca-Guedes, C.H., & Martins, M.A. (1999). Exercise-induced bronchospasm in children: effects of asthma severity. *Am J Respir Crit Care Med* Vol. 159, No. 6 (June 1999), pp. 1819-1823, ISSN 1073-449X

Carraro, S., Corradi, M., Zanconato, S., Alinovi, R., Pasquale, M.F., Zacchello, F., & Baraldi, E. (2005). Exhaled breath condensate cysteinyl leukotrienes are increased in children with exercise-induced bronchoconstriction. *J Allergy Clin Immunol*, Vol. 115, Vol. 4, (April 2005), pp. 764-770, ISSN 0091-6749

Chapman, D.G., Berend, N., King, G.G., & Salome, C. (2010). Can we cure airway hyperresponsiveness with a gym membership? *J Appl Physiol*, Vol. 109, No. 2, (August 2010), pp. 267-268, ISSN 0363-6143

Chimenti, L., Morici, G., Paternò, A., Bonanno, A., Siena, L., Licciardi, A., Veca, M., Guccione, W., Macaluso, F., Bonsignore, G. & Bonsignore, M.R. (2007). Endurance training damages small airway epithelium in mice. *Am J Respir Crit Care Med*, Vol. 175, No. 5, (March 2007), pp. 442-449, ISSN 1073-449X

Chimenti, L., Morici, G., Paternò, A., Bonanno, A., Vultaggio, M., Bellia, V. & Bonsignore M.R. (2009). Environmental conditions, air pollutants, and airway cells in runners: a longitudinal field study. *J Sports Sci*, Vol. 27, No. 9, (July 2009), pp. 925-935, ISSN 0264-0414

Chimenti, L., Morici, G., Paternò, A., Santagata, R., Bonanno, A., Profita, M., Riccobono, L., Bellia, V. & Bonsignore, M.R. (2010). Bronchial epithelial damage after a Half-Marathon race in non-asthmatic amateur runners. *Am J Physiol Lung Cell Mol Physiol*, Vol. 298, No. 6, (June 2010), L857-L862, ISSN 1040-0605

Crimi, E., Pellegrino, R., Smeraldi, A., & Brusasco, V. (2002). Exercise-induced bronchodilation in natural and induced asthma: effects on ventilatory response and performance. *J Appl Physiol*, Vol. 92, No. 6, (June 2002), pp. 2353-2360, ISSN 0363-6143.

Davis, M.S. & Freed, A.N. (2001). Repeated hyperventilation causes peripheral airways inflammation, hyper-reactivity, and impaired bronchodilation in dogs. *Am J Respir Crit Care Med*, Vol. 164, No. 5, (September 2001), pp. 785-789, ISSN 1073-449X

Davis, M.S., Lockard, A.J., Marlin, D.J. & Freed, A.N. (2002). Airway cooling and mucosal injury during cold weather exercise. *Equine Vet J Suppl*, Vol. 34, (September 2002), pp. 413-416, ISSN 2042-3306

Davis, M.S., Schoefield, B. & Freed, A.N. (2003). Repeated peripheral airway hyperpnea causes inflammation and remodelling in dogs. *Med Sci Sports Exerc*, Vol. 35, No. 4, (April 2003), pp. 608-616, ISSN 0195-9131

Denguezli, M., Ben Chiekh, I., Ben Saad, H., Zaouali-Ajina, M., Tabka, Z. & Zbidi, A. (2008) One-year endurance training: Effects on lung function and airway inflammation. *J Sports Sci*, Vol. 26, No. 12, (October 2008), pp. 1351-1359, ISSN 0264-0414

Dogra, S., Kuk, J.L., Baker, J., & Jamnik, V. (2011). Exercise is associated with improved asthma control in adults. *Eur Respir J*, Vol. 37, No. 2, (February 2011), pp. 010-020, ISSN 0903-1936

Durand, F., Kippelen, P., Ceugniet, F., Gomez, V.R., Desnot, P., Poulain, M. & Préfaut, C. (2005). Undiagnosed exercise-induced bronchoconstriction in ski-mountaineers. *Int J Sports Med*, Vol. 26, No. 3, (April 2005), pp. 233-237, ISSN 0172-4622

Fanelli, A., Cabral, A.L., Neder, J.A., Martins, M.A., & Carvalho, C.R. (2007). Exercise training on disease control and quality of life in asthmatic children. *Med Sci Sports Exerc*, Vol. 39, No. 9, (September 2007), pp. 1474-1480, ISSN 0195-9131

Fitch, K.D., Sue-Chu, M., Anderson, S.D., Boulet, L.P., Hancox, R.J., McKenzie, D.C., Backer, V., Rundell, K.W., Alonso, J.M., Kippelen, P., Cummiskey, J.M., Garnier, A. & Ljungqvist, A. (2008). Asthma and the elite athlete: summary of the International Olympic Committee's consensus conference, Lausanne, Switzerland, January 22-24, 2008. *J Allergy Clin Immunol,*Vol. 122, No. 2, (August 2008), pp. 254-260, 260.e1-7, ISSN 0091-6749

Font-Ribera, L., Villanueva, C.M., Nieuwenhuijsen, M.J., Zock, J.-P.,Kogevinas, M. & Henderson, J. (2011). Swimming pool attendance, asthma, allergies, and lung function in the Avon Longitudinal Study of Parents and Children Cohort. *Am J Respir Crit Care Med*, Vol. 183, No. 5, (1 March 2011), pp. 582-588, ISSN 1073-449X

Fredberg, J., Jones, K., Nathan, M., Raboudi, S., Prakash, Y.S., Shore, S.A., Butler, J.P., & Sieck, G.C. (1996). Friction in airway smooth muscle: mechanism, latch and implications in asthma. *J Appl Physiol*, Vol. 81, No. 6, (December 1996), pp. 2703-2712, ISSN 0363-6143

Fredberg, J., Inouye, D., Miller B., Nathan, M., Jafari, S., Raboudi, S.H., Butler, J.P., & Shore, S.A. (1997). Airway smooth muscle, tidal stretches, and dynamically determined contractile states. *Am J Respir Crit Care Med*, Vol. 156, No. 6, (December 1997), pp. 1752-1759, ISSN 1073-449X

Freed, A.N., Bromberger-Barnea, B. & Menkes, H.A. (1985). Dry air-induced constriction in lung periphery: a canine model of exercise-induced asthma. *J Appl Physiol*, Vol. 59, No. 6, (December 1985), pp. 1986-1990, ISSN 8750-7587

Freed, A.N. (1995). Models and mechanism of exercise-induced asthma. *Eur Resp J*, Vol. 8, No. 10, (October 1995), pp. 1770-1785, ISSN 0903-1936

Freed, A.N. & Davis, M.S. (1999). Hyperventilation with dry air increases airway surface fluid osmolarity in canine peripheral airways. *Am J Respir Crit Care Med*, Vol. 159, No. 4 Pt 1, (April 1999), pp. 1101-1107, ISSN 1073-449X

Freedman, S. (1992). Exercise as a bronchodilator. *Clin Sci*, Vol. 83, No. 4, (October 1992), pp. 383-389, ISSN 0143-5221

Garcia-Aymerich, J., Lange, P., Benet M., Schnohr, P., & Antó, J.M. (2006). Regular physical activity reduces hospital admission and mortality in chronic obstructive pulmonary disease: a population based cohort study. *Thorax* Vol. 61, No. 9, (September 2006), pp. 772-778, ISSN 0040-6376

Garcia-Aymerich, J., Lange, P., Benet, M., Schnohr, P., & Antó, J.M. (2007). Regular physical activity modifies smoking-related lung function decline and reduces risk of chronic obstructive pulmonary disease: a population-based cohort study. *Am J Respir Crit Care Med*, Vol. 175, No. 5, (1 March 2007), pp. 458-463, ISSN 1073-449X

Garcia-Aymerich, J., Varraso, R., Antó, J.M., & Camargo. C.A. Jr. (2009). Prospective study of physical activity and risk of asthma exacerbations in older women. *Am J Respir Crit Care Med*, Vol. 179, No. 11, (1 June 2009), pp. 999-1003, ISSN 1073-449X

Gelb, A.F., Tashkin, D.P., Epstein, J.D., Gong, H. Jr., & Zamel, N. (1985). Exercise-induced bronchodilation in asthma. *Chest*, Vol. 87, No. 2, (February 1985), pp. 196-201, ISSN 0012-369

Gilbert, I.A., Lenner, K.A., & McFadden, E.R. Jr. (1988). Sympathoadrenal response to repetitive exercise in normal and asthmatic subjects. *J Appl Physiol*, Vol 64, No. 6, (June 1988), pp. 2667-2674, ISSN 0363-6143

Gotshall, R.W. (2002). Exercise-induced bronchoconstriction. *Drugs*, Vol. 62, No. 12, (June 2002) pp. 1725-1739, ISSN 0012-6667

Gump, A., Haughney, L., & Fredberg, J.J. (2001). Relaxation of activated airway smooth muscle: relative potency of isoproterenol versus tidal stretch. *J Appl Physiol*, Vol. 90, No. 6, (June 2001), pp. 2306-2310, ISSN 0363-6143

Gunst, S., & Tang, D. (2000). The contractile apparatus and mechanical properties of airway smooth muscle. *Eur Respir J*, Vol. 15, No. 3, (March 2000), pp. 600-616, ISSN 0903-1936

Gunst, S., & Wu, M. (2001). Selected contribution: plasticity of airway smooth muscle stiffness and extensibility: role of length-adaptive mechanisms. *J Appl Physiol*, Vol. 90, No. 2, (February 2001), pp. 741-749, ISSN 0363-6143

Haahtela, T., Malmberg, P., & Moreira, A. (2008). Mechanisms of asthma in Olympic athletes - practical implications. *Allergy*, Vol. 63, No. 6 (June 2008), pp. 685-694, ISSN 0105-4538.

Haas, F., Pasierski, S., Levine, N., Bishop, M., Axen, K., Pineda, H., & Haas, A. (1987). Effect of aerobic training on forced expiratory airflow in exercising asthmatic humans. *J Appl Physiol*, Vol. 63, No. 3, (September 1987), pp. 1230-1235, ISSN 0363-6143

Hallstrand, T.S., Bates, P.W., & Schoene, R.B. (2000). Aerobic conditioning in mild asthma decreases the hyperpnea of exercise and improves exercise and ventilatory capacity. *Chest*, Vol. 118, No. 5, (November 2000); pp.1460-1469, ISSN 0012-3692

Hallstrand, T.S., Moody, M.W., Aitken, M.L., & Henderson, W.R. Jr. (2005a). Airway immunopathology of asthma with exercise-induced bronchoconstriction. *J Allergy Clin Immunol*, Vol. 116, No. 3, (September 2005), pp. 586-593, ISSN ISSN 0091-6749

Hallstrand, T.S., Moody, M.W., Wurfel, M.M., Schwartz, L.B., Henderson, W.R. Jr, & Aitken, M.L. (2005b). Inflammatory basis of exercise-induced bronchoconstriction. *Am J Respir Crit Care Med*, Vol. 172, No. 6, (15 September 2005), pp. 679-686, ISSN 1073-449X

Hallstrand, T.S., & Henderson, W.R. Jr. (2010). An update on the role of leukotrienes in asthma. *Curr Opin Allergy Clin Immunol*, Vol. 10, No. 1, (February 2010), pp. 60-66, ISSN 1528-4050

Hashimoto, S., Matsumoto, K., Gon, Y., Nakayama, T., Takeshita, I. & Horie, T. (1999). Hyperosmolarity-induced interleukin-8 expression in human bronchial epithelial cells through p38 mitogen-activated protein kinase. *Am J Respir Crit Care Med*, Vol. 159, No. 2, (February 1999), pp. 634-640, ISSN 1073-449X

Hashimoto, S., Gon, Y., Matsumoto, K., Takeshita, I., Maruoka, S. & Horie, T. (2000). Inhalant corticosteroids inhibit hyperosmolarity-induced, and cooling and rewarming-induced interleukin-8 and RANTES production by human bronchial epithelial cells. *Am J Respir Crit Care Med*, Vol 162, No. 3 Pt 1, (September 2000), pp. 1075-1080, ISSN 1073-449X

Helenius, I.J., Rytila, P., Metso, T., Haahtela, T., Venge, P. & Tikkanen, H.O. (1998a). Respiratory symptoms, bronchial responsiveness, and cellular characteristics of induced sputum in elite swimmers. *Allergy*, Vol. 53, No. 4, (April 1998), pp. 346-352, ISSN 0105-4538

Helenius, I.J., Tikkanen, H.O., Sarna, S., Haahtela, T. (1998b). Asthma and increased bronchial responsiveness in elite athletes: atopy and sport event as risk factors. *J Allergy Clin Immunol*, Vol. 101, No. 5, (May 1998), pp. 646-652, ISSN 0091-6749

Helenius, I.J., & Haahtela, T. (2000). Allergy and asthma in elite summer sports athletes. *J Allergy Clin Immunol*, Vol. 106, No. 3, (March 2000), pp. 444-452, ISSN 0091-6749

Helenius I., Rytilä, P., Sarna, S., Lumme, A., Helenius, M., Remes, V., & Haahtela, T. (2002). Effect of continuing or finishing high-level sports on airway inflammation, bronchial hyperresponsiveness, and asthma: A 5-year prospective follow-up study of 42 highly trained swimmers. *J Allergy Clin Immunol*, Vol. 109, No. 6, (June 2002), pp. 962-968, ISSN 0091-6749

Hermans, C., Knoops, B., Vieding, M., Arsalane, K., Toubeau, G., Famagne, P. & Bernard, A. (1999). Clara cell protein as marker of Clara cell damage and bronchoalveolar blood barrier permeability. *Eur Respir J*, Vol. 13, No. 5, (May 1999), pp. 1014-1021, ISSN 0903-1936

Hewitt, M., Creel, A., Estell, K., Davis, I.C. & Schwiebert, L.M., (2009). Acute exercise decreases airway inflammation, but not responsiveness, in an allergic asthma model. *Am J Respir Cell Mol Biol*, Vol. 40, No. 1, (January 2009), pp. 83–89, ISSN 1044-1549

Hewitt, M., Estell, K., Davis, I.C. & Schwiebert, L.M., (2010). Repeated bouts of moderate intensity aerobic exercise reduce airway reactivity in a murine asthma model. *Am J Respir Cell Mol Biol*, Vol. 42, No. 2, (February 2010), pp. 243–249, ISSN 1044-1549

Hirayama, F., Lee, A.H., & Hiramatsu, T. (2010). Life-long physical activity involvement reduces the risk of chronic obstructive pulmonary disease: a case-control study in Japan. *J Phys Act Health* Vol. 7, No. 5, (September 2010), pp. 622-626, ISSN 1543-3080

Holzer, K., Anderson, S.D., Chan, H.K., & Douglass, J. (2003). Mannitol as a challenge test to identify exercise-induced bronchoconstriction in elite athletes. *Am J Respir Crit Care Med*, Vol. 167, No. 4, (February 15, 2003), pp. 534-537

Hulks, G., Mohammed, A.F., Jardine, A.G., Connell, J.M., & Thomson, N.C. (1991). Circulating plasma concentrations of atrial natriuretic peptide and catecholamines in response to maximal exercise in normal and asthmatic subjects. *Thorax*, Vol. 46, No. 11, (November 1991), pp. 824-828, ISSN 0040-6376

Inman, M.D., Watson, R.M., Killian, K.J., & O'Byrne, P.M. (1990). Methacholine airway responsiveness decreases during exercise in asthmatic subjects. *Am Rev Respir Dis*, Vol. 141, No. 6, (June 1990), pp. 1414-1417, ISSN 0003-0805

Kanazawa, H., Asai, K., Hirata, K., & Yoshikawa, J. (2002). Vascular involvement in exercise-induced airway narrowing in patients with bronchial asthma. *Chest*, Vol. 122, No. 1, (July 2002), pp. 166-170, ISSN 0012-3692

Kapsali, T., Permutt, S., Laube, B., Scichilone, N., & Togias, A. (2000). The potent bronchoprotective effect of deep inspiration and its absence in asthma. *J Appl Physiol*, Vol. 89, No. 2, (August 2000), pp. 711-720, ISSN 0363-6143

Karjalainen, E.M., Laitinen, A., Sue-Chu, M., Altraja, A., Bjermer, L. & Laitinen, L.A. (2000). Evidence of airway inflammation and remodeling in ski athletes with and without bronchial hyperresponsiveness to methacholine. *Am J Respir Crit Care Med*, Vol. 161, No. 6, (June 2000), pp. 2086-2091, ISSN 1073-449X

Kippelen, P., Caillaud, C., Coste, O., Godard, P. & Préfaut, C. (2004). Asthma and exercise-induced bronchoconstriction in amateur endurance-trained athletes. *Int J Sports Med*, Vol. 25, No. 2, (February 2004), pp. 130-132, ISSN 0172-4622

Kippelen, P., Caillaud, C., Robert, E., Connes, P., Godard, P. & Préfaut, C. (2005). Effect of endurance training on lung function. *Br J Sports Med*, Vol. 39, No. 9, (September 2005), pp. 617-621, ISSN 0306-3674

Kuo, K.H., Wang, L., Paré, P.D., Ford, L.E., & Seow, C.Y. (2001). Myosin thick filament lability induced by mechanical strain in airway smooth muscle. *J Appl Physiol*, Vol. 90, No. 5, (May 2001), pp. 1811-1816, ISSN 0363-6143

Kyle, J.M., Walzer, R.B., Hanshaw, S.L., Leaman, J.R. & Frobase, J.K. (1992). Exercise-induced bronchospasm in the young athlete: guidelines for routine screening and initial management. *Med Sci Sports Exerc*, Vol. 24, No. 8, (August 1992), pp. 856-859, ISSN 0195-9131

Langdeau, J.B., Turcotte, H., Bowie, D.M., Jobin, J., Desgangé, P., & Boulet, L.P. (2000). Airway hyperresponsiveness in elite athletes. *Am J Respir Crit Care Med*, Vol 161, No. 5, (May 2000), pp. 1479–1484, ISSN 1073-449X

Langdeau, J.B., Turcotte, H., Thibault, G. & Boulet, L.P. (2004). Comparative prevalence of asthma in different groups of athletes: a survey. *Can Respir J*, Vol. 11, No. 6, (September 2004), pp. 402-406, ISSN 1198-2241

Langdeau, J.B., Day, A., Turcotte, H. & Boulet, L.P. (2009). Gender differences in the prevalence of airway hyperresponsiveness and asthma in athletes. *Respir Med*, Vol. 103, No. 3, (March 2009), pp. 401-406, ISSN 0954-6111

Lee, T.H. & Anderson, S.D. (1985). Heterogeneity of mechanisms in exercise induced asthma. *Thorax*, Vol. 40, No. 7, (July 1985), pp. 481-487, ISSN 0040-6376

Leith, D.E., & Bradley, M. (1976). Ventilatory muscle strength and endurance training. *J Appl Physiol*, Vol. 41, No. 4, (October 1976), pp.508-516, ISSN 0363-6143

Loughlin, C.E., Esther, C.R. Jr., Lazarowski, E.R., Alexis, N.E., Peden, D.B. (2010). Neutrophilic inflammation is associated with altered airway hydration in stable asthmatics. *Respir Med*, Vol.104, No. 1, (January 2010), pp. 29-33, ISSN 0954-6111

Lowder, T., Dugger, K., Deshane, J., Estell, K. & Schwiebert, L.M. (2010). Repeated bouts of aerobic exercise enhance regulatory T cell responses in a murine asthma model. *Brain Behav Immun*, Vol. 24, No. 1, (January 2010), pp. 153–159, ISSN 0889-1591

Lumme, A., Haahtela, T., Ounap, J., Rytilä, P., Obase, Y., Helenius, M., Remes, V., & Helenius, I. (2003). Airway inflammation, bronchial hyperresponsiveness and asthma in elite ice hockey players. *Eur Respir J*, Vol. 22, No. 1, (July 2003), pp. 113-117, ISSN 0903-1936

Lund, T.K., Pedersen, L., Anderson, S.D., Sverrild, A. & Backer, V. (2009). Are asthma-like symptoms in elite athletes associated with classical features of asthma?. *Br J Sports Med*, Vol. 43, No. 14, (December 2009), pp. 1131-1135, ISSN 0306-3674

Macklem, P. (1989). Mechanical factors determining maximum bronchoconstriction. *Eur Respir J Suppl*, Vol. 6 (June 1989), pp. 516S-519S, ISSN 0904-1850

Mansfield, L., McDonnell, J., Morgan, W., & Souhrada, J.F. (1979). Airway response in asthmatic children during and after exercise. *Respiration*, Vol. 38, No. 3, (March 1979), pp. 135-143, ISSN 0025-7931

Matsumoto, I., Araki, H., Tsuda, K., Odajima, H., Nishima, S., Higaki, Y., Tanaka, H., Tanaka, M., & Shindo, M. (1999). Effects of swimming training on aerobic capacity and exercise induced bronchoconstriction in children with bronchial asthma. *Thorax*, Vol. 54, No. 3, (March 1999), pp.196-201, ISSN 0040-6376

McFadden, E.R. Jr. (1990). Hypothesis: exercise-induced asthma as a vascular phenomenon. *Lancet*, Vol. 335, No. 8694, (April 1990), pp. 880-883, ISSN 0140-6736

McClean, M.A., Matheson, M.J., McKay, K., Johnson, P.R., Rynell, A.C., Ammit, A.J., Black, J.L., & Berend, N. (2003). Low lung volume alters contractile properties of airway smooth muscle in sheep. *Eur Respir J*, Vol. 22, No. 1, (July 2003), pp. 50-56, ISSN 0903-1936

Mendes, F.A., Gonçalves, R.C., Nunes, M.P., Saraiva-Romanholo, B.M., Cukier, A., Stelmach, R., Jacob-Filho, W., Martins, M.A., & Carvalho, C.R. (2010). Effects of aerobic training on psychosocial morbidity and symptoms in patients with asthma: a randomized clinical trial. *Chest*, Vol. 138, No. 2(August 2010), pp. 331-337, ISSN 0903-1936

Mendes, F.A., Almeida, F.M., Cukier, A., Stelmach, R., Jacob-Filho, W., Martins, M.A. & Carvalho CR. (2011). Effects of aerobic training on airway inflammation in asthmatic patients. *Med Sci Sports Exerc*, Vol. 43, No. 2, (February 2011), pp. 197-203, ISSN 0195-9131

Milanese, M., Saporiti, R., Bartolini, S., Pellegrino, R., Baroffio, M., Brusasco, V., & Crimi, E. (2009). Bronchodilator effects of exercise hyperpnea and albuterol in mild-to-moderate asthma. *J Appl Physiol*, Vol. 107, No. 2, (August 2009), pp. 494-499, ISSN 0363-6143

Moreira, A., Delgado, L., Palmares, C., Lopes, C., Jacinto, T., Rytilä, P., Silva, J.A., Castel-Branco, M.G., & Haahtela, T. (2008). Competitive swimmers with allergic asthma show a mixed type of airway inflammation. *Eur Respir J* Vol. 31, No. 5, (May 2008), pp. 1139-1141, ISSN 0903-1936

Moreira, A., Delgado, L., & Carlsen, K.H. (2011a). Exercise-induced asthma : why is it so frequent in Olympic athletes ? *Expert Rev Resp Med*, Vol. 5, No. 1, (February 2011), pp.1–3, ISSN 1747-6348

Moreira, A., Palmares, C., Lopes, C. & Delgado, L. (2011b). Airway vascular damage in elite swimmers. *Respir Med*, (2011 Jun 11), Epub ahead of print, DOI: 10.1016/j.rmed.2011.05.011, ISSN 0954-6111

Morici, G., Bonsignore, M.R., Zangla, D., Riccobono, L., Profita, M., Bonanno, A., Paternò, A., Di Giorgi, R., Mirabella, F., Chimenti, L., Benigno, A., Vignola, A.M., Bellia, V., Amato, G. & Bonsignore, G. (2004). Airway cell composition at rest and after an all-out test in competitive rowers. *Med Sci Sports Exerc*, Vol. 36, No. 10, (October 2004), pp. 1723-1729, ISSN 0195-9131

Munakata, M., Mitzner, W., & Menkes, H. (1988). Osmotic stimuli induce epithelial-dependent relaxation in the guinea pig trachea. *J Appl Physiol*, Vol. 64, No. 1, (January 1988), pp. 466-471, ISSN 0363-6143

Neder, J.A., Nery, L.E., Silva, A.C., Cabral, A.L., & Fernandes, A.L. (1999). Short-term effects of aerobic training in the clinical management of moderate to severe asthma in children. *Thorax*, Vol. 54, No. 3, (March 1999), pp. 202-206, ISSN 0040-6376

Parson, J.P., & Mastronarde, J.G. (2005). Exercise-induced bronchoconstriction in athletes. *Chest*, Vol. 128, No. 12 (December 2005), pp. 3966-3974, ISSN 0012-3692

Parsons, J.P., Baran, C.P., Phillips, G., Jarjoura, D., Kaeding, C., Bringardner, B., Wadley, G., Marsh, C.B. & Mastronarde, J.G. (2008). Airway inflammation in exercise-induced bronchospasm occurring in athletes without asthma. *J Asthma*, Vol.45, No. 5, (June 2008), pp. 363-367, ISSN 0277-0903

Parsons, J.P. (2009). Exercise-induced bronchospasm: symptoms are not enough. *Expert Rev Clin Immunol*, Vol. 5, No. 4, (July 2009), pp. 357-359, ISSN 1744-666X

Pastva, A., Estell, K., Schoeb, T.R., Atkinson, T.P. & Schwiebert, L.M., (2004). Aerobic exercise attenuates airway inflammatory responses in a mouse model of atopic asthma. *J. Immunol*, Vol. 172, No. 7, (April 2004), pp. 4520–4526, ISSN 0022-1767

Pedersen, L., Lund, T.K., Barnes, P.J., Kharitonov, S.A. & Backer, V. (2008). Airway responsiveness and inflammation in adolescent elite swimmers. *J Allergy Clin Immunol*, Vol. 122, No. 2, (August 2008), pp. 322-7, 327.e1, ISSN 0091-6749

Piacentini, G.L., & Baraldi, E. (2011). Pro: Swimming in chlorinated pools and risk of asthma. We can now carry on sending our children to swimming pools!. *Am J Respir Crit Care Med*, Vol. 183, No. 5, (1 March 2011), pp. 569-570, ISSN 1073-449X

Pratusevich, V.R., Seow, C.Y., & Ford, L.E. (1995). Plasticity in canine airway smooth muscle. *J Gen Physiol*, Vol. 105, No. 1, (January 1995), pp. 73-94, ISSN 0022-1295

Provost-Craig, M.A., Arbour, K.S., Sestili, D.C., Chabalko, J.J. & Ekinci, E. (1996). The incidence of exercise-induced bronchospasm in competitive figure skaters. *J Asthma*, Vol. 33, No. 1, (January 1996), pp. 67-71, ISSN 0277-0903

Romberg, K., Bjermer, L., & Tufvesson, E. (2011). Exercise but not mannitol provocation increases urinary Clara cell protein (CC16) in elite swimmers. *Respir Med*, Vol. 105, No. 1, (January 2011), pp. 31-36, ISSN 0954-6111

Rundell, K.W., Im, J., Mayers, L.B., Wilber, R.L., Szmedra, L., & Schmitz, H.R. (2001). Self-reported symptoms and exercise-induced asthma in the elite athlete. *Med Sci Sports Exerc*, Vol. 33, No. 2, (February 2001), pp. 208-213, ISSN 0195-9131.

Rundell, K.W. & Jenkinson, D.M., (2002). Exercise-induced bronchospasm in the elite atlete. *Sports Med*, Vol. 32, No. 9, (2002), pp. 583-600, ISSN 0112-1642

Scichilone, N., Permutt, S., & Togias, A. (2001). The lack of the bronchoprotective and not the bronchodilatory ability of deep inspiration is associated with airways hyperresponsiveness. *Am J Respir Crit Care Med*, Vol. 163, No. 2 (February 2001), pp. 413-419, ISSN 1073-449X

Scichilone, N., Morici, G., Marchese, R., Bonanno, A., Profita, M., Togias, A. & Bonsignore, M.R. (2005). Reduced airway responsiveness in nonelite runners. *Med Sci Sports Exerc*, Vol. 37, No. 12, (December 2005), pp. 2019-2025, ISSN 0195-9131

Scichilone, N., Marchese, R., Soresi, S., Interrante, A., Togias, A., & Bellia, V. (2007). Deep inspiration-induced changes in lung volume decrease with severity of asthma. *Respir Med*, Vol. 101, No. 5, (May 2007), pp. 951-956, ISSN 0954-6111

Scichilone, N., Morici, G., Zangla, D., Chimenti, L., Davì, E., Reitano, S., Paternò, A., Santagata, R., Togias, A., Bellia, V. & Bonsignore, M.R. (2010). Effects of exercise training on airway responsiveness and airway cells in healthy subjects. *J Appl Physiol*, Vol. 109, No. 2, (August 2010), pp. 288-294, ISSN 0363-6143

Shaaban, R., Leynaert, B., Soussan, D., Anto, J.M., Chinn, S., De Marco, R., Garcia-Aymerich, J., Heinrich, J., Janson, C., Jarvis, D., Sunyer, J., Svanes, C., Wjst, M., Burney, P.G., Neukirch, F., & Zureik, M. (2007). Physical activity and bronchial hyperresponsiveness: European Community Respiratory Health Survey II. *Thorax*, Vol 62, No. 5, (May 2007), pp. 403-410, ISSN 0040-6376

Silva, R.A., Vieira, R.P., Duarte, A.C., Lopes, F.D., Perini, A., Mauad, T., Martins, M.A., & Carvalho, C.R. (2010). Aerobic training reverses airway inflammation and remodelling in an asthma murine model. *Eur Respir J*, Vol. 35, No. 5, (May 2010), pp. 994-1002, ISSN 0903-1936

Skloot, G., Permutt, S., & Togias, A. (1995). Airway hyperresponsiveness in asthma: a problem of limited smooth muscle relaxation with inspiration. *J Clin Invest*, Vol. 96, No. 5, (November 1995), pp. 2393-2403, ISSN 0021-9738

Speelberg, B., van der Berg, N.J., Oosthoek, C.H., Verhoeff, N.P. & van der Brick, W.T. (1989). Immediate and late asthmatic response induced by exercise in patients with reversible airflow limitation. *Eur Respir J*, Vol. 2, No. 5, (May 1989), pp. 402-408, ISSN 0903-1936

Stenfors, N. (2010). Self-reported symptoms and bronchial hyperresponsiveness in elite cross-country skiers. *Respir Med*, Vol. 104, No. 11, (November 2010), pp. 1760-1763, ISSN 0954-6111

Stirling, D.R., Cotton, D.J., Graham, B.L., Hodgson, W.C., Cockcroft, D.W., & Dosman, J.A. (1983). Characteristics of airway tone during exercise in patients with asthma. *J Appl Physiol*, Vol. 54, No. 4, (April 1983), pp. 934-942, ISSN 0363-6143

Sue-Chu, M., Larsson, L., & Bjermer, L. (1996). Prevalence of asthma in young cross-country skiers in central Scandinavia: differences between Norway and Sweden. *Respir Med*, Vol. 90, No. 2, (February 1996), pp. 99-105, ISSN 0954-6111

Sue-Chu, M., Karjalainen, E.-M., Altraja, A., Laitinen, A., Laitinen, L.A., Næss, A.B., Larsson, L., & Bjermer, L. (1998). Lymphoid aggregates in endobronchial biopsies from young elite cross-country skiers. *Am J Respir Crit Care Med*, Vol. 158, No. 2, (August 1998), pp. 597–601, ISSN 1073-449X

Sue-Chu, M., Larsson, L., Moen, T., Rennard, S.I. & Bjermer, L. (1999). Bronchoscopy and bronchoalveolar lavage findings in cross-country skiers with and without "ski asthma". *Eur Respir J*, Vol. 13, No. 3, (March 1999), pp. 626-632, ISSN 0903-1936

Sue-Chu, M., Karjalainen, E.M., Laitinen, A., Larsson, L., Laitinen, L.A. & Bjermer, L. (2000). Placebo-controlled study of inhaled budesonide on indices of airway inflammation in bronchoalveolar fluid and bronchial biopsies in cross-country skiers. *Respiration*, Vol. 67, No. 4, (April 2000), pp. 417-425, ISSN 0025-7931

Toledo, A.C., Magalhaes, R.M., Hizume, D.C., Vieira, R.P., Biselli, P.J., Moriya, H. T., Mauad, T., Lopes, F.D., & Martins, M.A. (2011). Aerobic exercise attenuates pulmonary injury induced by exposure to cigarette smoke. *Eur Respir J*, (23 Jun, 2011), doi: 10.1183/09031936.00003411, ISSN 0903-1936

Turcotte, H., Langdeau, J.B., Thibault, G., & Boulet, L.P. (2003). Prevalence of respiratory symptoms in an athlete population. *Resp Med*, Vol. 97, No. 8, (August 2003), pp. 955–963, ISSN 0954-6111

Vergès, S., Devouassoux, G., Flore, P., Rossini, E., Fior-Gozlan, M., Levy, P. & Wuyam, B. (2005). Bronchial hyperresponsiveness, airway inflammation, and airflow limitation in endurance athletes. *Chest*, Vol. 127, No. 6, (June 2005), pp. 1935-1941, ISSN 0012-3692

Vieira, R.P., Claudino, R.C., Duarte, A.C.S., Santos, A.B., Perini, A., Faria Neto H.C.C., Mauad, T., Martins, M.A., Dolhnikoff, M. & Carvalho, C.R.F. (2007). Aerobic exercise decreases chronic allergic lung inflammation and airway remodeling in mice. *Am J Respir Crit Care Med*, Vol. 176, No. 9, (November 2007), pp. 871–877, ISSN 1073-449X

Vieira, R.P., de Andrade, V.F., Duarte, A.C.S., Dos Santos, A.B., Mauad, T., Martins, M.A., Dolhnikoff, M. & Carvalho, C.R.F. (2008). Aerobic conditioning and allergic pulmonary inflammation in mice. II. Effects on lung vascular and parenchymal inflammation and remodeling. *Am J Physiol Lung Cell Mol Physiol*, Vol. 295, No. 4, (October 2008), pp. L670–L679, ISSN 1040-0605

Vieira, R.P., Toledo, A.C., Ferreira, S.C., Santos, A.B., Medeiros, M.C., Hage, M., Mauad, T., Martins, Mde. A., Dolhnikoff, M. & Carvalho C.R.F. (2011). Airway epithelium mediates the anti-inflammatory effects of exercise on asthma. *Respir Physiol Neurobiol*, Vol. 175, No. 3, (March 2011), pp. 383-389, ISSN 1569-9048

Voisin, C., Sardella, A., Marcucci, F., & Bernard, A. (2010). Infant swimming in chlorinated pools and the risks of bronchiolitis, asthma and allergy. *Eur Respir J*, Vol. 36, No. 1 (July 2010), pp. 41-47, ISSN 0903-1936

Vorrink, S.N., Kort, H.S., Troosters, T., & Lammers, J.W. (2011). Level of daily physical activity in individuals with COPD compared with healthy controls. *Respir Res* Vol. 12, (22 March 2011), p. 33, ISSN 1465-9921

Yoshikawa, T., Shoji, S., Fujii, T., Kanazawa, H., Kudoh, S., Hirata, K., & Yoshikawa, J. (1998). Severity of exercise-induced bronchoconstriction is related to airway eosinophilic inflammation in patients with asthma. *Eur Respir J*, Vol. 12, No. 4, (October 1998), pp. 879-884, ISSN 0903-1936

WADA (October 18, 2010), available from http://www.wada-ama.org/en/Download-Centers/Medical-info-to-support-TUECs-decisions/Asthma/

Xue, Z., Zhang, L., Liu, Y., Gunst, S.J., & Tepper, R.S. (2008). Chronic inflation of ferret lungs with CPAP reduces airway smooth muscle contractility in vivo and in vitro. *J Appl Physiol*, Vol. 104, No. 3, (March 2008), pp. 610-615, ISSN 0363-6143

12

Aquatic Sports Dermatoses: Clinical Presentation and Treatment Guidelines

Jonathan S. Leventhal and Brook E. Tlougan

NYU School of Medicine, Department of Dermatology New York, NY, USA

1. Introduction

Aquatic sport dermatoses include a variety of skin conditions that occur in athletes who participate in sporting activities in or on the water. Chemicals and microbes inhabiting the aquatic environment are often responsible for the development of these cutaneous conditions. We review common water sports dermatoses and divide them based on activities that occur in saltwater, freshwater and activities outside the water. Some of the water sports represented in the review include swimming, diving, scuba diving, snorkeling and water polo which are mainly based in the water, as well as sailing, rowing, fishing, surfing, whitewater rafting and water-skiing which are based on the water and outside the water. Aquatic sports dermatoses are presented according to their etiology including infectious and organism-related, contact dermatitis and miscellaneous causes. We also describe conditions specifically associated with water sports including sailing, rowing, fishing and surfing. This comprehensive review focuses on the key recognizable clinical features and principles of management of aquatic sports dermatoses. Our aim is to help sports medicine physicians, dermatologists and other health care providers recognize and treat water sport dermatoses in athletes.

2. Freshwater

2.1 Infectious and organism-related

2.1.1 Swimming pool granuloma

Swimming pool granuloma, also known as fish tank granuloma or fish fancier's granuloma is caused by infection with atypical mycobacteria, including *Mycobacterium marinum* and *Mycobacterium scrofulaceum*. Swimmers may be infected from exposure to freshwater or saltwater. Fish, dolphins, snails and water fleas are proposed vectors of disease transmission (Huminer *et al.*, 1986).

Clinical presentation. Individuals present with verrucous nodules or plaques that occasionally ulcerate approximately 6 weeks after inoculation. The lesions commonly manifest in the upper extremities, particularly the fingers, and may spread linearly demonstrating a sporotrichoid pattern along the route of lymphatics (Ang *et al.*, 2000; Gluckman, 1995). Diagnosis is best made with biopsy of skin lesions for histopathologic examination and culture. Rare and severe infection may occur from direct extension from the skin to the bones and joints resulting in osteomyelitis, arthritis and tenosynovitis

(Clark *et al.*, 1990; Collins *et al.*, 1988). Disseminated infection typically occurs in immunosuppressed hosts and may be fatal (Tchornobay *et al.*, 1992; King *et al.*, 1983).

Management. The first-line treatment includes oral clarithromycin 500 mg twice daily for 6 weeks. Oral minocycline 100 mg twice daily may also be used, but mycobacterial resistance to minocycline has been reported (Adams, 2006).

2.1.2 Hot tub folliculitis

Hot tub folliculitis, also known as *Pseudomonas aeruginosa* folliculitis and "splash rash" is an infection caused by *Pseudomonas aeruginosa* after exposure to contaminated water. Swimming pools, showers, baths, hot tubs, saunas and water slides are associated with this condition (Chandrasekar *et al.*, 1984; Fox & Hambrick, 1984; Zichini *et al.*, 2000).

Clinical presentation. Individuals present with follicular-based macules and papulopustules that typically manifest 8–48 hours after exposure with contaminated water (Fox & Hambrick, 1984; Highsmith *et al.*, 1985). The lesions usually heal without scaring, although post-inflammatory hyperpigmentation and desquamation of the skin may occur less commonly. Systemic symptoms occasionally occur and include fever, malaise, sore throat, otalgia, lymphadenopathy, nausea and diarrhea. Rare complications which typically occur in immunosuppressed individuals include abscess formation, ecythma gangrenosum, subcutaneous nodules and cellulitis (Berger *et al.*,1995; El Baze *et al.*, 1985). Use of a Wood's lamp may help detect hot tub folliculitis in the early stages by visualizing a pale green fluorescence (Amichai *et al.*, 1994).

Management. In immunocompetent individuals treatment is not required and infection typically resolves spontaneously in less than 2 weeks. Supportive treatment includes acetic acid 5% compresses used for 20 minutes 2-4 times daily for symptomatic relief (Tlougan *et al.*, 2010a). Only in severe cases should the use of antibiotics be considered.

2.1.3 Diving suit dermatitis

Diving suit dermatitis is an infection caused by *Pseudomonas aeruginosa* serotypes O:10 and O:6, which are different from the serotypes associated with hot tub folliculitis.

Clinical presentation. Individuals present with erythematous papules that are diffusely scattered on the trunk and extremities. Rarely, systemic symptoms may manifest including fever, headache and malaise (Tlougan *et al.*, 2010a).

Management. First-line treatment consists of oral antibiotics such as ciprofloxacin 500 mg twice daily. Preventive methods include cleaning diving suits with 0.45% lactic acid after each use and showering immediately after diving (Tlougan *et al.*, 2010a).

2.1.4 Pitted keratolysis

Pitted keratolysis is an infection caused by *Corynebacterium* or *Kytococcus sedentarius*. This condition is usually seen in individuals who walk barefoot and is associated with excessive sweating (Shelley & Shelley, 1982; Zaias, 1982).

Clinical presentation. Individuals present with superficial pinpoint or ringed erosions with multiple shallow and sharply punched-out (1-3 mm) pits. The lesions have a "dirty" appearance and a foul odor (Tlougan *et al.*, 2010a)

Management. The infection generally responds well to topical or oral erythromycin, topical clindamycin or topical 5% benzoyl peroxide (Pharis *et al.*, 1997). Pitted keratolysis may clear on its own with elimination of excess moisture.

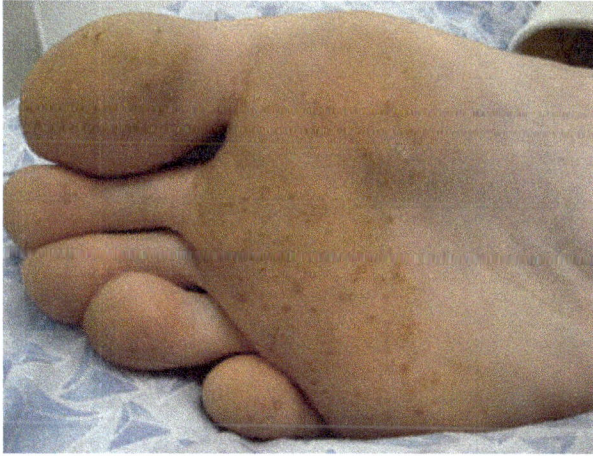

Fig. 1. Pitted keratolysis. Multiple shallow punched-out pits on anterior sole of foot (Tlougan *et al.*, 2010a). Reproduced with permission from *International Journal of Dermatology.*

2.1.5 Bikini bottom
Bikini bottom is a deep bacterial folliculitis typically caused by *Streptococcus* or *Staphylococcus aureus.* It usually occurs in swimmers who wear tight-fitted wet swimwear for prolonged periods of time (Saltzer *et al.*, 1997).
Clinical presentation. Individuals present with firm nodules that manifest along the inferior gluteal crease (Basler *et al.*, 1998).
Management. First-line treatment includes a course of oral antibiotics for 10 days, such as Cephalexin (Basler *et al.*, 1998). Prevention of this condition includes prompt removal of wet swimwear.

2.1.6 Swimmer's Itch
Swimmer's itch, also known as Schistosome dermatitis, clam-digger's itch or cercarial dermatitis, is caused by infection with larvae from the fluke family Schistosomatidae. The condition typically occurs in swimmers exposed to freshwater, but may also occur in saltwater (Mulvihill & Burnett 1990). Rodents and birds are the primary hosts that release ova containing the immature larvae which mature in snails (Wolf *et al.*, 1995). The larvae infect humans through penetration of the skin and eventually die causing an immunologic reaction and sensitization two weeks after initial contact. Further exposures result in lesions within hours (Wolf *et al.*, 1995).
Clinical presentation. Individuals present with multiple erythematous pruritic papules (3-5 mm) with occasional urticarial plaques (Adams, 2006; Hicks, 1977). Systemic symptoms occur rarely and include fever, chills and lymphadenopathy (Cort, 1950; Wall, 1976).
Management. Lesions typically resolve spontaneously within 3 to 7 days, but topical corticosteroids and antihistamines may help relieve pruritus. Only severe cases require systemic corticosteroids (Adams, 2006).

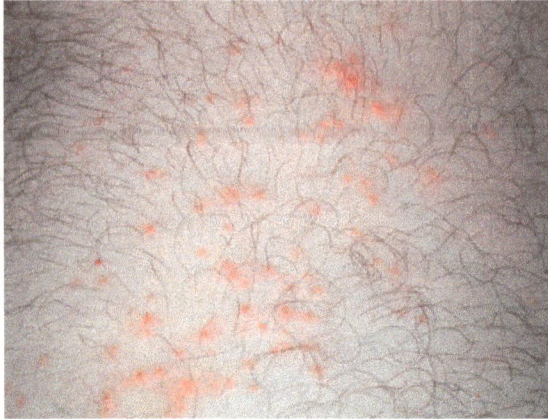

Fig. 2. Swimmer's itch. Scattered erythematous papules on thigh of a swimmer (Tlougan et al., 2010a). Reproduced with permission from *International Journal of Dermatology*.

2.1.7 Molluscum contagiosum

Molluscum contagiosum, also known as "water warts" is a cutaneous viral infection caused by the poxvirus *Molluscum contagiosum* (Gottlieb & Myskowski, 1994). Various studies have documented an association between this infection and water exposure (Niizeki *et al.*, 1984; Weismann *et al.*, 1973).

Clinical presentation. Individuals present with pearly-white or skin-colored papules and nodules that may demonstrate a central dimple or umbilication (Tlougan *et al.*, 2010a).

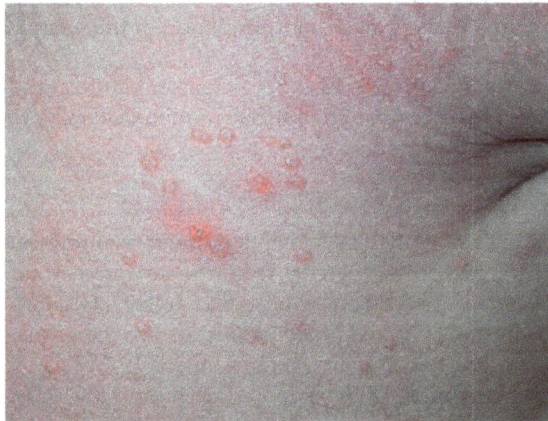

Fig. 3. Molluscum contagiosum. Several 1-2 mm pearly dome-shaped papules with central umbilication (Tlougan *et al.*, 2010a). Reproduced with permission from *International Journal of Dermatology*.

Management. Lesions usually resolve spontaneously without scarring within one year but may persist longer. Therapeutic options to facilitate the resolution of lesions include curettage, liquid nitrogen, trichloroacetic acid and cantharidin. Other off-label options include topical 5-FU or imiquimod (Tlougan *et al.*, 2010a).

2.1.8 Warts

Verrucae or warts are caused by human papillomavirus (HPV) and are common in swimmers and individuals that use communal showers (Gentles & Evans, 1973; Johnson, 1995; Penso-Assathiany *et al.*, 1999).

Clinical presentation. Individuals present with well-defined, papillomatous or verrucous papules with a roughened surface. Plantar warts appear as endophytic papules or plaques of the soles with black specs at the center (Tlougan *et al.*, 2010a).

Management. Therapeutic options include mechanical destruction with liquid nitrogen, laser and curettage. Methods of chemical destruction include salicylic acid, cantharidin and trichloroacetic acid. Athletes may apply imiquimod, 5-FU, squaric acid (SADBE) and diphenylcyclopropenone (DPCP) for self-management of these lesions. (Tlougan *et al.*, 2010a). Recalcitrant warts may be treated with injected *Candida antigen*, mumps antigen or bleomycin. (Tlougan *et al.*, 2010a). Oral cimetidine has been shown to be effective in some studies, although its clinical utility remains debated (Orlow & Paller, 1993; Tlougan et al, 2010a).

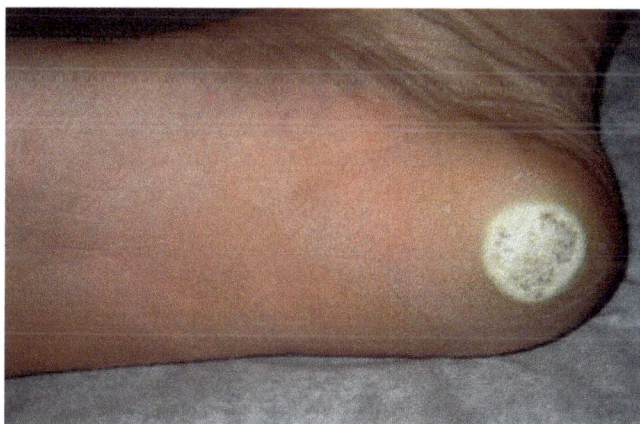

Fig. 4. Verrucae. Plantar wart with roughened surface and black specs at the center (Tlougan et al, 2010a). Reproduced with permission from *International Journal of Dermatology*.

2.1.9 Athlete's foot

Athlete's foot, also known as tinea pedis, is a common cutaneous fungal infection caused by dermatophytes. Infection may be transmitted through swimming pools, pool decks and shower floors (Bolanos, 1991; Kamihama *et al.*, 1997).

Clinical presentation. Individuals typically present with the interdigital subtype that manifests as erythema and scaling with or without pruritus. Other clinical forms include the moccasin subtype with plantar erythema, scaling and hyperkeratosis and the inflammatory subtype with painful bullae or pruritic vesicles (Tlougan et al., 2010a).

Management. First-line therapy includes topical antifungal agents used twice daily to affected areas for one to several months. Systemic antifungal agents such as terbinafine 250 mg daily or itraconazole 200 mg daily for 2 weeks may be required for more extensive or refractory lesions. Infection may be prevented by wearing protective sandals in public showers or pool decks. Athletes may prophylactically apply topical antifungal agents twice weekly to prevent reinfection (Adams, 2006).

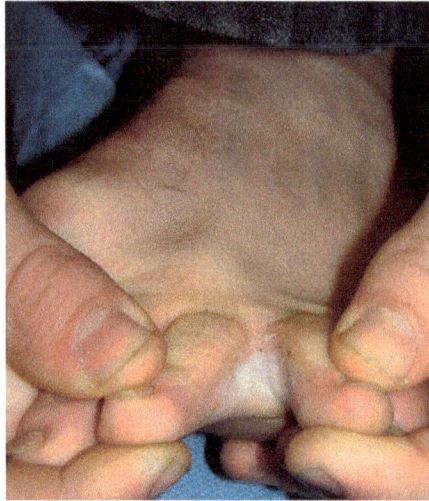

Fig. 5. Athlete's foot. Interdigital subtype of tinea pedis with erythema and scaling between digits (Tlougan *et al.*, 2010a). Reproduced with permission from *International Journal of Dermatology*.

2.2 Contact dermatoses

Contact	Dermatosis	Offending Agent
Allergic	Swim goggles dermatitis	dibutylthiourea (rubber accelerator)
	Nose clip & ear plug dermatitis	rubber accelerator compounds
	Diving mask dermatitis	isopropylparaphenylenediamine (IPPD)
	Wet suit dermatitis	diethylthiourea dibutylthiourea diphenylthiourea ethyl butylthiourea para-tertiary-butylphenol-formaldehyde resin
	Swim fin dermatitis	dibutylthiourea diethylthiourea IPPD
	Swim cap dermatitis	mercaptobenzothiazole
	Pool water dermatitis	bromine chlorine potassium peroxymonosulfate (PPMS)
Irritant	Pool dermatitis	bromine chlorine

Table 1. Freshwater contact dermatoses

2.2.1 Swimming gear

Athletes may develop contact dermatitis to a variety of components found in swimming gear. Swim goggles, nose clips and ear plugs may result in dermatitis from exposure to rubber accelerators with dibutylthiourea (Azurdia & King, 1998; Cronin & Rubber, 1980; Goette, 1984; Romaguiera *et al.*, 1988). Diving mask dermatitis, also known as scuba diver facial dermatitis, may result from exposure to isopropylparaphenylenediamine (IPPD), a rubber antioxidant in face masks (Maibach, 1975; Maibach, 1975; Tuyp, 1983). Swim fin dermatitis may also occur from contact sensitivity to IPPD, in addition to other components including dibutylthiourea and diethylthiourea (Balestrero *et al.*, 1999; Fisher, 1999). Swim cap dermatitis may result from contact sensitivity to mercaptobenzothiazole (Cronin & Rubber, 1980). Other components of swim gear that may elicit a contact allergy include diphenylthiourea, para-tertiary-butylphenol-formaldehyde resin and ethyl butylthiourea found in swim suits, as well as Tego103G, a disinfectant of wet suits (Boehncke *et al.*, 1997; Munro *et al.*, 1989; Nagashima *et al.*, 2003; Reid *et al.*, 1993).

Clinical presentation. Individuals with swim goggles dermatitis present with pruritic, periorbital erythema with vesicles, and yellow exudative lesions in severe cases (Tlougan *et al.*, 2010a). Diving mask dermatitis presents with redness and pruritus over areas of direct contact (Fisher, 1980; Maibach, 1975; Tuyp, 1983). Individuals with contact dermatitis to swim caps, ear plugs and nose clips present with well-defined, erythematous, scaling plaques and occasionally vesicles over areas in direct contact with the offending agent. Wet suit dermatitis manifests as a pruritic, vesicular or eczematous eruption on the neck, trunk and extremities (Tlougan *et al.*, 2010a).

Management. Mainstay treatment for swim goggle dermatitis includes the use of medium-potency topical corticosteroids, while systemic steroids may be required in severe cases. Topical immunomodulators may also be effective in mild and chronic conditions (Tlougan *et al.*, 2010a). For contact allergies to other types of swim gear described above, avoidance of the offending allergen and use of silicone based gear is recommended (Fisher, 1980; Goette, 1984; Taylor & Rubber, 1986).

2.2.2 Pool and pool water dermatitis

Pool dermatitis is an irritant dermatitis to chemicals in swimming pools, particularly chlorine and bromine.

Fig. 6. Pool dermatitis. Eczematous plaques in uncovered areas in a swimmer (Tlougan *et al.*, 2010a). Reproduced with permission from *International Journal of Dermatology*.

One study found that swimmers developed more severe cutaneous eruptions after swimming in brominated pools compared to chlorinated pools (Penny, 1991). In contrast to pool dermatitis, pool water dermatitis is an allergic contact dermatitis to chlorinated or brominated compounds in the water. Potassium peroxymonosulfate (PPMS) which is another decontaminant used in pools and hot tubs may also cause pool water dermatitis (Gilligan et al., 2010).

Clinical presentation. Individuals with pool dermatitis present with pruritic, urticarial or eczematous plaques in uncovered areas of skin (Penny, 1991; Rycroft & Penny, 1983). Individuals with pool water dermatitis present with pruritic, erythematous, scaling plaques in uncovered areas of the skin (Fitzgerald et al., 1995; Sasseville et al., 1999).

Management. Avoidance of the offending irritant and halogenated water is recommended for sensitized athletes (Penny, 1991). Diligent use of emollients is also imperative.

2.3 Miscellaneous
2.3.1 Purpura gogglorum

Purpura gogglorum or periocular purpura induced by goggles is thought to be caused by collision forces, suction trauma or pressure of the goggles on the periocular soft tissue (Jonasson, 1997; Jowett & Jowett, 1997; Metzer & Berlob, 1992).

Clinical presentation. Individuals present with purpura around the eyes.

Management. These lesions usually heal spontaneously. In severe cases with vision changes and extensive swelling and facial tenderness, referral to the emergency department to evaluate for possible fracture of facial bones is warranted (Tlougan et al., 2010a).

2.3.2 Platform purpura

Platform purpura is a skin condition that occurs during a missed dive in which the forces upon entering the pool are transmitted to the skin of the thighs (Tlougan et al., 2010a).

Clinical presentation. Individuals present with symmetrical, erythematous plaques on the thighs that may be painful (Tlougan et al., 2010a).

Management. Supportive care includes nonsteroidal anti-inflammatory drugs and application of warm compresses for 5–10 minutes two or three times daily for pain relief. The lesions typically resolve within a few days (Tlougan et al., 2010a).

2.3.3 Aquagenic pruritus

Aquagenic pruritus occurs after brief exposure to water at any temperature and is associated with mast cell degranulation, elevated blood levels of histamine and local release of acetylcholine in the skin (Greaves, 1992).

Clinical presentation. Individuals present with pruritus or a tingling, burning or stinging sensation after exposure to water without any apparent skin changes. The symptoms last between 10 minutes and a couple of hours (Steinman & Greaves, 1985).

Management. Phototherapy, particularly PUVA and narrow-band UVB may help relieve pruritus, while some patients may respond to antihistamines (Greaves, 1992; Xifra et al., 2005).

2.3.4 Aquagenic, cold and cholinergic urticaria

Aquagenic urticaria is a rare type of physical urticaria that occurs upon contact with any form of water at any temperature (Hide et al., 2000; Shelley & Rawnsley, 1964). In contrast, cold urticaria occurs in athletes exposed to cold water and is also associated with winter sports (Sarnaik *et al.*, 1986). While essential acquired cold urticaria is the most common type of cold urticaria, secondary causes include cryoglobulinemia and connective tissue disorders (Sarnaik *et al.*, 1986). Familial cold autoinflammatory syndrome is another condition that manifests with cold urticaria in addition to periodic fever and joint pain (Hoffman *et al.*, 2001). Cholinergic urticaria is the most common subtype of physical urticaria found in athletes, and is typically induced by physical exertion, exposure to heat or emotional stress (Jorizzo, 1987).

Clinical presentation. Individuals with aquagenic urticaria present with urticarial wheals on any submerged skin surface shortly after contact with water. Occasionally, only a focal urticarial eruption may occur (Shelley & Rawnsley, 1964). Systemic symptoms occur rarely and include headache and respiratory distress (Baptist & Baldwin, 2005; Luong & Nguyen, 1998). Cold urticaria presents with erythematous, edematous papules along cold-exposed skin surfaces that are very pruritic. Individuals may also present with systemic symptoms including anaphylaxis and loss of consciousness which may result in drowning (Sarnaik *et al.*, 1986).Cold urticaria may be differentiated from aquagenic urticaria by placement of an ice cube on the forearm for several minutes, with resulting development of a square urticarial plaque during rewarming of the skin (Blanco *et al.*, 2000). Individuals with cholinergic urticaria typically present initially with itching or burning, with subsequent development of flushing and hives minutes after the onset of physical activity (Jorizzo, 1987). The diagnosis is supported by exercise testing, sauna test or hot bath challenge with a resulting urticarial eruption (Jorizzo, 1987).

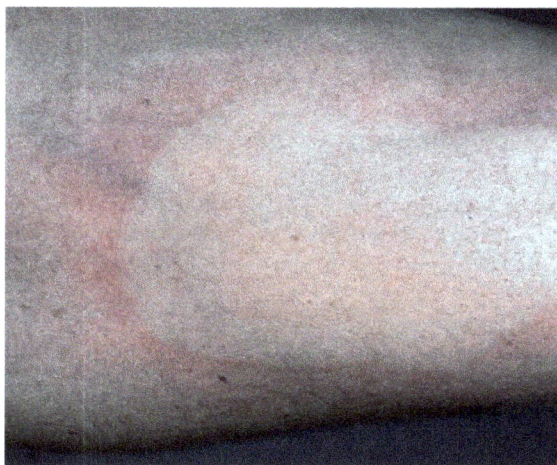

Fig. 7. Cold urticaria. Square urticarial plaque develops after placement of an ice cube on the forearm skin during rewarming of the skin (Tlougan *et al.*, 2010a). Reproduced with permission from *International Journal of Dermatology*.

Management. Individuals with aquagenic urticaria may respond to antihistamines and anticholinergic agents. Other alternative treatment options include PUVA and UVB (Juhlin & Malmros-Enander, 1986; Parker *et al.*, 1992). Individuals with cold urticaria generally respond well to antihistamines (Juhlin, 2004; Zuberbier *et al.*, 2006). Health care providers should also consider secondary causes of cold urticaria including cryoglobulinemia and connective tissue disorders and treat the underlying conditions (Sarnaik *et al.*, 1986). It is recommended that affected athletes wear protective clothing when exposed to cold environments. Traditional therapy for cholinergic urticaria includes antihistamines and leukotriene inhibitors (Otto & Calabria, 2009).

2.3.5 Green hair

Green hair occurs in swimmers with blonde, gray or white hair after exposure to copper in pool water. Frequent hot air drying, brushing, sun exposure, peroxide bleaching and use of alkaline or tar shampoos increases the likelihood of developing green hair (Carson, 1977; Holmes & Goldsmith, 1974).

Clinical presentation. Individuals present with green-colored hair after swimming (Goette, 1978).

Management. Effective treatment options for green hair include 3-5% hydrogen peroxide and copper chelating shampoos (Adams, 2001).

2.3.6 Swimmer's shoulder

Swimmer's shoulder typically occurs during the crawl stroke in which the athlete's chin rubs against the shoulder while turning the head to breathe, with the development of irritation dermatitis (Koehn, 1991).

Clinical presentation. Individuals present with erythematous and slightly roughened plaques on the anterior aspect of the shoulder after swimming (Tlougan *et al.*, 2010a).

Management. Lesions typically heal without treatment, while application of petroleum jelly or polysporin ointment may provide additional relief (Tlougan *et al.*, 2010a).

2.3.7 Pool palms

Pool palms describe a type of frictional dermatitis resulting from repetitive rubbing of the skin surfaces against rough surfaces in the pool (Blauvelt *et al.*, 1992; Wong & Rogers, 2007).

Clinical presentation. Individuals present with symmetric erythematous plaques on the convexities of the palmar hands and fingers (Lacour, 1995).

Management. This condition usually resolves spontaneously after cessation of the irritating activity (Tlougan *et al.*, 2010a).

3. Saltwater

3.1 Infectious and organism-related
3.1.1 Cnidarial dermatoses

Cnidarial dermatoses result from contact with marine invertebrates of the phylum *Cnidaria*. These organisms contain nematocysts on their tentacles which may pierce the skin and release toxins that may result in cutaneous as well as systemic reactions. Several organisms known to affect water athletes and swimmers include Portuguese man-of-war, jelly fish, sea anemones, fire corals and red sea corals.

Clinical presentation. Individuals stung by Portuguese man-of-war present with pain after the initial sting, followed by development of a pruritic, erythematous, urticarial eruption that subsides after a few days. Violaceous lesions and vesicles occasionally occur, while systemic symptoms including anaphylaxis are rare (Adams, 2006). Similarly, jellyfish stings present with initial stinging sensation followed by urticarial or papulovesicular lesions in a linear distribution (Burnett, 1992; Currie & Jacups, 2005).Delayed reactions including hyperpigmentation, lipodystrophy, keloid-like scars and erythema nodosum may result, while severe reactions including respiratory distress and cardiac arrest rarely occur (Burnett *et al.*, 1986; Manowitz & Rosenthal, 1979; Tamanaha & Izumi, 1996; Veraldi & Carrera, 2000).

Individuals stung by sea anemones present with an initial stinging or burning sensation with erythema, edema, petechial hemorrhages and ecchymoses. Eventually, an erythematous, papulovesicular eruption develops and local necrosis, ulceration and desquamation may occur (Halstead, 1988). Bathing or showering exacerbates the stinging or burning sensation. Severe side effects include acute renal failure and fulminant hepatic failure (Garcia *et al.*, 1994; Mizuno *et al.*, 2000). Seabather's eruption results from contact with larvae of the adult sea anemone and the thimble jellyfish and presents similarly with systemic symptoms occurring in up to 10% of cases. (Freudenthal & Joseph, 1993; MacSween & Williams, 1996; Sams, 1949; Tomchik *et al.*, 1993).

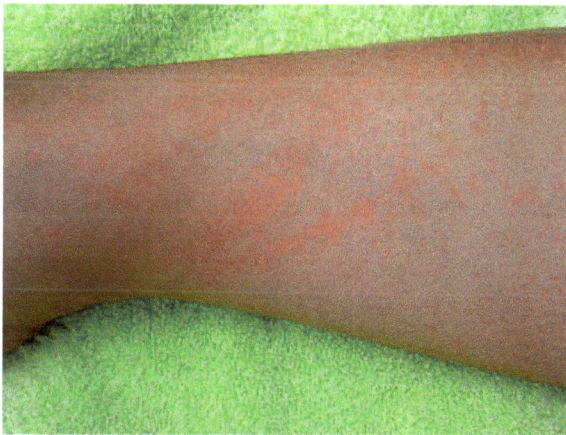

Fig. 8. Jellyfish sting. Linear erythematous plaques, which may be vesicular or urticarial (Tlougan *et al.*, 2010b). Reproduced with permission from *International Journal of Dermatology*.

Individuals stung by the fire coral present with erythematous, burning lesions caused by formic acid on the coral's outer shell. Individuals stung by the red soft coral present with urticarial eruption of the hands and arms with vesicular-bullous lesions, in addition to conjunctivitis, rhinitis and asthma from release of a toxin (Addy, 1991; Canarasa *et al.*, 1993; Fisher, 1999; Miracco *et al.*, 2001; Onizuka *et al.*, 2001).

Management. Supportive care for Cnidarial dermatoses includes application of warm compresses, topical corticosteroids and antihistamines for symptomatic relief. Some authors recommend applying sand to the affected areas to facilitate removal of the nematocysts. Severe anaphylactic reactions require epinephrine. Clinicians should consider pain management and tetanus prophylaxis as well (Tlougan *et al.*, 2010b).

For jellyfish stings, application of vinegar may provide relief. Some authors recommend prompt placement of meat tenderizer to help inactive toxins (Freiman *et al.*, 2004). It is important to note that swimmers should not immerse themselves in freshwater after being stung by saltwater Cnidaria because this may activate nematocysts (Tlougan *et al.*, 2010b). Treatment of fire coral dermatitis includes application of ammonium to neutralize formic acid (Tlougan *et al.*, 2010b).

3.1.2 Echinodermata dermatoses

Echinodermata dermatoses result from contact with marine invertebrates from the phylum *Echinodermata*. Organisms which may result in injury to aquatic athletes and swimmers include sea stars, sea urchins and sea cucumbers.

Clinical presentation. Individuals in contact with the spines of seastars may present with puncture wounds and a burning sensation which may persist for one month (Auerbach, 1991). Contact with sea urchin spines may result in a painful puncture wound with surrounding erythema and edema, while broken spines may remain lodged in the skin. Rarely, tenosynovitis and systemic reactions including nausea, syncope and respiratory distress may occur (Baden, 1987). Contact with sea cucumbers may present as a burning irritant dermatitis. The sea cucumber toxin holothurin, a potent cardiac glycoside, may cause a chemical conjunctivitis and even blindness, while ingestion may result in death (Tlougan *et al.*, 2010b).

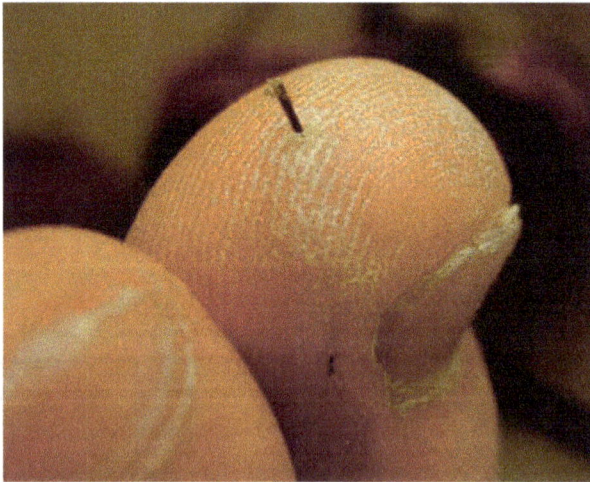

Fig. 9. Sea urchin spine. Spine punctured through the skin with resulting pain, redness and swelling (Tlougan *et al.*, 2010b). Reproduced with permission from *International Journal of Dermatology*.

Management. Symptomatic relief for individuals affected by seastars and sea urchins includes warm compresses, topical corticosteroids and antihistamines. Anaphylaxis should be promptly treated with epinephrine. Athletes affected by sea cucumbers should immediately irrigate the wound with warm water, soap, vinegar or isopropyl alcohol to rinse off the holothurin toxin. Healthcare providers should treat eye injury with topical anesthesia, irrigation and consultation with an ophthalmologist (Tlougan *et al.*, 2010b).

3.1.3 Sponge dermatitis

Marine sponge dermatitis results from contact with marine invertebrates of the phylum *Porifera*. Marine sponges with sharp spicules can cause minor abrasions upon contact with swimmers. In addition, marine sponges may cause an irritant dermatitis as well as local and systemic reactions from the production of crinitoxins by some species (Brown & Shepherd, 1992; Sims & Irci, 1979).

Clinical presentation. Individuals present with a stinging sensation followed by pain, pruritus, and swelling shortly after contact with the organism. Severe effects may result from the crinitoxins with cutaneous manifestations including vesiculations, bullae, desquamation, in addition to delayed allergic contact reactions, erythema multiforme and rarely anaphylaxis (Brown & Shepherd, 1992).

Management. Similar to Cnidarial dermatoses, management includes symptomatic relief as described above and epinephrine for anaphylactic reactions (Tlougan et al., 2010b).

3.2 Contact dermatitis
3.2.1 Seaweed dermatitis

Seaweed dermatitis is a type of contact dermatitis that results from irritants produced from *Lyngbya majuscula*, a blue-green alga that is prevalent in the Pacific, Indian, and Caribbean oceans (Chu, 1959; Osborne et al., 2001).

Clinical presentation. Individuals present with blisters and desquamation with associated stinging, burning, or pruritic sensation within 24 hours after contact (Gauer & Arnold, 1961; Izumi & Moore, 1987). The lesions progress to an erythematous dermatitis that commonly surrounds the perineal and perianal areas lasting for about one week. Ingestion or inhalation of the irritants may result in burning of the upper gastrointestinal tract and respiratory irritation (Anderson et al., 1988; Marshall & Vogt, 1994).

Management. Supportive therapy includes symptomatic relief with cool compresses, treatment with topical corticosteroids, antihistamines and analgesics (Izumi & Moore, 1987).

4. On the water

4.1 Sailing/rowing
4.1.1 Pulling boat hands

Pulling boat hands is due to a combination of mechanical injury and exposure to cold, and is usually seen in sailors, rowers and crew team members (Toback et al., 1985). There is a strong association between this condition and Raynaud's phenomenon, which causes pallor and numbness of the distal digits with resulting color changes from white to blue to red (Toback et al., 1985).

Clinical presentation. Individuals present with erythematous papules, macules, nodules and blisters that may be painful and pruritic. The lesions typically manifest over the distal dorsal aspect of the hands and proximal phalanges, with sparing of the skin over the metacarpophalangeal (MCP) joints and fingertips (Tlougan et al., 2010c).

Management. The mainstay treatment includes topical corticosteroids, while supportive care includes use of moisturizers, gloves and freshwater soaks (Tlougan et al., 2010c).

4.1.2 Sailor's marks

Sailor's marks are associated with repetitive contact and friction between the rope and hands of sailors, with resulting thickening of the skin (Unal et al., 2005).

Clinical presentation. Individuals present with hyperkeratotic thickening of the superficial skin, with band-shaped calluses that manifest bilaterally on the dorsolateral and palmar regions of the first MCP joint and the mediopalmar site of the fifth MCP joint (Tlougan *et al.*, 2010c).

Management. Prevention of the condition includes wearing protective gloves while sailing (Tlougan *et al.*, 2010c).

4.1.3 Rowing blisters
Rowing blisters result from friction between rower's hands and the oar handles (Rumball *et al.*, 2005).

Clinical presentation. Individuals present with painful blisters that typically manifest on the anterior surfaces of the fingers and palms (Tlougan *et al.*, 2010c).

Management. Treatment consists of supportive care of the blisters by draining the lesions without disruption of the roof of the blister up to three times in the first day, and application of petroleum jelly and occlusive dressing (Tlougan *et al.*, 2010c).

4.2 Fishing
4.2.1 Fishing rod dermatitis
Fishing rod dermatitis is a contact dermatitis that results from exposure to isopropylparaphenylenediamine (IPPD) or other closely related components of carbon-fiber fishing rods (Minciullo *et al.*, 2004).

Clinical presentation. Individuals present with unilateral erythematous, scaly hand plaques (Tlougan *et al.*, 2010c).

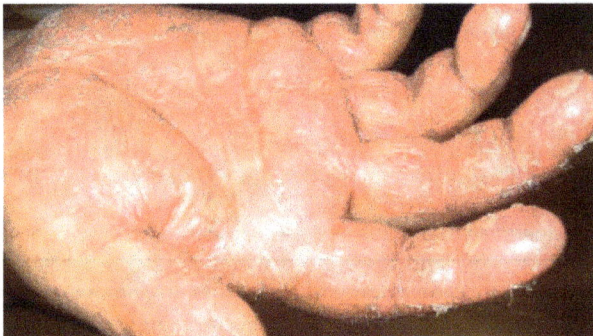

Fig. 10. Fishing rod dermatitis. Erythematous, scaly plaques on the hand (Tlougan *et al.*, 2010c). Reproduced with permission from *International Journal of Dermatology*.

Management. Treatment consists of topical corticosteroids and oral antihistamines. Preventive methods include using a protective cover and insulating tape over the fishing handles and avoidance of IPPD fishing rods (Tlougan *et al.*, 2010c).

4.2.2 Live fish bait allergy
Live fish bait allergy occurs from exposure to the insects and worms used as fish bait. Contact dermatitis may result from exposure to various species of worms such as *Lumbrinereis latreilli*, *Nereis versicolor* and *Chironomus thummi thummi*, as well as larvae of the maggot *Calliphora*

vomitoria (Camarasa & Serra-Baldrich, 1993; De Jaegher & Goossens, 1999; Janssens *et al.*, 1995; Usamentiaga *et al.*, 2005; Virgili *et al.*, 2001). Additionally, fisherman may develop allergic contact dermatitis to azo compounds used to dye maggots (Warren & Marren, 1997).
Clinical presentation. Individuals typically present with bilateral pruritus and edema of the hands, and occasionally with hyperkeratotic lesions of the thumbs and index fingers (Virgili *et al.*, 2001). Fish bait allergy may cause an urticarial eruption, respiratory reactivity or rhinoconjunctivitis (Bernstein *et al.*, 1983; Siracusa *et al.*, 1994).
Management. Individuals gradually improve with avoidance of the offending allergens (Tlougan *et al.*, 2010c).

4.2.3 Erysipeloid

Erysipeloid, also known as "fish poison", "shrimp poison", "crab poison" and "scallop poison" is a bacterial infection of traumatized skin by *Erysipelothrix rhusiopathiae*, mostly seen in fisherman (Burke *et al.*, 2006; Reboli & Farrar, 1989). Infection most commonly results in localized cutaneous disease, while disseminated cutaneous disease and generalized systemic infections may occur as well (Barnett *et al.*, 1983).
Clinical presentation. Patients typically present with well-circumscribed, violaceous, edematous plaques on the fingers and hands that are painful and tender to palpation. The lesions generally display central clearing over time and vesicles may develop as well (Gorby & Peacock, 1998; Reboli & Farrar, 1989). Systemic infection may manifest with constitutional symptoms such as fever and malaise, as well as septicemia, arthritis, empyemas, endocarditis and cerebral abscesses (Gorby & Peacock, 1998; Reboli & Farrar, 1989).
Management. Mainstay treatment of localized cutaneous and diffuse cutaneous forms of disease includes a one week course of penicillin (Varella & Nico, 2005). Severe systemic reations require larger doses of penicillin G (Reboli & Farrar, 1989). Erythromycin may be used in individuals with penicillin allergy.

4.2.4 Rubber boot dermatitis

Rubber boot dermatitis is an allergic contact dermatitis that fisherman develop after exposure to rubber fishing boots (Ross, 1969).
Clinical presentation. Individuals present with a diffuse eczematous eruption throughout the leg. If the lesions progress without treatment, a pompholyx-like eruption may manifest on the palms and soles with scaling, thickening, fissures and exfoliation of the skin (Tlougan *et al.*, 2010c).
Management. Topical corticosteroids and antihistamines are the mainstay treatment. Oral steroids may be required for severe infections. Prevention includes avoidance of rubber boots in sensitized fisherman (Tlougan *et al,* 2010c).

4.3 Surfing
4.3.1 Surfer's nodules

Surfer's nodules are a type of athlete's nodules and occur from repetitive contact and pressure between the surfboard and surfer's bony prominences such as the knees and ankles (Basler., 1989; Erickson & Von Gemmingen, 1967). Some authors also propose that this condition may represent a foreign body reaction to sand or other foreign material (Pharis *et al.*, 1997).
Clinical presentation. Individuals usually present with nontender, fibrotic nodules on the pretibial surface of the leg or the mid-dorsum of the foot (Cohen *et al.*, 1990).

Management. Treatment consists of topical keratolytics such as salicylic acid and lactic acid. Other therapeutic modalities include intralesional corticosteroids, topical corticosteroids and excision of the lesions (Adams *et al.*, 2006). Prevention of this condition includes the use of protective padding on the knees and ankles (Cohen *et al.*, 1990).

4.3.2 Surf rider's dermatitis

Surf rider's dermatitis is a type of irritant contact dermatitis that is generally seen in surfers and users of belly boards, boogie boards and body boards. Friction, shearing forces and pressure between the athlete's body and the surfing board contribute to the development of the eruption (Bischof, 1995). Allergic reactions to surfing board polymers and wax may also occur (Tennstedt *et al.*, 1981).

Clinical presentation. Individuals present with painful erythematous and edematous lesions on the nipples. Surfers may also present with small abrasions and fissures (Tlougan *et al.*, 2010c).

Management. The lesions resolve spontaneously without treatment. Supportive care includes analgesics for pain relief as well as protective dressings and soft clothing (Tlougan *et al.*, 2010c).

5. Conclusion

Aquatic sports dermatoses consist of a variety of cutaneous conditions that occur in athletes who participate in activities on or in the water. Certain conditions are specifically associated with freshwater or saltwater, while others may occur in both settings. Furthermore, participation in particular sporting activities predisposes athletes to certain dermatoses. The approach to athletes with water-related dermatoses consists of taking an appropriate history to recognize the type of water sport, nature of the water exposure with regards to duration in or on the water, saltwater versus freshwater, and any related equipment or contact with organisms. The etiologies of water-related dermatoses are usually infectious and organism-related or result from contact dermatitis. Our review highlights the key physical findings that are most consistent with particular aquatic sports dermatoses. We discuss first-line treatment guidelines and preventive measures that should help guide healthcare providers in the management of athletes with water-related skin conditions.

6. References

Adams BB. Sports Dermatology. New York, NY: Springer, 2006.

Adams BB. Skin infections in athletes. Dermatol Nurs 2008; 20: 39–44.

Addy JH. Red sea coral contact dermatitis. Intl J Derm 1991; 30: 271–273.

Amichai E, Finkelstein E, Halevy S. Early detection of pseudomonas infection using a Wood's lamp (letter). Clin Exp Dermatol 1994; 19: 449.

Anderson B, Sims J, Liang A, et al.. Outbreak of eye and respiratory irritation in Lahaina, Maui, possibly associated with Microcoleus lyngbyaceus. J Environ Health 1988; 50: 205–209.

Ang P, Rattana-Apiromyakij N, Goh CL. Retrospective study of Mycobacterium marinum skin infections. Int J Dermatol 2000; 39: 343–347.

Auerbach PS. Marine envenomations. N Engl J Med 1991; 325: 486–493.

Azurdia RM, King CN. Allergic contact dermatitis due to phenolformaldehyde resin and benzoyl peroxide in swimming goggles. Contact Derm 1998; 38: 234–235.

Baden HP. Injuries from sea urchins. Clin Dermatol 1987; 5: 112–117.

Balestrero S, Cozzani E, Ghigliotti G, et al.. Allergic contact dermatitis from a wet suit. J Eur Acad Dermatol Venereol 1999; 13: 228–229.

Baptist AP, Baldwin JL. Aquagenic urticaria with extracutaneous manifestations. Allergy and Asthma Proc 2005; 26: 217–220.

Barnett JH, Estes AS, Wirman JA, et al.. Erysipeloid. J Am Acad Dermatol 1983; 9: 116–123.

Basler RS. Skin injuries in sports medicine. J Am Acad Dermatol 1989; 21: 1257–1262.

Basler RSW, Basler DL, Basler GC, et al.. Cutaneous injuries in women athletes. Dermatol Nurs 1998; 10: 9–18.

Berger TG, Kaveh S, Becker D, et al.. Cutaneous manifestations of pseudomonas infections in AIDS. J Am Acad Dermatol 1995; 32: 279–280.

Bernstein DI, Gallagher JS, Bernstein IL. Mealworm asthma: clinical and immunologic studies. J Allergy Clin Immunol 1983; 72: 475–480.

Bischof RO. Surf rider's dermatitis. Contact Derm 1995; 32: 247.

Blanco J, Ramirez M, Garcia F, et al.. Localized aquagenic urticaria. Contact Derm 2000; 42: 303–304.

Blauvelt A, Duarte AM, Schachner LA. Pool palms. J Am Acad Dermatol 1992; 27: 92.

Boehncke WH, Wessman D, Zollner TM, et al.. Allergic contact dermatitis from diphenylthiourea in a wet suit. Contact Derm 1997; 36: 271.

Bolanos B. Dermatophyte feet infection among students enrolled in swimming courses at a university pool. Bol Asoc Med P R 1991; 83: 181–184.

Brown CK, Shepherd SM. Marine trauma, envenomation and intoxications. Emerg Med Clin N Am 1992; 10: 385–408.

Burke WA, Griffith DC, Scott CM, et al.. Skin problems related to the occupation of commercial fishing in North Carolina. N C Med J 2006; 67: 260–265.

Burnett JW, Galton GJ, Burnett HW. Jellyfish envenomation syndromes. J Am Acad Dermatol 1986; 14: 100–104.

Burnett JW. Human injuries following jellyfish stings. Md Med J 1992; 41: 509–513.

Burton GRN, et al.. Microbiology for the Health Sciences, 5th edn. Philadelphia, PA: JB Lippincott, 1996; 18.

Camarasa JG, Serra-Baldrich E. Contact urticaria from a worm (Nereis versicolor). Contact Derm 1993; 28: 248–249.

Camarasa JG, Nugues AE, Serra-Baldrich E. Red sea coral contact dermatitis. Contact Derm 1993; 29: 285–286.

Carson TE. Green hair. JAMA 1977; 238: 1025.

Chandrasekar PH, Rolston KVI, Kannangara DW, et al.. Hot tub associated dermatitis due to Pseudomonas aeruginosa. Arch Dermatol 1984; 120: 1337–1340.

Chu GWTC. Seaweed dermatitis apparently caused by a marine alga. Laboratory Observations. Proceedings of the 34th Annual Meeting of the Hawaiian Academy of Science, 1959:19.

Clark RB, Spector H, Friedman DM, et al.. Osteomyelitis and synovitis produced by Mycobacterium marinum in a fisherman. J Clin Microbiol 1990; 28: 2570–2572.

Cohen PR, Eliezri YD, Silvers DN. Athlete's nodules. Sports Med 1990; 10: 198–203.

Collins RJ, Chow SP, Ip FK, et al.. Synovial involvement by Mycobacterium marinum. A histopathological study of 25 culture-proven cases. Pathology 1988; 20: 340–345.

Cort WW. Studies on schistosome dermatitis: XI. Status of knowledge after more than twenty years. Am J Hyg 1950; 52: 251–307.

Cronin E. Rubber. In: CroninE, ed. Contact Dermatitis. New York: Churchill Liingstone, 1980: 752.

Currie BJ, Jacups SP. Prospective study of Chironex fleckeri and other box jellyfish stings in the "Top end"of Australia's Northern Territory. Med J Aust 2005; 183: 631–636.

De Jaegher C, Goossens A. Protein contact dermatitis from midge larvae (Chironomus thummi thummi). Contact Derm 1999; 41: 173.

El Baze P, Thyss A, Caldani C, et al.. Pseudomonas aeruginosa o-II folliculitis. Development into ecthyma gangrenosum in immunosuppressed patient. Arch Dermatol 1985; 121: 873–876.

Erickson JG, Von Gemmingen GR. Surfer's nodules and other complications of surfboarding. JAMA 1967; 201: 134–136.

Fisher AA. Water-related dermatoses: Part I. Cutis 1980; 136: 139–140.

Fisher AA. Sports-related cutaneous reactions: Part II. Allergic contact dermatitis to sports equipment. Cutis 1999; 63: 202–204.

Fitzgerald DA, Wilkinson SM, Bhaggoe R, et al.. Spa pool dermatitis. Contact Derm 1995; 33: 53.

Folster-Holst R, Disko R, Rowert J, et al.. Cercarial dermatitis contracted via contact with an aquarium: case report and review. Br J Dermatol 2001; 145: 638–640.

Fox AB, Hambrick GW Jr. Recreationally associated Pseudomonas aeruginosa folliculitis. Arch Dermatol 1984; 120: 1304–1307.

Freiman A, Barankin B, Elpern DJ. Sports dermatology. Part 2: swimming and other aquatic sports. CMAJ 2004; 171: 1339–1341.

Freudenthal AR, Joseph PR. Seabather's eruption. N Engl J Med 1993; 329: 542–544.

Garcia PJ, Schein RM, Burnett JW. Fulminant hepatic failure from a sea anemone sting. Ann Intern Med 1994; 120: 665–666.

Gauer FH, Arnold HL Jr. Seaweed dermatitis: first report of a dermatitis-producing marine alga. Arch Dermatol 1961; 84: 720–732.

Gentles JC, Evans EG. Foot infections in swimming baths. Br Med J 1973; 3: 260–262.

Gilligan P, Vander Horst A, Zirwas MJ. Allergy to a Hot Tub Water Treatment Chemical: An Unexpectedly Common Cause of Generalized Dermatitis in Men. J Clin Aesthetic Dermatol 2010; 3: 54–56.

Gluckman SJ. Mycobacterium marinum. Clin Dermatol 1995; 13: 273–276.

Goette DK. Swimmer's green hair. Arch Dermatol 1978; 114: 127–128.

Goette DK. Raccoon-like periorbital leukoderma from contact with swim goggles. Contact Derm 1984; 0: 129–131.

Gorby GL, Peacock JE Jr. Erysipelothrix rhusiopathiae endocarditis: microbiologic, epidemiologic, and clinical features of an occupational disease. Rev Infect Dis 1998; 10: 317–318.

Gottlieb SL, Myskowski PL. Molluscum contagiosum. Int J Dermatol 1994; 33: 453–461.

Greaves MW, Handfield-Jones SE. Aquagenic pruritus: pharmacological findings and treatment. Eur J Dermatol 1992; 2: 482–484.

Halstead BW. Poisonous and Venomous Marine Animals of the World. Princeton, NJ, USA: Darwin Press, 1988.

Handzel O, Halperin D. Necrotizing (malignant) external otitis. Am Fam Physician 2003; 68: 309–312.

Harries MJ, Lear JT. Occupational skin infections. Occup Med (Lond) 2004; 54: 441–449.

Headly AW, Knight DE. Scanning sports. Physician Sports Med 1976; 4: 102.

Hicks JH. Swimming and the skin. Cutis 1977; 19: 448–450.

Hide M, Yamamura Y, Sanada S, et al.. Aquagenic urticaria: a case report. Acta Derm Venereol 2000; 80: 148–149.

Highsmith AK, Le PN, Khabbaz RF, et al.. Characteristics of Pseudomonas aeruginosa isolated from whirlpools and bathers. Infect Control 1985; 6: 407–412.

Hoffman HM, Wanderer AA, Broide DH. Familial cold autoinflammatory syndrome: phenotype and genotype of an autosomal dominant periodic fever. J Allergy Clin Immunol 2001; 108: 615–620.

Holmes LB, Goldsmith LA. The man with green hair. N Engl J Med 1974; 291: 1037.

Huminer D, Pitlik SD, Block C, et al.. Aquarium-borne Mycobacterium marinum skin infection. Report of a case and review of the literature. Arch Dermatol 1986; 122: 698–703.

Izumi AK, Moore RE. Seaweed (Lyngbya majuscula) dermatitis. Clin Dermatol 1987; 5: 92–100.

Janssens V, Morren M, Dooms-Goossens A, et al.. Protein contact dermatitis: myth or reality? Br J Dermatol 1995; 132: 1–6.

Johnson LW. Communal showers and the risk of plantar warts. J Fam Pract 1995; 40: 136–138.

Jonasson F. Swimming goggles causing severe eye injuries. Br Med J 1997; 1: 881–883.

Jorizzo JL. Cholinergic urticaria. Arch Dermatol 1987; 123: 455-7.

Jowett NI, Jowett SG. Ocular purpura in a swimmer. Postgrad Med J 1997; 73: 819–820.

Juhlin L, Malmros-Enander I. Familial polymorphous light eruption with aquagenic urticaria: successful treatment with PUVA. Photo-dermatology 1986; 3: 346–349.

Juhlin L. Inhibition of cold urticaria by desloratadine. J Dermatolog Treat 2004; 15: 51–59.

Kamihama T, Kimura T, Hosokawa JI, et al.. Tinea pedis outbreak in swimming pools in Japan. Public Health 1997; 111: 249–253.

King A, Fairley J, Rasmussen J. Disseminated cutaneous Mycobacterium marinum infections. Arch Dermatol 1983; 119: 268–270.

Koehn GG. Skin injuries in sports medicine. J Am Acad Dermatol 1991; 24: 152.

Kush BJ, Hoadley AW. A preliminary survey of the association of Pseudomonas aeruginosa with commercials whirlpool bath waters. Am J Public Health 1980; 70: 279–281.

Lacour JP, El Baze P, Castanet J, et al.. Diving suit dermatitis caused by Pseudomonas aeruginosa: two cases. J Am Acad Dermatol 1994; 31: 1055–1056.

Lacour JP. Dermatite palmaire juvenile des piscines. Ann Dermatol Venereol 1995; 122: 695–696.

Luong KV, Nguyen LT. Aquagenic urticaria: report of a case and review of the literature. Ann Allergy Asthma Immunol 1998; 80: 483–485.

MacSween RM, Williams HC. Seabather's eruption – a case of Caribbean itch. Br Med J 1996; 312: 957–958.

Maibach H. Scuba diver facial dermatitis: allergic contact dermatitis to N-isopropyl-N-phenylpara-phenylenediamine. Contact Derm 1975; 1: 330.

Manowitz NR, Rosenthal RR. Cutaneous-systemic reactions to toxins and venoms of common marine organisms. Cutis 1979; 23: 450–454.

Mantoux F, Hass H, Lacour JP. Wet suit-related Pseudomonas aeruginosa dermatitis in a child. Pediatr Dermatol 2003; 20: 458–459.

Marshall KL, Vogt RL. Illness associated with eating seaweed, Hawaii, 1994. West J Med 1998; 169: 293–295.

Metzer A, Berlob P. Suction purpura. Arch Dermatol 1992; 128: 822–824.

Minciullo PL, Patafi M, Ferlazzo B, et al.. Contact dermatitis from a fishing rod. Contact Derm 2004; 50: 322.

Miracco C, Lalinga AV, Sbano P, et al.. Delayed skin reaction to red sea coral injury showing superficial granulomas and atypical CD30+ lymphocytes: report of a case. Br J Derm 2001; 145: 849–851.

Mizuno M, Nishikawa K, Yuzawa Y, et al.. Acute renal failure after a sea anemone sting. Am J Kidney Dis 2000; 36: E10.

Mulvihill CA, Burnett JW. Swimmer's itch: a cercarial dermatitis. Cutis 1990; 46: 211–213.

Munro CS, Shields TG, Lawrence TM. Contact allergy to Tego 103G disinfectant in a deep-sea diver. Contact Derm 1989; 21: 278–279.

Nagashima C, Tomitaka-Yagami A, Matsunaga K. Contact dermatitis due to para-tertiary-butylphenol-formaldehyde resin in a wetsuit. Contact Derm 2003; 49: 267–268.

Niizeki K, Kano O, Kondo Y. An epidemic study of molluscum contagiosum. Relationship to swimming. Dermatologica 1984; 169: 197–198.

Onizuka R, Kamiya H, Muramoto K, et al.. Purification of the major allergen of red soft coral (Dendronephthya nipponica). Int Arch Allergy Immunol 2001; 125: 135–143.

Orlow SJ, Paller A. Cimetidine therapy for multiple viral warts in children. J Am Acad Dermatol 1993; 28: 794-6.

Osborne NJT, Webb PM, Shaw GR. The toxins of Lyngbya majuscula and their human and ecological effects. Environ Int 2001; 27: 381–392.

Otto HF, Calabria CW. A case of severe refractory chronic urticaria: a novel method for evaluation and treatment. Allergy Asthma Proc 2009; 30: 333-7.

Parker RK, Crowe MJ, Guin JD. Aquagenic urticaria. Cutis 1992; 50: 283–284.

Penny PT. Hydrotherapy pools of the future – the avoidance of health problems. J Hosp Infect 1991; 18(Suppl.1): 535–542.

Penso-Assathiany D, Flahault A, Roujeau JC. Warts, swimming pools and atopy: a case control study conducted in a private dermatology practice. Ann Dermatol Venereol 1999; 126: 696–698.

Pharis DB, Teller C, Wolf JE Jr. Cutaneous manifestations of sports participation. J Am Acad Dermatol 1997; 36: 448–459.

Reboli AC, Farrar WE. Erysipelothrix rhusiopathiae: an occupational pathogen. Clin Microbiol Rev 1989; 2: 354–359.

Reid CM, Van Grutten M, Rycroft RJ. Allergic contact dermatitis from ethylbutylthiourea in neoprene. Contact Derm 1993; 28: 193.

Romaguiera C, Grimalt F, Vilaplana J. Contact dermatitis from swimming goggles. Contact Derm 1988; 18: 178–179.

Ross JB. Rubber boot dermatitis in Newfoundland: a survey of 30 cases. Can Med Assoc J 1969; 100: 13–19.

Rumball JS, Lebrun CM, Di Ciacca SR, et al.. Rowing injuries. Sports Med 2005; 35: 537–555.

Rycroft RJG, Penny PT. Dermatoses associated with brominated swimming pools. BMJ 1983; 287: 462.

Saltzer KR, Schutzer PJ, Weinberg JM, et al.. Diving suit dermatitis: a manifestation of Pseudomonas folliculitis. Cutis 1997; 59: 245–246.

Sarnaik AP, Vohra MP, Sturman SW, et al.. Medical problems of the swimmer. Clin Sports Med 1986; 5: 47–64.

Sams WM. Seabather's eruption. Arch Dermatol Syph 1949; 60: 227–237.

Sasseville D, Geoffrion G, Lowry RN. Allergic contact dermatitis from chlorinated swimming pool water. Contact Derm 1999; 41: 347–348.

Sausker WF. Pseudomonas aeruginosa folliculitis ("splash rash"). Clin Dermatol 1987; 5: 62–67.

Shelley WB, Rawnsley HM. Aquagenic urticaria: contact sensitivity reaction to water. JAMA 1964; 189: 406–408.

Shelley WB, Shelley ED. Coexistent erythrasma, trichomycosis axillaries, and pitted keratolysis: an overlooked corynebacterial triad? J Am Acad Dermatol 1982; 7: 752–757.

Sims JK, Irei MY. Human Hawaiian marine sponge poisoning. Hawaii Med J 1979; 38: 263–270.

Sinnott JT, Trout T, Berger L. The swimming-pool granuloma that wouldn't heal. Hosp Pract 1988; 23: 82–84.

Siracusa A, Bettini P, Bacoccoli R, et al.. Asthma caused by live fish bait. J Allergy Clin Immunol 1994; 93: 424–430.

Spitalny KC, Vogt RL, Witherell LE. National survey on outbreaks associated with whirlpool spas. Am J Public Health 1984; 74: 725–726.

Steinman HK, Greaves MW. Aquagenic pruritus. J Am Acad Dermatol 1985; 13: 91–96.

Taylor JS. Rubber. In: FisherAA, ed. Contact Dermatitis, 3rd edn. Philadelphia: Lea and Febiger, 1986: 603–643.

Tamanaha RH, Izumi AK. Persistent cutaneous hypersensitivity reaction after a Hawaiian box jellyfish sting (Carybdea alata). J Am Acad Dermatol 1996; 35: 991–993.

Tchornobay AM, Claudy AL, Perrot JL, et al.. Fatal disseminated Mycobacterium marinum infection. Int J Dermatol 1992; 31: 286–287.

Tennstedt D, Lachapelle JM. Windsurfer dermatitis from black rubber components. Contact Derm 1981; 7: 160–161.

Tlougan BE, Podjasek JO, Adams BB. Aquatic sports dermatoses: Part 1 - In the Water: Freshwater Dermatoses. Int J Dermatol. 2010; 49: 874-885

Tlougan BE, Podjasek JO, Adams BB. Aquatic Sports Dematoses. Part 2 - In the Water: Saltwater Dermatoses. Int J Dermatol. 2010; 49: 994-1002.

Tlougan BE, Podjasek JO, Adams BB. Aquatic sports dermatoses: Part 3 - On the water. Int J Dermatol. 2010; 49: 1111-1120.

Toback AC, Korson R, Krusinski PA. Pulling boat hands: a unique dermatosis from coastal New England. J Am Acad Dermatol 1985; 12: 649–655.

Tomchik RS, Russell MT, Samant AM, et al.. Clinical perspectives on Seabather's eruption, also known as 'sea lice'. JAMA 1993; 269: 1669–1672.

Tuyp E, Mitchell JC. Scuba diver facial dermatitis. Contact Derm 1983; 9: 334–335.

Unal VS, Sevin A, Dayican A. Palmar callus formation as a result of mechanical trauma during sailing. Plast Reconstr Surg 2005; 115: 2161–2162.

Usamentiaga P, Rodriguez F, Martin-Gil D, et al.. Protein contact dermatitis by fishing bait (Lumbrinereis latreilli). Contact Derm 2005; 53: 236–237.

Varella TCN, Nico MMS. Erysipeloid. Int J Dermatol 2005; 44: 497–498.

Veraldi S, Carrera C. Delayed cutaneous reaction to a jellyfish. Int J Dermatol 2000; 38: 28–29.

Virgili A, Ligrone L, Bacilieri S, et al.. Protein contact dermatitis in a fisherman using maggots of a flesh fly as bait. Contact Derm 2001; 44: 262–263.

Walker N. Molluscum contagiosum and its distribution. Br J Dermatol 1910; 22: 284–286.

Wall RC. An analysis of the current status of the schistosome dermatitis problem in Michigan. Sterkiana 1976; 1: 63–64.

Warren LJ, Marren P. Textile dermatitis and dyed maggot exposure. Contact Derm 1997; 36: 106.

Watts RW, Dall RA. An outbreak of Pseudomonas aeruginosa folliculitis in women after leg-waxing (letter). Med J Aust 1986; 144: 163–164.

Weismann K. An epidemic of molluscum contagiosum originating in an outdoor public swimming-pool. An analysis of 125 consecutive cases. Ugeskr Laegr 1973; 135: 2151–2156.

Wolf P, Schaffler K, Cerroni L, et al.. Cercarial dermatitis in Styria. Z Hautkr 1995; 70: 136–140.

Wong L, Rogers M. Pool palms. Pediatr Dermatol 2007; 24: 95.

Xifra A, Carrascosa JM, Ferrandiz C. Narrow-band ultraviolet B in aquagenic pruritus. Br J Derm 2005; 153: 1233–1234.

Zaias N. Pitted and ringed keratolysis. J Am Acad Dermatol 1982; 7: 787–791.

Zichichi L, Asta G, Noto G. Pseudomonas aeruginosa folliculitis after shower/bath exposure. Int J Dermatol 2000; 39: 270–273.

Zuberbier T, Bindslev-Jensen C, Canonica W, et al. EAACI/GA2LEN/EDF guideline: management of urticaria. Allergy 2006; 61: 321–331.

13

Evaluation of Neural Networks to Identify Types of Activity Among Children Using Accelerometers, Global Positioning Systems and Heart Rate Monitors

Francisca Galindo-Garre and Sanne I. de Vries
TNO
The Netherlands

1. Introduction

There is a growing awareness of the health benefits of physical activity during childhood and adolescence. However, there is still much to be learned about the nature of children's physical activity patterns and the mechanisms underlying these benefits (Rowland, 2007; Twisk, 2001). The physical activity pattern of children is very different from that of adults. Children's physical activity pattern is characterized by frequent spasmodic bursts of short duration (Baquet et al., 2007). They participate in intermittent and unstructured activities and the type of activities children engage in changes as they develop, going from informal active play during early childhood to activities that begin to mirror those of adults during adolescence (Salmon & Timperio, 2007). The understanding of children's physical activity pattern has been hampered by the lack of satisfactory instruments for measuring it.

Children's physical activity has traditionally been measured with self-reports. Self-reports are easily administered, low-cost measurements. However, they do not capture the sporadic short-burst nature of children's physical activity very well (Baquet et al., 2007). Furthermore, self-reports are influenced by recall bias or social desirability. Accelerometers have therefore, in recent times, become the method of choice in physical activity research. These lightweight, unobtrusive devices provide objective information about the frequency, intensity, and duration of physical activity. In most studies, the raw acceleration signal is converted into activity counts. Total or mean activity counts per day and minutes per day spent above a certain intensity threshold are reported. Activity counts are linearly related to energy expenditure. This does not value the richness of accelerometer data (Esliger et al., 2005) because this approach is unable to correctly distinguish between different types of activities with different levels of energy expenditure but that produce similar mean activity counts over time. A solution for this problem is to use not only the mean counts over a certain time period, but also more information about the distribution of these counts (i.e. standard deviation, percentiles) over time.

Recently, statistical models have been developed to identify specific types of physical activities based on a new methodology for processing accelerometer data. The most common classification algorithms have been developed by using the pattern-recognition or "machine-learning" approach. These algorithms are decision trees (Bonomi et al., 2009a, Bonomi et al., 2009b), neural networks (Staudenmayer et al., 2009; De Vries et al., 2011a), and hidden Markov models (Pober et al., 2006), and they use several descriptive statistics calculated over non overlapping segments of accelerometer data as input variables of the models to classify a set of previously registered physical activities. Pattern-recognition approaches have shown to be successful in classifying a number of controlled physical activities among adults and elderly but not many studies apply these approaches to accelerometer data from children.

Our research group has developed several neural network algorithms to classify a number of controlled physical activities among children (De Vries et al., 2011b). The study population was a group of 58 healthy children between the age of 9 and 12 years. The physical activities observed were sitting, standing still, walking, running, rope skipping, playing soccer, and cycling. The children were wearing uni-axial and three-axial accelerometers on the hip and on the ankle. Our results showed that algorithms based on data from three-axial accelerometers worn on the hip performed better (77%) than models based on uni-axial accelerometers (72%), and models based on accelerometers worn on the ankle (57% and 68% for the uni-axial and the three-axial model respectively). However, the developed algorithms could not discriminate between two self-paced speeds of cycling, and there were misclassification errors when classifying the activities playing soccer and cycling. Discriminating between activities performed with different intensity is important to accurately estimate energy expenditure.

The classification performance of pattern-recognition models to discriminate between activities performed with different intensity may be improved by including information about the intensity of physical activities assessed with other sensors than accelerometers such as global positioning systems (GPS) and heart rate monitors. GPS not only provides information about the geographic location of physical activity, but also provides a precise time reference, which can be used in combination with location information to assess velocity. Until now, GPS measurements have only been combined with accelerometer data to provide insight into the location of the physical activity. Maddison and Mhurchu (2009) describe several studies in which accelerometer data are integrated with location GPS data to map participant's neighborhood to identify where physical activity took place, to describe physical activity pattern, and to discriminate between active and inactive transportation. Velocity measurements assessed by GPS can be included in a pattern-recognition model to discriminate between physical activities performed at different speeds (for example, regular walking or cycling versus brisk walking or cycling).

Another objective assessment methods that may be valuable in relation to accelerometer based pattern-recognition models are heart rate monitors. Heart rate monitors do not register physical activity directly; their assessment of physical activity is based on the linear relationship between oxygen uptake and heart rate. When the intensity of an activity increases, the heart rate increases. Eston et al. (1998) showed that models that combine three-axial accelerometer data and heart rate data assessed a better prediction of energy expenditure than models based on three-axial accelerometers alone. Recent evidence suggests that the Actiheart, an integrated accelerometer and heart rate unit, provides a more accurate prediction of children's energy expenditure than either heart rate or accelerometry alone. However, there are no studies combining accelerometer and heart rate data to improve the classification performance of pattern-recognition models. Therefore, the purpose of this study was to examine whether the accuracy of the previously developed

ANN models based on three-axial accelerometer data from the hip might be improved by including more information about the intensity of activities by means of heart rate data or by adding information about the velocity of activities fromGPS.

2. Methods

2.1 Subjects and data collection

Children between the age of 9 and 12 years were recruited from three elementary schools in the Netherlands by sending written information about the purpose and nature of the study to their parents. Finally 58 healthy children (31 boys, 27 girls) were permitted by one of their parents to participate in the study. Data from 52 children (27 boys, 25 girls) had measurements from all devices (accelerometer, GPS and heart rate monitors), and could be used for the analyses. The characteristics of these children are shown in Table 1. Each child was observed by a research assistant while performing a fixed sequence of 20 minutes comprising the following activities: sitting during a writing task, standing, walking, running, rope skipping, playing soccer (i.e., kicking the ball back and forth to the research assistant), regular cycling and brisk cycling. The research assistant recorded the starting and the finishing time of each activity with a stopwatch. In order to imitate real-life, all activities were performed at a self-paced speed. With the exception of sitting, all activities were conducted outdoors in the direct vicinity of the subject's school in similar weather conditions (i.e., no rain, mild wind). For cycling, the subjects used their own bicycle. All subjects wore various measurement instruments: a heart rate receiver unit (Polar Electro S610i, Finland) on the wrist with the transmitter (Polar T61 Coded Transmitter, Finland) worn on the chest, a three-axial ActiGraph accelerometer (ActiGraph GT3X, Pensicola, FL) and a GPS (QSTARZ travel recorder V4.3, Taipei, Taiwan) on the right hip. The ActiGraph is the most validated and widely used accelerometer. It has good reproducibility, validity, and feasibility when used to assess physical activity in children (De Vries et al., 2009). The axes senses of the three-axial accelerometer are vertical, medio-lateral and anterior-poterior direction. Accelerometer data (counts) were collected for each axis in one second epochs. The default sample-rate frequency setting of the GPS (kilometer per hour) is also 1 Hz and the Polar heart rate monitor (beats per minute) sampled at 0.2 Hz (once in every 5 seconds). Children's body height and body weight were measured with a portable stadiometer (Seca 225, Vogel & Halke GmbH & Co, Germany) and a digital scale (Soehnle 62882, Leifheit AG, Germany).

	Boys (n = 27)	Girls (n = 25)	Total (n = 52)
Age (years)	10.9 (0.8)	11.1 (0.7)	11.0 (0.7)
Height (cm)	151.6 (5.7)	148.0 (5.5)	149.9 (5.8)
Weight (kg)	43.5 (9.2)	41.1 (5.4)	42.3 (7.7)
BMI (kg/m^2)	18.8 (3.2)	18.8 (2.5)	18.8 (2.9)

Table 1. Children's characteristics (mean and standard deviation).

2.2 Data processing

When the data collection was complete, the accelerometer data were downloaded to a personal computer and processed using the ActiLifeGT3X software program. GPS data were also downloaded to the computer and processed using Qstarz Travel Recorder PC Utility V4 software. Polar Precision Performance software was used to read the Polar Electro S610i receiver. Next, the data was labeled to one of the eight physical activities according to the starting and the finishing time of each activity. Data from the physical activity sitting were eliminated because this activity was performed inside of the school and the GPS monitors cannot receive an accurate signal inside of buildings. For each of the seven remaining activities the first and the last four seconds of the signals were deleted to eliminate any noise in the data of the transition period between activities. This time buffer was determined by visually inspecting the data set. If the activity (e.g., standing) was carried out several times, the signal was cleaned for each period. The cleared data for the physical activities were then used for further analyses.

2.3 Statistical analysis

First, descriptive statistics were used to characterize the sample and to study signal differences between activity types. Second, correlations between accelerometer counts (3-axes) and GPS data and between accelerometer counts (3-axes) and heart rate data were computed to study the relationship between these variables. Third, differences in the mean accelerometer counts from different axes, GPS speed, and heart rate per child between activities types were tested with an ANOVA. Finally, post hoc tests comparing all pairs of physical activity were performed. Values were considered statistically significant when the two-sided P value was lower than 0.05.

To classify the activity type, four artificial neural networks (ANN) models were developed; a model based on: three-axial accelerometer data (Model 1), three-axial accelerometer data and GPS data (Model 2), three-axial accelerometer data and heart rate data (Model 3), and three-axial accelerometer data, GPS data and heart rate data (Model 4).

ANNs provide a flexible non-linear extension of multiple regression. Feed-forward neural network models were used for the analyses (Ripley, 1996). They consist of a function with a set of predictors or input variables that represent characteristics or statistical summaries describing the signals, a single hidden layer with several hidden units, and one discrete dependent or output variable with several categories that represent physical activity types. Figure 1 presents an illustration of a feed-forward ANN model with five hidden units. The mathematical equations of the model are also provided. If x_i denotes an input variable, y_k an output variable with k categories and f_j and f_k denote the transformation functions, then this model can be written as

$$y_k = f_k\left(\alpha_k + \sum_{j \to k} w_{jk} f_j\left(\alpha_j + \sum_{i \to j} w_{ij} x_i\right)\right) \tag{1}$$

The transformation functions f_j and f_k are taken to be the logistic function

$$f(x) = \frac{\exp(x)}{1 + \exp(x)} \tag{2}$$

since this transformation performed better than other alternative functions. Alternative transformation functions are described in Ripley (1996). The parameters w_{ij} and w_{jk} are known as weights, and they are linear combinations of the inputs or the hidden units. Finally, the intercepts α_j and α_k are known as biases.

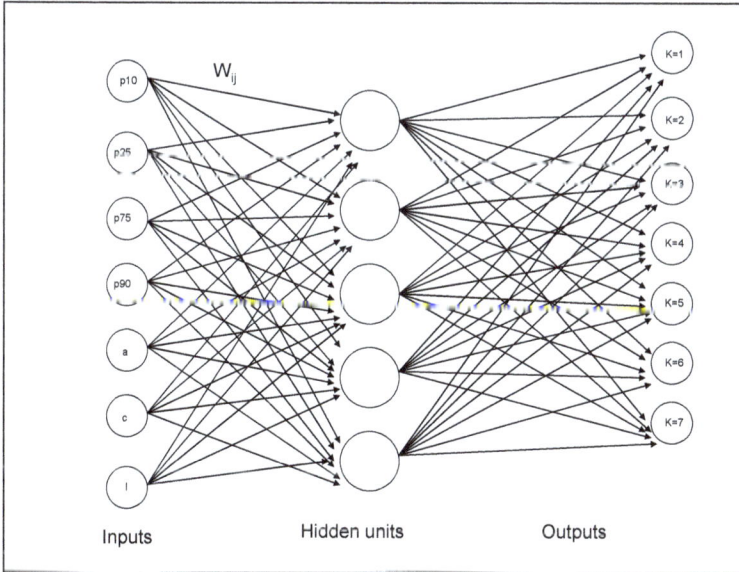

Note: The input variables represent the characteristics of the acceleration signal: p10 = 10th percentile; p25 = 25th percentile; p75 = 75th percentile; p90 = 90th percentile; a = absolute deviation; c = coefficient of variability; and l = lag-one autocorrelation; the hidden units are weighted combinations of the input variables; in the output, each k represents a physical activity.

Fig. 1. Feed-forward neural network model for k=7 activities

Before estimating the ANN models, all signals were segmented into non overlapping intervals of 10 seconds. For heart rate the intervals only contained two data points because the sampling interval was 5 seconds. Next, several signal characteristics or statistical summaries were computed for each 10 second segment. The statistical summaries used in this study were selected from the set of characteristics used by Rothney et al. (2007), Bonomi et al. (2009), and Staudenmayer et al. (2009). For the accelerometer data, we used the following signal characteristics: 10th, 25th, 75th, and 90th percentiles, absolute deviation (i.e., the sum of the absolute difference between each element of the interval and the mean), coefficient of variability (i.e., the ratio of the standard deviation and the mean), and lag-one autocorrelation (i.e., the correlation between consecutive elements within intervals). These statistics were computed for each axis independently. For the GPS signal, the features mean and absolute deviation were included as input variables for the two models with GPS data. For the heart rate signal, only the mean was computed because of the reduced number of data points per interval.

The accuracy of the four models was evaluated by leave-one-subject-out cross-validation (Venables & Ripley, 2002). In this method a set of n-1 subjects was used as a training set and the subject left out was used as a test set. This process was repeated for all n subjects. Feed-forward ANN models with a single hidden layer, five hidden units, and a weight decay[1] equal to 0.006 showed the highest classification accuracy. Next, contingency tables were built to evaluate the classification errors of the models in more detail.

---

[1] In order to use a weight decay as penalty, the input variables were rescaled to range between 0 and 1.

All statistical analyses were performed using the software package R version 2.8.0 (R Development Core Team, 2008). The classification models were developed with the function nnet (Venables & Ripley, 2002). Both R and nnet are freely available.

3. Results

3.1 Descriptive results

Figure 2a-c shows the main output per measurement instrument. Figure 2a reports accelerometer mean counts per second and standard deviations for the x-, y- and z-axes. The figure shows that the differences in mean counts between physical activities are larger for the x-axis than for the other two axes. Furthermore, it can be seen that the standard deviations are larger for the activity rope skipping than for the other activities. The differences in mean counts per second between standing and all other activities are significant for each axis (x-axis: $F(6,330)=401.03$, $p<.001$; y-axis: $F(6,330)=207.7$, $p<.001$; z-axis; $F(6,330)=72.01$, $p<.001$).

Figure 2b represents bar-charts of mean heart rate output and standard deviations in beats per minute (bpm) across children per physical activity. The mean heart rate is higher for standing (129.5 bpm) than for walking (114.9 bpm). This unexpected result most likely occurred because the recovery time of the heart rate returning to resting status between physical activities is larger than the eliminated data of the time buffer of 4 seconds. The activity standing was performed for short intervals of 1 minute after each activity. Because heart rate values for standing are very high, the differences in heart rate between standing and walking and between standing and regular cycling (136.7 bmp) are not significant. The global test was ($F(6,248)=54.02$ $p<.001$).

Figure 2c reports the mean speed in kilometers per hour (km/h) and standard deviation across children for each activity ($F(6,323)=742.4$, $p<.001$). Mean speed is higher for cycling than for all other activities and there is a significant difference between regular cycling (10.3

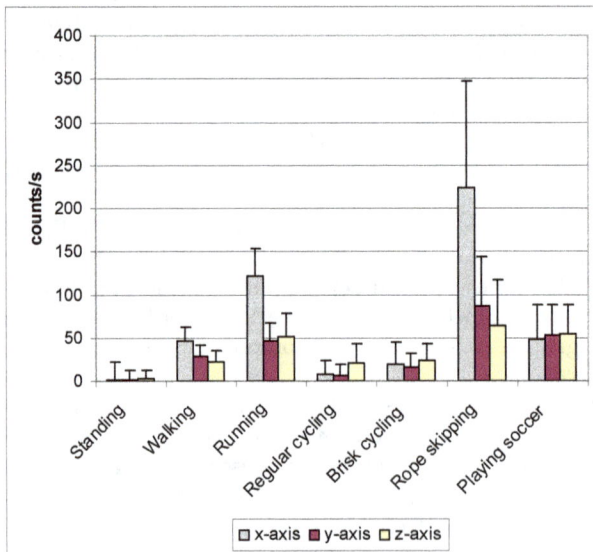

Fig. 2a. Three-axial accelerometer data in counts per second for seven physical activities (mean and standard deviation)

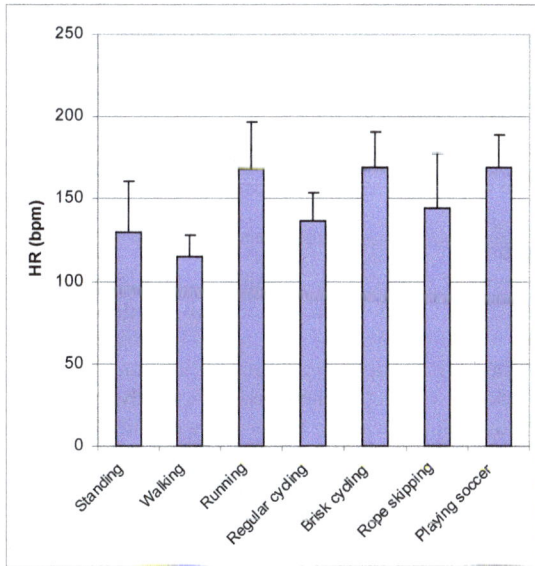

Fig. 2b. Heart rate in beats per minute for seven physical activities (mean and standard deviation)

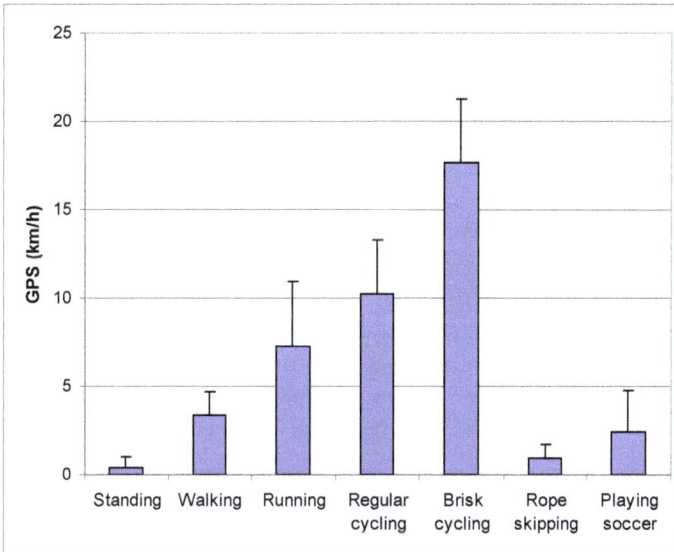

Fig. 2c. GPS velocity in kilometer per hour for seven physical activities (mean and standard deviation)

km/h) and brisk cycling (17.7 km/h). There is also a significant difference between walking (3.4 km/h) and running (7.3 km/h). The mean speed for playing soccer (2.4 km/h) is lower than the mean speed for walking. This unexpected result may be due to differences in intensity that children play soccer (i.e., long periods of standing still and short bursts of movement). The standard deviation for playing soccer (2.3) is also larger than the standard deviation for walking (1.3).

From Figure 2a-c it can be seen that the mean counts for regular cycling and brisk cycling are very similar while the differences in mean speed and mean heart rate suggest that the intensity of brisk cycling is higher than the intensity of regular cycling. This illustrates the additional value of these monitors to discriminate between two activities with similar means counts.

3.2 Activity classification

Table 2 reports the percentage of correctly classified activities of the cross-validated results for the four developed ANN models. In general all models performed well (>80%) in classifying the activities walking, standing still, rope skipping, running and playing soccer. Cycling was best classified by models including GPS data. Overall, the model based on accelerometer data (Model 1) correctly classified 82% of the activity types. When adding GPS data (Model 2), the overall percentage of correctly classified activities improved to 89%. The improvement was lower (from 82% to 84%) when heart rate data were added to the model (Model 3). Finally, the overall percentage of correctly classified activities with the complete model including accelerometer, GPS and heart rate data (Model 4) was 90%. This is 1% higher than the percentage of correctly classified activities achieved by Model 2.

	Model 1	Model 2	Model 3	Model 4
Standing	87	94	89	95
Walking	92	94	94	95
Running	89	84	87	85
Regular cycling	67	87	70	89
Brisk cycling	33	80	56	72
Rope skipping	91	91	90	90
Playing soccer	87	86	87	89
Total	82	89	84	90

Table 2. Percentage of correctly classified activity types for the fitted ANN models: Model 1 (accelerometer), Model 2 (accelerometer + GPS), Model 3 (accelerometer + heart rate), and Model 4 (accelerometer + GPS + heart rate).

In order to evaluate the classification errors of the four models in more detail, a contingency table was built for each model representing the relationship between the observed and the predicted physical activities. Table 3 shows that the highest percentage of misclassification errors occurred for allocation to the activities brisk and regular cycling. The percentages of misclassification were higher for brisk cycling than for regular cycling. Model 1 achieved the highest misclassification error for both cycling activities (53.6%) followed by Model 3 (31.2%). Furthermore, Model 1 and Model 3 could not discriminate between the activities regular cycling and standing very well. Model 2 achieved the highest misclassification errors between the activities standing and rope skipping.

4. Discussion

The purpose of this study was to investigate whether the accuracy of the previously developed ANN models from De Vries et al. (2011b) could be improved by the inclusion of data on the intensity of activities by means of heart rate data and/or inclusion of data on the speed of activities from GPS. The results have shown that the performance of the previously developed accelerometer based ANN model, which classified 82% of the activities correctly, improves by 2-8% when including other sensor data. The largest improvement was found when adding GPS data. Including GPS data seemed especially valuable for distinguishing between regular and brisk cycling. The percentages improved from 67% to 87% for regular

Observerd activities	Predicted activities						
	Standing	Walking	Running	Regular cycling	Brisk cycling	Rope skipping	Playing soccer
Standing							
Model 1	87.5	0.7	0.4	8.2	0.0	0.8	2.4
Model 2	94.4	0.7	0.0	1.0	0.4	1.1	2.5
Model 3	88.6	0.3	0.3	6.6	1.4	1.0	1.6
Model 4	94.8	0.5	0.3	1.0	0.5	0.9	1.9
Walking							
Model 1	0.7	92.3	0.9	1.0	2.6	0.0	2.6
Model 2	1.8	94.0	0.3	1.0	1.1	0.2	1.5
Model 3	0.7	94.0	0.0	3.5	0.6	0.0	1.2
Model 4	1.2	95.3	0.0	2.3	0.1	0.1	0.9
Running							
Model 1	1.0	2.5	89.2	1.2	0.6	1.5	3.9
Model 2	2.3	3.4	84.2	0.9	0.9	3.2	5.1
Model 3	0.5	2.4	86.9	1.6	1.6	2.4	4.6
Model 4	1.3	1.3	85.5	0.8	1.9	3.8	5.4
Regular cycling							
Model 1	13.7	2.6	1.1	67.4	10.8	0.5	4.0
Model 2	0.3	2.5	0.8	86.9	6.3	0.0	3.3
Model 3	13.9	2.7	1.6	70.3	8.0	0.6	2.9
Model 4	0.6	2.0	1.4	88.8	5.5	0.0	1.8
Brisk cycling							
Model 1	3.1	8.8	3.6	42.5	33.4	0.0	8.5
Model 2	0.0	3.2	1.9	13.8	80.4	0.0	0.8
Model 3	2.8	3.1	5.2	25.8	55.7	0.0	7.3
Model 4	0.0	3.8	4.5	16.4	72.5	0.0	2.8
Rope skipping							
Model 1	2.9	0.0	1.4	2.0	0.4	91.2	2.2
Model 2	4.9	0.0	0.6	0.3	0.0	91.2	3.0
Model 3	2.6	0.2	2.3	2.4	0.5	89.5	2.6
Model 4	4.5	0.5	0.8	0.5	0.0	90.4	3.4
Playing soccer							
Model 1	1.5	3.9	3.0	2.8	1.1	0.9	86.8
Model 2	3.0	4.0	3.4	1.3	0.9	1.0	86.4
Model 3	1.4	2.1	2.4	2.6	4.1	0.5	86.9
Model 4	2.6	2.4	2.7	0.6	1.8	1.1	88.7

Table 3. Cross-validation results for the classification of seven physical activities of Model 1 (accelerometer), Model 2 (accelerometer + GPS), Model 3 (accelerometer + heart rate), and Model 4 (accelerometer + GPS + heart rate) in percentages.

cycling, and from 33% to 80% for brisk cycling. Though the model based on data from all sensors (Model 4) produced the best overall classification, the gain in the percentage of activities correctly classified was only 1% higher that the improvement achieved by the model based on accelerometer and GPS data (Model 2), and the differences in performance per activity were very small (<−3%). Compared to Model 4, Model 2 could discriminate better between regular and brisk cycling, and it was simpler because it used less input variables. Therefore, the addition of GPS data to the model based on three-axial accelerometer data is sufficient to discriminate between activities performed with different intensity.

It is difficult to compare our results with those of previous studies because all the studies differ in the age groups studied, the type of accelerometer monitor the participants worn, the type of patter-recognition model used, the type of signal analyzed (raw data or counts), and also the type of physical activities classified (see Bonomi et al., 2009a, Khan et al., 2008; Liu & Chang, 2009; Staudenmayer et al., 2009). Staudenmayer et al. (2009) achieved a high percentage of correctly classified activities (89%) with an ANN model with a sample of adults. Bonomi et al. (2009) also achieved a high percentage of correctly classified activities (93%) with a decision tree model for a sample of adults. An advantage of the models proposed by Khan et al. (2008) and Liu & Chang (2009) could be that they used combined characteristics of the three-axial accelerometer signal as input variables in the models. However, our classification results did not improve when we performed additional analyses including combined characteristics of the three-axial accelerometer data.

To our knowledge, this is the first study that used ANN models with data from multiple sensors to classify children's physical activity type. We can only compare our results to the single sensor model proposed in De Vries et al. (2011b). Though the performance of the model based on three-axial accelerometer data presented in this paper (82%) is better than the performance of the equivalent model proposed in De Vries et al. (2011b) for children (77%), the differences in performance can be mainly explained by the differences in the type of activities classified. De Vries et al. (2011b) did not distinguish between regular and brisk cycling, and they included data from the activity sitting. In their model a high misclassification error was found between the activities sitting and standing. In this study, data from the activity sitting were not included because this activity was performed inside of the schools and accurate GPS data cannot be registered inside of buildings.

In previous studies, the output of multiple sensors has been combined to increase the prediction of energy expenditure. There are several monitors available that combine multiple sensors. For example, the Actiheart is an integrated accelerometer and heart rate unit and it provides a more accurate prediction of children's energy expenditure than either heart rate or accelerometry alone (Rowlands and Eston, 2007). Another device is the Intelligent Device for Energy Expenditure and Activity (IDEEA) which consists of five mini-accelerometers attached to the chest, to both thighs and under both feet (Rothney et al., 2007). However, these monitors cannot be used in large epidemiological studies because they are either very expensive or difficult to place. Heart rate monitors perform better in combination with other sensors than alone when classifying physical activity because their assessment of physical activity is based on the linear relationship between oxygen uptake and heart rate. If the intensity of an activity increases, the heart rate increases. Moreover, there are large inter-individual differences in the heart rate recovery time, and in rest heart rate levels. Therefore, heart rate data must be calibrated before including them in a pattern recognition model.

Beside heart rate units, GPS monitors have already been combined with accelerometer data in previous studies to assess physical activity. Mostly location GPS data were combined with accelerometer data to assess physical activity (Maddison & Mhurchu, 2009). Our study has showed that speed GPS data may help to discriminate between physical activities performed with different intensity, such as regular cycling and brisk cycling, better than heart rate data because GPS data do not need to be calibrated. Furthermore, other factors such as emotional stress can change the heart rate. A drawback of GPS monitors is that the GPS signal strength is not always sufficient, for example, when the monitors are worn inside of buildings.

This study had some weaknesses. First, it is known that children's activity pattern is different from the adults' activity pattern. In children's physical activity, there is more variance in intensity within and between activities. In addition they more often change of type of activity. In this study, all signals were segmented in non overlapping intervals of 10 seconds, and signal features were calculated for each interval. However, 10 seconds may be a too long time period when there are several transitions between activities within a few seconds. Therefore, it must be studied whether the classification performance of the models may increase when shorter time intervals are used.

Furthermore, future studies should determine whether the accuracy of the ANN models based on accelerometers and heart rate data could be further improved by increasing the measurement frequency of heart rate, by calibrating the heart rate signal or by computing other signal features. Alternative features could be the maximum peak per interval or the maximum deviation from the baseline heart rate.

5. Acknowledgment

This study was funded by the Dutch Ministry of Health, Welfare and Sport. We are grateful to Hannah Hofman and Marjolein Engels for giving assistance during data collection.

6. References

Baquet G, Stratton G, Praagh E van, Berthoin S. (2007). Improving physical activity assessment in prepubertal children with high-frequency accelerometry monitoring: a methodological issue. *Preventive Medicine*, Vol.44, No.2, (February 2007), pp. 143-147, ISSN 0091-7435

Bonomi AG, Goris AH, Yin B, Westerterp KR. (2009a). Detection of type, duration, and intensity of physical activity using an accelerometer. *Medicine & Science in Sports & Exercise*, Vol.41, No. 9 (September 2009), pp. 1770-1777, ISSN 0195-9131

Bonomi AG, Plasqui G, Goris AH, Westerterp KR. (2009b) Improving assessment of daily energy expenditure by identifying types of physical activity with a single accelerometer. *Journal of Applied Physiology*, Vol.107, No.3, (September 2009), pp. 655-661, ISSN 8750-7587

De Vries SI, Engels, M, Galindo Garre F. (2011b). Identification of children's activity type with accelerometer-based neural networks. *Medicine & Science in Sports & Exercise*, (in press 2011), ISSN 0195-9131

De Vries SI, Hirtum WJEM van, Bakker I, Hopman-Rock M, Hirasing RA, Mechelen W van. (2009). Validity and reproducibility of motion sensors in youth: a systematic update. *Medicine & Science in Sports & Exercise*, Vol. 41, No.4, (April 2009), pp. 817-827, ISSN 0195-9131

Esliger DW, Copeland JL, Barnes JD, Tremblay MS. (2005). Standardizing and optimizing the use of accelerometer data for free-living physical activity monitoring. *Journal of Physical Activity & Health, Vol.2, No.3, (July 2005)*, pp. 366-83, ISSN 1543-3080

Eston RG, Rowlands AV, Ingleden DK. (1998). Validity of heart rate, pedometry, and accelerometry for predicting the energy cost of children's activities. *Journal of Applied Physiology*, Vol.84, No.1, (January 1998), pp. 362-371, ISSN 8750-7587

Khan AM, Lee YK, Kim TS. (2008) Accelerometer signal-based human activity recognition using augmented autoregressive model coefficients and artificial neural nets. *Proceedings of 30 th Annual International Conference of the Engineering in Medicine and Biology Society*, ISBN 978-1-4244-1814-5, Vancouver, August 2008.

Liu SH, Chang YJ. (2009). Using accelerometers for physical actions recognition by a neural fuzzy network. *Telemedicine and E-Health*, Vol.15, No. 9, (November 2009) pp. 867-876, ISSN 1556-3669

Maddison R, Mhurchu CN. (2009) Global positioning system: a new opportunity in physical activity measurement. *International Journal of Behavioral Nutrition and Physical Activity*, Vol.6, No.73, (November 2009), pp.12-16, ISSN 1479-5868

Pober DM, Staudenmayer J, Raphael C, Freedson PS. (2006). Development of novel techniques to classify physical activity mode using accelerometers. *Medicine & Science in Sports & Exercise*, Vol.38, No.9, (September 2006), pp. 1626-1634, ISSN 0195-9131

Ripley BD. (1996). *Pattern recognition and neural networks*, Cambridge University Press, ISBN 0-521-46986-7, Cambridge, England.

Rothney MP, Neumann M, Beziat A, Chen KY. (2007). An artificial neural network model of energy expenditure using nonintegrated acceleration signals. *Journal of Applied Physiology*, Vol.103, No.4, (October 2007), pp.1419-1427, ISSN 8750-7587

Rowland TW. (2007). Promoting Physical Activity for Children's Health : Rationale and Strategies. *Sports Medicine*, Vol.37, No.11, (January 2007), pp. 929-36, ISSN 0112-1642

Salmon J, Timperio A. (2007). Prevalence, trends and environmental influences on child and youth physical activity. *Medicine Sport and Science*, vol.50, (January 2007), pp. 183-99, ISSN 0254-5020

Staudenmayer J, Pober D, Crouter SE, Bassett DR, Freedson P. (2009). An artificial neural network to estimate physical activity energy expenditure and identify physical activity type from an accelerometer. *Journal of Applied Physiology*, Vo.107, No.4, (October 2009), pp. 1300-1307, ISSN 8750-7587

Twisk JW. (2001). Physical activity guidelines for children and adolescents: a critical review. *Sports Medicine*, Vol.31, No.8, (August 2001), pp. 617-27, ISSN 0112-1642

Venables WN, Ripley BD. (2002). *Modern Applied Statistics with S (Fourth Edition)*, Springer-Verlag, ISBN 0-387-95457-0, New York, United States.

Vries SI, Galindo Garre F, Engbers LH, Hildebrandt VH, Buuren S van. (2011a). Evaluation of Neural Networks to Identify Types of Activity Using Accelerometers. *Medicine & Science in Sports & Exercise*, Vol.43, No.1, (Januari 2011), pp. 101-107, ISSN 0195-9131

14

The Involvement of Brain Monoamines in the Onset of Hyperthermic Central Fatigue

Cândido C. Coimbra[1], Danusa D. Soares[2] and Laura H. R. Leite[3]
[1]*Federal University of Minas Gerais, Department of Physiology and Biophysics,*
[2]*Federal University of Minas Gerais, Department of Physical Education,*
[3]*Federal University of Juiz de Fora, Department of Physiology,*
Brazil

1. Introduction

The fatigue that results from physical exercise is a multifactorial phenomenon that is comprised of complex interactions between physiological and psychological factors. Fatigue is assumed to be an inability to maintain the required force or power or an increasing difficulty to continue the work rate at a given exercise intensity. Taking into account that homeostasis disturbances may be harmful, fatigue should be considered a defense mechanism that prevents tissue damage by reducing the intensity of or even interrupting physical activity.

Fatigue is known to have peripheral and/or central origins. Although most studies focus peripheral factors, which include circulatory, metabolic, muscular, nutritional and thermoregulatory disorders, exercise-induced cerebral metabolism and neurohumoral or neurotransmitter turnover are also implicated in fatigue genesis. "Central fatigue" refers to these central nervous system alterations that may prevent muscular and neural damage by failing to drive the muscles appropriately.

Most authors consider central fatigue during prolonged exercise to be a consequence of the accumulation or depletion of neurotransmitters, serotonin in particular. Although the role of serotonergic neural trafficking on exercise performance has been well documented, dopamine and noradrenaline neurotransmissions also contribute to central fatigue. In addition to having their activity modified by exercise, all of these brain monoamines exhibit relevant thermoregulatory effects. These amines play an important role in the function of thermoregulatory centers, such as the preoptic area and the anterior hypothalamus, and it is hypothesized that changes in their turnover are associated with the development of fatigue as a consequence of heat imbalances.

The brain is especially endangered by hyperthermia. For this reason, the exacerbation of exercise-induced hyperthermia appears to diminish the central nervous system drive to the working muscles; this protects the brain from thermal damage while causing a detriment to physical endurance. This effect is more pronounced when hyperthermia occurs simultaneously with inhibitory signals from the central nervous system, as in the case of altered neurotransmitter metabolisms. Even though it has been stated that central fatigue coincides with critical high core body and brain temperatures, as well as increased heat storage, evidence indicates that complex and dynamic mechanisms are reliable regulators of exercise performance. In this way, the heat storage and the body heating rates associated with changes in neurotransmitter content in thermoregulatory centers emerge as important factors in determining fatigue.

The main focus of this section is to link serotonin, dopamine and noradrenaline brain levels and exercise-induced hyperthermia with the onset of central fatigue. It is improbable that central fatigue is caused by a unique pathway; therefore the interaction between these systems may play an important role in establishing hyperthermia-induced central fatigue. From a health perspective, fatigue should be considered a warning sign that prevents the organism from the harmful consequences of sports activities.

2. Fatigue as a defense mechanism during exercise

Fatigue can disturb performance in many occupations, including firefighting, the military, construction and laboring, and it can limit participation in most recreational activities and sports (McKenna & Hargreaves, 2008). Understanding fatigue has implications far from those circumscribed to sports performance. In ill patients, fatigue and, thus, exercise limitations can drastically restrict daily activities and lead to a poor quality of life. Therefore, it is not surprising that exercise-induced fatigue has gained so much attention among researchers in the fields of exercise science and medicine.

Exercise-induced fatigue has been traditionally defined as an elevation in the perception of effort to develop a desired force or power and also as an eventual inability to produce this force (Davis & Bailey, 1997; Enoka & Stuart, 1992). Many different models have been proposed in an attempt to understand the underlying mechanisms of fatigue. Since the early works by Fletcher and Hopkins (1907) and Hill et al. (1924), lactic acid production, cardiovascular system inefficiency, metabolic substrate depletion and waste product accumulation have been recognized as the main signs of fatigue. Until recently, most studies have dealt with exercise-induced fatigue under a failure perspective, which means that any limitation arising from exercising muscles would lead to an interruption in the motor task. In such an approach, the failure to maintain force depends on "peripheral" fatigue that occurs distal to the point of nerve stimulation and on "central" fatigue that results from a failure to voluntarily activate the muscle (Gandevia, 2001). However, it is important to emphasize that fatigue during exercise can occur without any signs of muscle dysfunction, substrate inadequacy within the exercised muscles or cardiovascular system overload; it may thus be under the influence of psychological factors such as arousal, mood and external motivation (Foley & Fleshner, 2008).

A more recent approach differs from the failure perspective and points to a more integrative scenario where fatigue should be seen as a defense mechanism. Thus, exercise is ended or its intensity is turned down to protect the individual from tissue damage (Marino, 2004). In 1996, Ulmer proposed the concept of teleoanticipation, where a feedback control system would exist for the optimal adjustment of the metabolic rate during exercise and would include a programmer that would take a finishing point into consideration. In this way, a marathon runner would consciously choose to run at a pace that would not pose a threat to himself. This assumption was further developed as the "Central Governor Model" that considers fatigue to be a sensation that results from a complex neural integration between afferent information and the brain (Noakes et al., 2005; Noakes & St Clair Gibson, 2004).

Peripheral information, such as substrate depletion and waste product accumulation, would act as a modulator of the cerebral control process in a dynamic, non-linear and integrated manner; this would cause an oscillatory behavior of the physiological responses and power output during exercise. This integrative model of fatigue proposes that a continuous interrelated control of feed-forward and feed-back mechanisms would exist and would be responsible for a secure system of homeostasis control during exercise (Noakes et al., 2005; Tucker, 2009; Tucker et al., 2006). This integration could be consciously and verbally manifested through the perception of effort, as measured by Borg's scale (1982) (St Clair Gibson et al., 2006; Tucker, 2009). Moreover, the teleoanticipatory central nervous system would be molded by previous exercise experiences and training (Noakes et al., 2005). Thus, fatigue may provide the cognitive system with a signal that encourages the organism to lower present goals and/or seek lower effort alternative strategies (Perrey et al., 2010).

In spite of being accepted by some research groups (Marino, 2010; Baron et al., 2009; Flouris & Cheung, 2009; Castle et al., 2006), this model has been criticized by others (Ament & Verkerke, 2009; Shephard, 2009). As discussed later in this chapter, our group has been working with a conception of fatigue that goes in this direction. We have shown that before any harm can occur, afferent information from different physiological systems must be centrally integrated, and exercise must be voluntarily interrupted (Balthazar et al., 2009, Leite et al., 2010; A. G. Rodrigues et al., 2004, 2009; Soares et al., 2004, 2007).

3. Central fatigue hypothesis

Although most studies have focused on the peripheral factors of fatigue, including circulatory, metabolic, muscular, nutritional, and thermoregulatory disorders (Bassett & Howley, 2000; Coyle et al., 1986; Coyle & González-Alonso, 2001; Febbraio, 2000; Hargreaves & Febbraio, 1998; Kreider et al., 1993; Noakes, 2000), exercise-induced cerebral metabolism and neurohumoral or neurotransmitter alterations are also implicated in the genesis of fatigue (Foley & Fleshner, 2008; Nybo & Secher, 2004; Roelands & Meeusen, 2010). This participation of central nervous system factors in the reduction of the voluntary activation of skeletal muscles during physical effort has been termed "central fatigue" (Foley & Fleshner, 2008; Gandevia, 2001). In this section, a focused discussion on the possible role of serotonin neurotransmission on exercise-induced central fatigue will be presented.

As first suggested by Newsholme et al. (1992), fatigue during prolonged exercise may be influenced by the activity of the brain serotonergic system; this has been commonly referred to as the "central fatigue hypothesis." Its major premise is that elevated central tryptophan availability increases serotonin activity during prolonged exercise, which may cause fatigue by increasing lethargy and loss of central drive/motivation (Newsholme et al., 1992). During resting periods, most tryptophan, the amino acid precursor of serotonin, circulates in the blood bound to albumin, the same transporter of free fatty acids. During prolonged exercise and as a response to metabolic demands, there is an increase in the plasma concentration of free fatty acids. This displaces tryptophan from the biding sites on albumin and causes an elevation in the free portion of this amino acid. As a consequence, tryptophan is readily available to cross the blood-brain barrier. Concomitantly, during prolonged exercise, the plasma concentrations of branched-chain amino acids either fall or do not change. Because these amino acids and tryptophan in its free form share the same transporter across the blood-brain barrier, a reduction in plasma concentrations of branched-chain amino acids during exercise could increase the uptake of tryptophan into the central nervous system and lead to an increase in serotonin synthesis during exercise. Thus, these two interrelated mechanisms underlie the "central fatigue hypothesis". Tryptophan increases induced by exercise have been described as occurring simultaneously with a significant rise in the concentration of 5-hydroxyindoleacetic acid, which is the main serotonin metabolite; these data indicate that exercise increases serotonin synthesis and turnover. Tryptophan alters serotonin within the brain, and there is a positive relationship between endogenous serotonin content and the activity of tryptophan transport mechanisms in hypothalamic brain slices or synaptosomal preparations. Electrolytic lesions of raphe nuclei or intracerebroventricular injections of 5,7-dihydroxytryptamine lead to a decrease in synaptosomal tryptophan accumulation with reduced nerve terminals (Denizeau & Sourkes,1977). In addition, both spontaneous and electrically evoked serotonin release from hypothalamic slices have been shown to be dependent on precursor availability, which causes parallel changes in brain serotonin levels and serotonin release (Schaechter & Wurtman, 1990).

Central serotonin activity can affect many physiological responses, such as pain tolerance (Prieto-Gomez et al., 1989), motor activity (Gerin & Privat, 1998), thermoregulation (Imeri et al., 2000; Lin et al., 1998; Myers, 1981, Soares et al., 2007) and hypothalamo–pituitary-adrenal axis activity (Chaouloff, 2000; Korte et al., 1991). Thus, alterations in one or more of the physiological responses mediated by the serotonergic system may decrease work capacity during exercise.

It has been shown that an increased availability of tryptophan, in the central nervous system reduces the mechanical efficiency and running time to fatigue, which are both related to serotonin content in the preoptic area (Soares et al., 2003, 2007). Moreover, serotonin content in the preoptic area is also associated with increased heat production and storage during exercise (Soares et al., 2007). Recently, it has been shown that alterations in the serotonin levels in the preoptic area and in the hypothalamus are also modulated by central angiotensinergic and cholinergic pathways (Leite et al., 2010; A. G. Rodrigues et al., 2009). For more details see section 7.

Serotonergic neurons have many important functions in the central nervous system, including motor activity control. However, the role of serotonin in the regulation of motor control is complex. There is widespread evidence that serotonin in the hippocampus is involved in locomotion (Meeusen et al., 1996; Takahashi et al., 2000). According to Soares et al. (2007), at fatigue, the hippocampal serotonin content was directly correlated with the exercise time of rats but not correlated with the heat storage rate. Data from A. G. Rodrigues et al. (2009) also showed that, at fatigue, the hippocampal serotonin content was not directly correlated with heat storage. Together, these results suggest that hippocampal serotonergic activity might also participate in fatigue during exercise through a mechanism other than thermoregulation. This is in agreement with reports that serotonergic neurons in the median raphe nuclei that project to the hippocampus are related to motor activity (Hillegaart & Hjorth, 1989; Jacobs et al., 1975).

Although the involvement of serotonin in central fatigue has been well documented, it has become evident that other neurotransmitters participate in the mechanisms of exercise-induced fatigue (Lacerda et al., 2006; A. G. Rodrigues et al., 2009). These data indicate that central fatigue is a more complex phenomenon than previously thought and that it involves the balance of at least two central aminergic neurotransmitter systems, as indicated by the serotonin/dopamine ratio (Balthazar et al., 2010; Foley & Fleshner 2008; Meeusen, 2006).

4. Proposed central mechanisms of fatigue

Fatigue should be seen as a multifaceted phenomenon influenced by both central and peripheral factors (Meeusen et al., 2006; Nybo & Secher, 2004). There is no doubt that alterations within the muscle contribute to exercise-induced fatigue; however, it is unlikely that alterations in muscle function are the sole mechanism of fatigue. In fact, the contribution of either central factors or factors upstream of the neuromuscular junction has been, for the most part, ignored in the literature (Foley & Fleshner, 2008).

At least three factors have been proposed to contribute to the delay in establishing the role of "central" factors in human muscle fatigue. First, it has simply been more convenient to assume that the muscle limits to produce force that have been established in reduced preparations of muscle that are devoid of effective neural input also apply to a conscious human subject. Second, the existing methods to gauge the central drive to muscles have not always been technically rigorous, and findings obtained with these methods have been easily criticized or ignored. Third, although changes in the central nervous system during exercise can be measured, it has been more demanding to show that they cause a deficit in force production (Gandevia, 2001).

Because muscle contractions are under the control of the central nervous system, it is likely that any significant alteration in the brain or the spinal cord would alter the neural drive to the neuromuscular junction, thus initiating fatigue (Taylor & Gandevia, 2008). In order to identify the adjustments that occur within the nervous system during fatiguing contractions, most studies have investigated the influence of afferent feedback, descending inputs, and spinal circuitry on the output of the motor neuron pool (Hunter et al., 2004). For example, the metabolites that accumulate in muscles during a prolonged exercise excite afferent fibers; these fibers enhance the central drive to maintain muscle perfusion by increasing the mean arterial pressure and modulating the motor neuron discharge rate (Gandevia, 2001). Such observations indicate that the decrement in force during a fatiguing contraction usually involves multiple neural mechanisms (Hunter et al., 2004).

During maximal voluntary isometric tasks, voluntary activation usually diminishes, and motor unit firing rates decline (Gandevia, 2001). However, it is not possible to clearly specify all of the putative sites within the central nervous system at which contributions to voluntary activation, central fatigue, and supraspinal fatigue occur. The traditional model indicates that there is a "chain", from higher levels within the central nervous system to the motoneuron via descending paths, and then through motor axons to the neuromuscular junction, the sarcolemma, T tubules, and, ultimately, to actin and myosin (Taylor & Gandevia, 2008).

Thus, central fatigue can be considered to be an impaired muscular performance that arises from decreased efferent signaling from the central nervous system. There are two general ways to study central fatigue. The first one seems to be a fairly direct way, and consists of using a technique where "added force" is determined. This occurs by overlaying a supramaximal electrical stimulus of a muscle onto a maximal voluntary contraction for that muscle. Any "added force" that may be generated that is in addition to that produced by the maximal voluntary contraction is indicative of an impairment from the central nervous system down to the level proximal to the neuromuscular junction. The second way to study central fatigue is to use an exogenous substance that is believed to induce central fatigue, and observe its effects on exercise capacity. However, unlike the first alternative, this method is indirect, because it cannot be exactly known if the substance had peripheral and/or central effects (Evans & Lambert, 2007).

4.1 Central nervous system biochemical changes and central fatigue

Given that intense exercise challenges the cardiovascular, respiratory, endocrine, and peripheral and central motor systems, changes in many central nervous system transmitter systems would be expected to accompany exercise and task failure or fatigue (Gandevia, 2001). All types of physical or psychological constraints lead to the activation of noradrenergic, dopaminergic and serotonergic systems at the brainstem level. These systems are particularly important for the global regulation of behavior, and they participate in the formulation of an adapted response of the central nervous system to an external stimulus (Sesboue & Guincestre, 2006).

The widespread central actions of many of these systems make it unlikely that any one is uniquely responsible for central fatigue. For example, there are serotonergic projections from the brain stem raphe nuclei to the cortex, hippocampus, hypothalamus, medulla, and spinal cord. There are noradrenergic projections from the locus coeruleus. Arousal, motivation, attention, tolerance to discomfort, and sensitivity to stress can all alter voluntary drive, at least subjectively, which suggests that many neural systems can modify central fatigue (Gandevia, 2001).

There is evidence of the roles of these neuromodulators on fatigue that will be minutely covered later in this chapter. However, it is important to first elucidate some aspects of the interrelatedness of central neuromodulators and fatigue. We have already discussed some aspects of serotonergic neurotransmission and its implication on the central fatigue during exercise.

Central noradrenergic neurons modulate humor and motivation, and when their activity is low, motivation decreases. This decrease leads to a diminishment of motor cortex activation and a subsequent decline in the stimulation of the descending path chain to the motoneurons (Sesboue & Guincestre, 2006). On the other hand, the response of cerebral dopamine to, for example, a physical constraint is biphasic. It has been shown that there is a small elevation in the levels of this neurotransmitter at the beginning of muscle work, which is followed by a reduction in its concentration as the intensity and duration of the effort increases; this reduction is most prominent at fatigue (Foley & Fleshner, 2008).

There are several other transmitters and their subtypes that need to be examined for their role in central fatigue. For example, it is already known that brain gamma-aminobutyric-acid (GABA) levels diminish with exercise (Gandevia, 2001) and that baclofen, a GABAergic agonist that acts on GABA B receptors, can postpone fatigue (Abdelmalki et al., 1997). Other humoral signals that must be considered to be involved in central fatigue are glutamine and ammonia, which are diminished and increased, respectively, after exercise (Gandevia, 2001). Another important proposed mechanism of central fatigue is related to hyperthermia during exercise. It is well known that hyperthermia reduces the central nervous system drive for exercise performance (Nielsen et al., 1993; Walters et al., 2000) and precipitates feelings of fatigue during exercise. However, this essential aspect of central fatigue will be discussed in detail in the next section.

5. Fatigue induced by exercise hyperthermia

It has been shown that hyperthermia reduces physical performance in many mammalian species (Bruck & Olschewski, 1987; Fuller et al., 1998; González-Alonso et al., 1999; Nielsen et al., 1993; Walters et al., 2000), reduces central nervous system drive for exercise performance (Nielsen et al., 1993; Walters et al., 2000) and precipitates feelings of fatigue at a sublethal threshold by establishing a safety level against heat stroke, thus protecting the brain, among other tissues, from thermal damage (Caputa et al., 1986; Marino,2004). The reduction in exercise performance as a consequence of hyperthermic stress has been described in isometric tasks (Nybo & Nielsen, 2001; Thomas et al., 2006; Todd et al., 2005), in dynamic exercises with fixed intensity, i.e., a constant workload (Nybo & Nielsen, 2001), and in self-paced prolonged exercises (Ely et al., 2010; Tatterson, 2000). Recently, from an evolutionary perspective, it has been suggested that physiological and (or) psychological safeguards should protect individuals by voluntarily reducing exercise and metabolic heat production before catastrophic hyperthermia (Cheung, 2007). In fact, various animals will cease exercise when their core temperatures exceed safe limits, and there must be a similar behavioral response in humans to reduce metabolic heat production and ultimately to protect the physiological integrity (Cheung & Sleivert, 2004).

5.1 Body temperature and thermoregulation

Humans possess efficient physiological and behavioral mechanisms for maintaining their internal temperature within narrow limits; these mechanisms allow survival even in diversified thermal environments such as tropical forests, deserts and very cold regions. Our body temperatures are carefully regulated at 37°C ± 1°C. However, our thermal physiology is "asymmetrical", which means that body temperature is placed very closely, within just a few degrees Celsius, to the upper existence limit (possibly related to the denaturation of regulatory proteins) but somewhat far, a few tens of degrees, from the lower survival limit (probably defined by the freezing temperature of water) (Romanovsky,2007).

The lowest values for body temperature occur in the morning, between 04:00 and 06:00 a.m., and the highest are observed between 17:00 and 20:00 h (Waterhouse et al., 2005). It should be noted that the temperature is not the same throughout the human body. There is a temperature gradient between the core (visceral) and body surface (cutaneous). With an elevation in body temperature to values over 42°C, there is an eminent risk of protein denaturating with subsequent cellular death. However, despite being more tolerant to hypothermia than to hyperthermia (see above) when the former is severe, i.e., when body temperature falls below 32°C, there are critical risks for life maintenance that include the loss of motor coordination, cardiac arrhythmias and even death by cardiac arrest (Kanosue, 2010).

Body temperature is the net result of the heat produced by metabolic actions and the heat dissipated to the environment. If the heat dissipation is smaller than heat production, excessive heat is stored and body temperature increases.

Metabolism generates heat from exergonic oxidative reactions that use adenosine triphosphate (ATP) as fuel. Basal metabolism is around 50% efficient, and the remaining energy is lost as heat. Exercising muscles are even less efficient, at no more than 25%. For example, given that the mean value for the specific heat of body tissue is 0.83 kcal.kg^{-1}.$^{\circ}$C^{-1}, a male adult weighting 70 kg with a body temperature of 37°C has around 2,150 Kcal of total heat stored in his body.

The basal metabolism produces 1 Kcal. kg^{-1}.h^{-1}, even in a thermoneutral environment, where temperature regulation is achieved only by means of sensible heat loss, i.e., without regulatory changes in metabolic heat production or evaporative heat loss. Because human tissues only need 0.83 kcal.kg^{-1} to increase the internal (core) temperature by 1°C, core temperatures would be elevated by 1°C.h^{-1}, even during rest periods, if no heat loss mechanisms are activated. Thus, losing heat to the environment is essential for survival. If there were no effective means by which body could lose heat, hyperthermia would be achieved very rapidly.

Thermoregulation is a typical example of an integrative hypothalamic function that generates autonomic, endocrine, motor and behavioral patterns as a response to an external challenge. Thermoregulation systems are composed of multiple independent neural pathways that have both feedback and feedforward mechanisms; these mechanism are activated by afferent information from peripheral temperature sensors and modulate the relationship between ambient and skin temperatures (Mekjavic & Eiken, 2006; Webb, 1995). The endothermic/homoeothermic animals are relatively independent from environmental conditions because they are able to regulate their body temperature through an association of autonomic and behavioral mechanisms (Mekjavic & Eiken, 2006; Schlader et al., 2009, 2010). The autonomic processes consist of involuntary thermoeffector responses, either to heat or cold, which modify heat production and dissipation rates, and include sweating, shivering and vasomotor alterations at the body surface (IUPS, 2001). However, as pointed out by some authors (Schalader et al, 2010; Romanovsky, 2007), those autonomic responses have a limited capacity to regulate body temperature. In contrast, behavioral mechanisms of thermoregulation are intended to establish a thermal environment that represents a preferred condition for heat exchange (heat gain, heat loss, or heat balance) between the organism and its environment. The responses involved in such regulation include moves to a different thermal ambiance, changes in posture, wetting of body surfaces, changes in microclimate by nest building, parental behavior (huddling), and, in humans, voluntary exercise and cultural achievements (e.g. clothing, housing, and air-conditioning) (IUPS, 2001).The association of behavioral and autonomic responses allows humans to survive in different and extreme environments (Mekjavi & Eiken, 2006).

Vasomotion and evaporation are the main mechanisms of heat defense. However, sweating (or panting) usually starts at a higher threshold temperature than skin vasodilation. Thus, sweating functions as a second line of defense for situations where an increase in skin blood flow alone is not sufficient to prevent a serious increase in body temperature. Cold defense processes operate in a parallel manner such that non-shivering thermogenesis is activated before shivering (Kanosue et al., 2010).

5.2 Exercise hyperthermia and fatigue

Because the mechanical efficiency of active muscles is around 25%, most of the remaining energy produced during exercise should be dissipated to the environment; otherwise, exercise may impose thermal stress to the organism. This dissipation can be hard if exercise takes place in a warm environment where heat dissipation mechanisms, such as conduction and radiation, are impaired. Dissipation can be even worse if it is associated with high humidity because heat lost by sweat evaporation would be severely compromised. In these environmental conditions, keeping up the same intensity effort during physical exercise could lead to a harmful situation in which the heat dissipation would be insufficient to compensate for the heat production. As a result, the body temperature would continuously increase, and a thermal equilibrium would not be reached.

To avoid serious injuries induced by excessive body heat storage and subsequent hyperthermia, it is imperative that the related activation of both the autonomic and behavioral responses, along with the different physiological systems, results in a decrease of exercise intensity or even in a termination of the activity (Cheung, 2007).

An elevation in internal body temperature and an increase in heat storage have been proposed as limiting factors to physical performance. Recent data support the hypothesis that both the heat storage rate and the internal body temperature seem to be the important determinants of fatigue during exercise (Balthazar et al., 2010; Coelho et al., 2010; Garcia et al., 2006; Lacerda et al., 2005; Leite et al., 2006; Magalhães et al., 2010; Nassif et al., 2008; A. G. Rodrigues et al., 2008; Soares et al., 2004, 2007). Thus, dissipation of heat from the body is thought to be more important than the control of heat production in the regulation of body temperature during exercise (Cheung & Sleivert, 2004).

Temperature regulation during exercise can be divided into two phases. During the first minutes of exercise, in what has been called the dynamic phase, there is a imbalance between heat production, which depends mainly on exercise intensity, and heat dissipation; this imbalance results in an abrupt increase in body (internal) temperature. Rapid peripheral vasoconstriction, mediated by the noradrenergic sympathetic system and observed at this earlier phase, impairs heat dissipation during this stage of exercise and leads to hyperthermia. Venous blood that drains exercising muscles brings excessive heat to the body core. Hypothalamic thermosensors detect the increase in blood temperature, and the thermal integrative center of the hypothalamus activates efferent heat loss mechanisms. The second phase of exercise, known as the steady phase of thermal balance, begins as thermal thresholds for heat dissipation mechanisms (vasodilation and sweating) are attained (Lacerda et al., 2006). From this point on, there is an increase in skin blood flow, mediated by the vasodilator cholinergic sympathetic system, which parallels the increase in the sweating rate. These autonomic actions increase the body heat dissipation and minimize the body temperature elevation. When heat storage reaches a critical limit, protective fatigue occurs independently of body energy stores. This excessive stored heat reduces the motivation for voluntary exercise before the individual integrity is compromised.

Neuromuscular control and hyperthermia have been widely investigated, and it has been consistently shown that hyperthermia diminishes neuromuscular activation (Morrison et al., 2004; Nybo & Nielsen, 2001; Todd et al., 2005). A model has been proposed that suggests that this impairment causes systemic failures in order to protect the organism from severe heat injuries (Cheung, 2007). A reduction in the central drive to the motor neuron pool during hyperthermia is thought to result from at least two possibilities. One considers that there is a reduction in the descending message from the higher brain impulses to the motor neurons. The other indicates that inhibition occurs subcortically, at the site of the motor neurons, where afferent feedback may decrease the excitability of those motor neurons (Cheung & Sleivert, 2004). The reduction in central drive may also result from both of these possibilities.

Brain function may also be altered during hyperthermia. Changes in behavior seen with overheating, such as confusion, a loss of coordination, syncope, and, in extreme hyperthermia, a loss of consciousness or seizures, have been consistently observed (Fuller et al., 1998; Schlader et al., 2010; Walters et al., 2000). These data indirectly suggest a change in central nervous system function with hyperthermia (Cheung & Sleivert, 2004; Nybo, 2008). Brain activity, specifically the ratio of low frequency (α: 8 –13 Hz) and high frequency (β: 13–30 Hz) brainwaves, is an indicator of arousal during hyperthermia. Exercise has been investigated in subjects cycling at 60% aerobic power in both a hot ($\cong$ 40°C) and cool ($\cong$19°C) environment (Nielsen et al., 2001). There was a reduction in β waves in the hot exercise condition such that the ratio of α to β waves increased, which indicates a reduced state of arousal in hyperthermic subjects. Moreover, the magnitude of the increase in the α to β wave ratio was correlated to elevated core temperatures. In the same study, subjects continually rated their perception of effort to be higher during hyperthermic condition (Nielsen et al., 2001).

Another important aspect regarding fatigue induced by exercise hyperthermia is cardiovascular function. It has been suggested that cardiovascular strain accompanying hyperthermia could indeed be one of the main factors underlying fatigue (Cheung & Sleivert, 2004). When heat production during exercise surpasses the capacity for heat dissipation to the environment and hyperthermia consequently develops, the ability to maintain cardiac output is jeopardized because stroke volume declines as the core temperature increases (Nybo, 2008). The competition between metabolic and thermoregulatory demands for blood flow during exercise may also accelerate the onset of fatigue through localized ischemia in specific tissues such as the brain or the gastrointestinal tract. Reduced blood flow to the gastrointestinal tract during exercise in heat may compromise the integrity of the intestinal walls (Sakurada & Hales 1998). As a result, the eventual leakage of lipopolysaccharides (endotoxins) into the circulation, a well-documented response to severe exercise-induced hyperthermia, can occur. It is important to point out that an occurrence of endotoxemia can trigger a cascade of detrimental physiological responses mediated by cytokines, which can induce a fever-like situation and can accelerate heat storage and heat stroke.

Neurohumoral factors, primarily disturbances in cerebral neurotransmitter levels, are part of the diverse mechanisms underlying fatigue induced by exercise hyperthermia. It is clear that several neurotransmitter systems are activated during exercise and that several of these systems affect the preoptic area and the anterior hypothalamus, which is of major importance for thermoregulation (Nybo, 2008). Therefore, it is important to highlight studies that correlate high heat storage and heating rates with elevated levels of serotonin in centers essential for thermoregulation (Leite et al., 2010; A. G. Rodrigues et al., 2009; Soares et al., 2007). However, there are only a few that have examined whether hyperthermia alters monoamines and other neurotransmitter levels in the brain during exercise. Although this subject will be discussed in detail in subsequent topics in this chapter, it is essential to first call attention to some aspects.

Among the monoamines, serotonin is of particular interest because it influences arousal levels. If serotonin levels increase, this could contribute to an increase in perceived effort and a reduction in work rate, actions that have often been observed during hyperthermia (Cheung & Sleivert, 2004). In contrast, because dopamine and noradrenaline have been associated with arousal, motivation, reinforcement and reward, control of motor behavior and mechanisms of addiction, some authors have investigated the role of these neurotransmitters on fatigue induced by exercise hyperthermia (Meeusen et al., 2006). Recently, it has been demonstrated that an alteration in dopamine transmission induced by the central blockade of dopamine D1 and D2 receptors impaired running performance in rats by decreasing the tolerance to heat storage. Furthermore, this blockade also impaired both the dissipation of exercise-induced heat and the recovery of the metabolic rate during the post-exercise period. These data provide evidence that the central activation of either dopamine D1 or D2 receptors may be essential for heat balance and exercise performance (Balthazar et al., 2010).

6. Ergogenic and ergolytic amines

Most theories consider central fatigue during prolonged exercise to be a consequence of changes in neurotransmitter turnover, particularly in the serotonergic system (Foley & Fleshner, 2008; Hasegawa et al., 2008; Nybo & Secher, 2004; Roelands & Meeusen, 2010).

Although the role of serotonergic neural traffic on exercise performance has been well-documented, evidence demonstrates that dopaminergic and noradrenergic neurotransmissions contribute to central fatigue as well (Foley & Fleshner, 2008; Hasegawa et al., 2008; Nybo & Secher, 2004; Roelands & Meeusen, 2010). Interestingly, all of these brain monoamines, in addition to having their activity modified by exercise, exhibit relevant thermoregulatory effects (Balthazar et al., 2009; Foley & Fleshner, 2008; Hasegawa et al., 2008; Roelands & Meeusen, 2010; Soares et al., 2004, 2007). It has been proposed that shifts in the turnover of these amines, which play an important role in the centers responsible for body temperature control, like the preoptic area and the anterior hypothalamus, may be associated with the development of fatigue coupled with heat imbalance.

6.1 Serotonin

Many authors have provided convincing evidence of the involvement of serotonin on the development of central fatigue (Blomstrand et al., 1989; Chaouloff, 1997; Fernstrom & Fernstrom, 2006; Gomez-Merino et al., 2001, Soares et al., 2007). The major premise is that increased brain serotonergic activity contributes to the onset of fatigue, possibly through its influence on many behavioral functions, such as elevated feelings of lethargy, tiredness and a loss of drive (Blomstrand, 2006; Meeusen et al., 2006; Roelands & Meeusen, 2010; Soares et al 2004, 2007). In contrast, low serotonin brain levels would favor improved exercise performance through the maintenance of motivation and arousal.

One the first studies that associated physical activity with elevated levels of serotonin in the central nervous system is Barchas & Freedman (1963), who reported high brain serotonin activity in rats who swam until exhaustion. Since then, many findings have confirmed that serotonin levels in the central nervous system increase during exercise and peak at the fatigue point (Blomstrand et al., 1989; Chaouloff, 1997; Fernstrom & Fernstrom, 2006; Gomez-Merino et al., 2001, Soares et al., 2007). Exercising until fatigue has been shown to cause an increase in the levels of both serotonin and its metabolite 5-hydroxyindoleacetic acid (5-HIAA) in the brain stem and hypothalamus and an additional increase in the level of 5-HIAA in the hippocampus and striatum. The authors concluded that because there was an increase in the turnover of serotonin in some parts of the brain, these may play a role in physical performance (Blomstrand et al., 1989). Gomez-Merino et al. (2001) examined the impact of acute intensive treadmill running on serotonin levels in the hippocampus and the frontal cortex and observed high levels of the monoamine in both regions after 90 minutes of exercise. In these same regions, as well as in the hippocampus, Soares et al. (2007) and A. G. Rodrigues et al. (2009) reported elevated concentrations of serotonin after running until fatigue. More recently, Caperuto et al. (2009) reported that although swimming training induced similar hypothalamic serotonin concentrations as sedentarism, its concentration in this brain region increased after an exhaustive training program with an insufficient recovery period. The data led to the hypothesis that elevated serotonin content may contribute to poor exercise performance during periods of excessive training.

A special focus has been given to the pharmacological manipulations used to elucidate the relationship between increased serotonergic activity and the early onset of fatigue (Bailey et al., 1993; Roelands et al., 2009). A study by Bailey et al. (1993) demonstrated that exercise performance benefitted from the use of a serotonin antagonist, while treatment with a serotonin agonist led to a detriment in exercise performance. Similarly, increased brain serotonin availability during exercise results in poor physical performance (Soares et al.,

2004, 2007). Reduced exercise performance related to higher serotonin content in the preoptic area and the hypothalamus was also verified after a central blockade of angiotensinergic synapses (Leite et al., 2010). Serotonin reuptake inhibitors have also been widely used, with the purpose of investigating the relationship between the neurotransmitter and central fatigue (Meeusen et al., 2001; Pannier et al., 1995; Parise et al., 2001; Struder et al., 1998; W. M. Wilson et al., 1992). However, the results are contradictory and inconclusive. Although data have demonstrated no effect of different serotonin reuptake inhibitors (pizotifen, fluoxetine, citalopam) on exercise performance in humans (Meeusen et al., 2001; Pannier et al., 1995; Parise et al., 2001; Roelands et al., 2009; Strachan et al., 2004), findings from Struder et al. (1998) and W. M. Wilson et al. (1992) indicate that fatigue occurs sooner with pharmacological augmentation of the brain's serotonergic activity by serotonin re-uptake inhibitor (paroxetine) supplements. These different outcomes might be explained by divergent exercise protocols, pharmacological manipulations, drug receptor specificity and drug dosages.

Recent evidence indicates that serotonin neurotransmission also contributes to the development of central fatigue through its interference with thermoregulation. Particularly in the preoptic area/anterior hypothalamus, increased serotonin availability has been associated with hyperthermia that was brought about by an increase in metabolic heat production and a decrease in heat loss (Lin et al., 1998; Soares et al., 2004, 2007).The central treatment with tryptophan during exercise results in the precipitation of fatigue due to a disruption of the thermal balance, which accelerates the increase in exercise-induced hyperthermia (Soares et al., 2004, 2007). This finding indicates an important role of serotonin in thermoregulation during exercise and agrees with the observation that the rate of body heating reduces the central nervous system drive for exercise performance (Soares et al., 2004, 2007). In fact, the data show that tryptophan-induced central fatigue due to hyperthermia and increased heat storage was intimately related to enhanced serotonin content in the preoptic area. In other words, increased serotonergic tonus in the preoptic area contributed to the aggravation of hyperthermia during exercise and the earlier settlement of central fatigue (Soares et al., 2007). This assumption is also true after the central manipulation of angiotensinergic transmissions (Leite et al., 2010). The central fatigue due to intense hyperthermia that was induced by central angiotensinergic inhibition was related to higher serotonin content in the preoptic area and the hypothalamus. In contrast, central cholinergic stimulation was associated with a decreased elevation in body temperature during exercise by abolishing the exercise-induced increase in serotonin content in the preoptic area (A. G. Rodrigues et al., 2009). These data emphasize that the onset of hyperthermic central fatigue seems to depend greatly on serotonin trafficking in thermoregulatory centers.

6.2 Dopamine

Although the role of serotonin in central fatigue has been well-documented, there is data that shows that dopamine also influences central fatigue (Balthazar et al., 2009, 2010; Foley & Fleshner, 2008; Hasegawa et al., 2008). Dopamine neurotransmission is associated with many physiological functions that could modify running performance, such as arousal, motivation, reinforcement, reward, motor behavior control and mechanisms of addiction (Balthazar et al., 2009, 2010; Foley & Fleshner, 2008; Hasegawa et al., 2008; Meeusen et al., 2007).

Central dopamine metabolism has been shown to increase in several brain regions during exercise (Balthazar et al., 2009; Foley & Fleshner, 2008; Hasegawa et al., 2008; Meeusen et al., 2007). Meeusen et al. (1997) showed that 60 min of exercise significantly increased dopamine content in the striatum. The same increase in dopamine concentration was seen in the midbrain, hypothalamus and hippocampus during exercise (Balthazar et al., 2009, 2010; Chaouloff et al., 1987). On the other hand, Bailey et al. (1993) reported reduced cerebral dopamine levels after prolonged running, which indicates that low dopamine levels during intense exercise may contribute to the reduction in physical capacity through an interference with motivation, arousal and the motor drive. It is important to point out that recent studies reveal that the variation in the brain dopamine content during exercise exhibits a dynamic profile; the levels increase between exercises and return to basal levels at the point of fatigue, which is the same time that serotonin content is at its peak (Bailey et al., 2003; Balthazar et al., 2009; Foley & Fleshner, 2008; Struder & Weicker, 2001a,b). Therefore, it seems that exercise continuation is favored by the increase in dopamine brain levels in between exercises, while central fatigue is a consequence of the reduced central dopamine concentrations along with other factors, such as the increased brain serotonin concentrations.

Findings that elevations in brain dopamine levels are associated with a delay in fatigue come primarily from pharmacological manipulations (Hasegawa et al., 2005; Watson et al., 2005). The administration of amphetamine, a potent dopamine releaser (Chandler & Blair, 1980), has been shown to significantly increase running time until exhaustion (Gerald, 1978). Acute inhibition of dopamine reuptake with bupropion has also been shown to result in exercise performance improvements (Hasegawa et al. 2008; Watson et al., 2005). Similarly, central dopamine activation prior to running until fatigue has also been shown to increase exercise time (Balthazar et al., 2009). In contrast, the blockade of brain dopaminergic receptors markedly reduces exercise tolerance (Balthazar et al., 2010). Interestingly, all of these changes in physical capacity were followed by an elevation in body temperature. In fact, various studies provide evidence that central dopamine activation plays an important role in thermoregulatory mechanisms; this leads to heat loss and body temperature reduction by inducing central temperature set-point adjustments and increasing heat dissipation through skin vasodilation (Balthazar et al., 2010; Barros et al., 2004; Chaperon et al., 2003; Nunes et al., 1991; Varty & Higgins, 1998). Nevertheless, there is evidence that an increase in dopamine levels in the preoptic area/anterior hypothalamus is followed by hyperthermic responses during exercise (Balthazar et al., 2009, 2010; Hasegawa et al. 2005, 2008; Watson et al., 2005). Watson et al. (2005) reported that bupropion, despite enabling subjects to maintain a greater time-trial power output while in the heat, led to a higher body temperature. Hasegawa et al. (2008) showed further evidence that the improved physical performance that was a result of bupropion treatment was accompanied by increased brain and body temperatures and related to an increase in the concentration of dopamine in the preoptic area/anterior hypothalamus. The central activation of dopaminergic transmissions also induces a longer time of running until fatigue, despite a higher heat storage and body temperature at the fatigue point (Balthazar et al., 2009). In contrast, a central blockade of D1 or D2 dopaminergic receptors impairs the dissipation of the exercise-induced heat stored during running, and results in persistent hyperthermia and markedly reduced exercise tolerance (Balthazar et al., 2010). Because the ergogenic response is affected by thermoregulation, the preoptic area/anterior hypothalamus seem to be the brain areas in which dopamine exerts its thermoregulatory actions; dopamine modulates heat production and dissipation during exercise, thus affecting running performance (Balthazar et al., 2009; Hasegawa et al. 2008; Watson et al., 2005). Another possible locus for the effects of central dopaminergic stimulation seems to be the dopaminergic reward circuits (Koob & Moal, 2008). Dopamine, acting on the mesolimbic reward system, could overrule the inhibitory signals arising from the central nervous system that normally compromise running performance (Balthazar et al., 2009; Hasegawa et al. 2008; Watson et al., 2005). The results of the interaction between thermoregulatory and reward adjustments that are induced by central dopamine may be an increase in the drive and motivation to continue exercise; this increased drive could dampen or override the inhibitory signals that arise from the central nervous system that end exercise due to hyperthermia. Therefore, it seems that the interference of central dopamine with the development of hyperthermic central fatigue depends mainly on the activation of reward circuitries that could overrule the hyperthermic inhibitory pathways (Balthazar et al., 2009; Hasegawa et al. 2008; Watson et al., 2005).

6.3 Noradrenaline

Little data has been reported on the contribution of noradrenaline in central fatigue. Although noradrenaline is associated with arousal, consciousness and reward mechanisms in the brain (Roelands & Meeusen, 2010), researchers have shown that elevated brain levels of this catecholamine has a negative effect on exercise performance (Piacentini et al., 2002; Roelands et al., 2008; Roelands & Meeusen, 2010). The administration of reboxetine, a noradrenaline reuptake inhibitor, led to a trend towards a decrease in exercise performance in well-trained endurance athletes (Piacentini et al., 2002). This response was later confirmed by Roelands et al. (2008), who suggested that an increase in the concentration of noradrenaline could be unfavorable for exercise performance because treatment with the noradrenaline reuptake inhibitor decreased physical capacity in both normal and high ambient temperatures. The inhibitory effect exerted by noradrenaline on physical performance, even though it was not accompanied by a significant change in body temperature, induced a tendency for hypothermia. This inclination was further corroborated by thermal stress scale scores that indicated a cold sense by the subjects after noradrenaline reuptake inhibition (Roelands et al., 2008).

Studies have provided conflicting data about the role of noradrenaline in thermoregulation. The literature points out that the divergent thermal effects of noradrenaline depend on the type of receptor that is being stimulated. Therefore, it seems that α-1 noradrenergic receptors mediate a rise in body temperature, while α-2 noradrenergic receptors are involved in a fall in body temperature (Feleder et al., 2004; Imbery et al., 2008; Quan et al., 1991, 1992). Noradrenaline administered in the preoptic area induces a hypothermic response because of a reduction in the metabolic rate (Quan et al., 1991). This response has been shown to be mediated by α-2 receptors, as demonstrated by the fact that an α-2 agonist evoked a dose-dependent decrease in body temperature that was abolished by an α-2 antagonist (Quan et al., 1992). Similar results were found after noradrenaline activation in the anterior hypothalamus during rest and exercise (Feleder et al., 2004; Gisolfi & Christman, 1980). On the other hand, Myers et al. (1987) suggested that both α-1 and α-2 noradrenergic receptors in the hypothalamus are required to evoke hypothermia. Moreover, it has been shown that α-1 activation of hypothalamic neurons results in a rapid hyperthermia (Feleder et al., 2004) and that α-1 agonists infused into the preoptic area evoke a quick rise in body temperature (Imbery et al., 2008).

The involvement of brain noradrenergic transmission in the onset of hyperthermic central fatigue is still uncertain. A study from Hasegawa et al. (2008) showed the most convincing evidence of the role of noradrenaline on the development of fatigue due to hyperthermia. The administration of a dopamine/noradrenaline reuptake inhibitor (bupropion) in the heat, prior to exercise until exhaustion, induced an increase in brain and body temperature; both were associated with a decreased heat loss response and a better physical capacity (Hasegawa et al., 2008). These responses were followed by similar level of increases in the concentrations of dopamine and noradrenaline in the preoptic area/anterior hypothalamus. Therefore, although bupropion has a higher potency for dopamine than noradrenaline (Holm & Spencer, 2000), the results demonstrate that the drug acts in the brain by enhancing the concentration of both dopamine and noradrenaline in a nucleus of major importance for thermoregulation. The interaction of dopamine and noradrenaline in the preoptic area/anterior hypothalamus likely extends the safe limits of hyperthermia. Nonetheless, the brain noradrenergic contribution to hyperthermic central fatigue needs to be investigated further. Special attention should be given to the interaction between noradrenaline and dopamine, in addition to serotonin, on the onset of central fatigue related to hyperthermia.

7. Brain monoamines and other neurotransmitters on the development of central fatigue: Balance between serotonin and dopamine?

It would be simplistic to assume that central fatigue is a result of the altered metabolism of a single neurotransmitter. On the contrary, data indicate that the phenomenon is much more complex and includes the interaction between many neurotransmitters that interfere with exercise performance, together with thermoregulation, through the modulation of brain monoamine concentrations (Bhattacharya & Sen, 1992, Foley & Fleshner, 2008; Leite et al., 2010; Meeusen et al., 2006, A. G. Rodrigues et al., 2004, 2009). In light of the facts that central fatigue is coincident with high body temperature and/or high rates of body heating and heat storage and that serotonergic, dopaminergic and noradrenergic transmissions are in command of fatigue, the interaction between such systems and with other neurotransmitters implicated in thermoregulation seems to affect physical capacity by influencing heat balance in important thermoregulatory centers.

The most commonly described interaction is between serotonin and dopamine (Davis & Bailey, 1997; Foley & Fleshner, 2008; Leite et al., 2010; Meeusen et al., 2006). The precursor of dopamine, tyrosine, competes with other amino acids, including tryptophan, for entry into the brain (Blomstrand, 2006; Fernstrom & Fernstrom, 2006; Foley & Fleshner, 2008; Meeusen et al., 2006). The interaction between serotonin and dopamine may be an important factor affecting the central component of fatigue (Foley & Fleshner, 2008; Leite et al., 2010; Meeusen et al., 2006). Both serotonin and dopamine transmissions increase in the central nervous system due to exercise; however, while serotonin concentration peaks at the fatigue point, dopaminergic activity increases in between exercises and returns to resting levels at fatigue (Bailey et al., 1993; Balthazar et al., 2009; Foley & Fleshner, 2008; Struder & Weicker, 2001a,b). On the basis of this data, the "central fatigue hypothesis" postulates that a high serotonin/dopamine ratio is associated with poor exercise performance, being the converse also true i.e. improvement of exercise performance (Foley & Fleshner, 2008; Leite et al., 2010;

Meeusen et al., 2006). In the first case, the increase in the brain activity of serotonin during physical activity seems to contribute to fatigue through an inhibition of the central dopaminergic system (Foley & Fleshner, 2008; Leite et al., 2010; Meeusen et al., 2006). To support such an assumption, it has been demonstrated that the administration of a serotonin agonist blocked the exercise-induced increase in brain dopamine concentrations; it has also been shown that treatment with a serotonin antagonist prevented a decrease in central dopamine levels at exhaustion (Bailey et al., 1993). Therefore, a decline in exercise performance seems to depend primarily on a serotonin level increase that could override the ergogenic effect of dopamine. Taking into account these data and data that show that both dopamine and serotonin mediate thermoregulation, it has been demonstrated that another factor that contributes to premature central fatigue is the association of high serotonin/dopamine ratio in the hypothalamus with intense hyperthermia (Leite et al., 2010).

Many studies have focused on analyzing the effects of the relationships between brain catecholamines on the development of hyperthermic central fatigue, particularly in regards to dopamine and noradrenaline (Hasegawa et al., 2005, 2008; Watson et al., 2005). Both neurotransmitters have been implicated in thermoregulation, and both have their activity elevated during exercise, likely as a function of the increased sympathetic tonus (Balthazar et al., 2009; Davies & Bailey, 1997; Hasegawa et al., 2008). The administration of bupropion has been the most commonly used drug to investigate such catecholaminergic interactions (Hasegawa et al., 2005, 2008; Watson et al., 2005). The acute administration of bupropion during rest has been shown to increase dopamine and noradrenaline levels in the hippocampus and in the preoptic area/anterior hypothalamus, and this effect was followed by hyperthermic responses (Hasegawa et al., 2005; Piacentini et al., 2003). During exercise, the acute ingestion of the drug in humans has been shown to improve time-trial exercise performance in a warm environment, despite higher body temperatures (Watson et al., 2005). In contrast to acute bupropion administration, the chronic ingestion of the drug does not influence time-trial exercise performance under the same environmental conditions, aside from inducing lower body temperature values than the temperatures observed during the acute bupropion study (Roelands et al., 2009; Watson et al., 2005). The mechanism for these observed discrepancies in bupropion administration seems to be the possible adaptation of central neurotransmitter homeostases during the treatment (Roelands et al., 2009). Hasegawa et al. (2008) showed further evidence that acute bupropion treatment prior to exercise until exhaustion in the heat induces increased brain and body temperatures and better physical capacity; these effects are both accompanied by similar increases in the concentrations of dopamine and noradrenaline in the preoptic area/anterior hypothalamus throughout exercise. Therefore, although bupropion has a higher affinity for dopamine than noradrenaline (Holm & Spencer, 2000), these results demonstrate that the drug acts in the brain by increasing the concentrations of both dopamine and noradrenaline in nuclei of major importance for thermoregulation; their interaction probably extends the safe limits of hyperthermia. The communication between these catecholamines seems to potentiate motivation, arousal and reward, thus enabling subjects to continue to sustain a high power output, despite approaching critical levels of body temperatures that could contribute to central fatigue development (Balthazar et al., 2009; Hasegawa et al., 2008; Watson et al., 2005). Nevertheless, the nature of such interplay between dopamine and noradrenaline is still uncertain.

Brain serotonergic activity has been demonstrated to be affected by cholinergic neurotransmission (Bhattacharya & Sen, 1992). The administration of muscarinic receptor agonists induces a dose-related decrease in the brain concentrations of serotonin. In contrast, the muscarinic receptor antagonist, pirenzepine, increases the central levels of this monoamine. These results indicate that an inverse relationship exists between the cholinergic and serotonergic neurotransmitter systems in the brain (Bhattacharya & Sen, 1992). More recent reports show evidence that central cholinergic activation also influences central fatigue through interactions with the serotonergic system (A. G. Rodrigues et al., 2004, 2009). Studies have shown that the stimulation of heat dissipation mechanisms is related to cholinergic activation and produces hypothermia when cholinoceptor agonists are injected centrally (Lin et al., 1980, Pires et al., 2007; Prímola-Gomes et al., 2007; A. G. Rodrigues et al., 2004, 2009). This effect was seen during exercise after central activation of the cholinergic system with physostigmine (an acetylcholinesterase inhibitor). The treatment decreased body heating rate and heat storage due to improved heat loss (A. G. Rodrigues et al., 2004, 2009). As a consequence, body temperature increases attenuated, which enabled fatigue to be established at a lower body temperature without exercise performance improvement. In such a situation, the cardiovascular overload was the main inductor of fatigue, prevailing over the hypothermic excitatory signals from the central nervous system that could ultimately favor physical work performance (Pires et al., 2007). It is important to note that the lower heat storage, as a product of central physostigmine treatment, was closely associated with decreased serotonin levels in the preoptic area at the moment of fatigue (A. G. Rodrigues et al., 2009). These data indicate that cholinergic stimulation abolishes the exercise-induced increase in serotonin content in the main thermoregulatory site. Moreover, these data support the idea that central cholinergic stimulation promotes decreases in heat storage during exercise by altering the activation of the brain serotonergic system.

Adding to the hypothesis that central fatigue is determined by interactions between neuronal signal substances, it has been demonstrated that a central angiotensinergic blockade during exercise affects serotonin concentration in the preoptic area and hypothalamus, in association with excessive hyperthermia and premature central fatigue (Leite et al., 2010). Acting centrally, angiotensin II exerts thermoregulatory effects that are characterized by hypothermia (Fregly & Rowland, 1996; K. M. Wilson & Fregly, 1985).Central treatment with losartan (angiotensin II AT_1 receptor antagonist) worsens hyperthermia and increases the body heating rate and heat storage rate that are indirectly related to the time to fatigue. This hyperthermic response is due to a heat imbalance that is characterized by higher heat production and lower peripheral heat loss (Leite et al., 2006, 2007). These effects of angiotensin II on heat balance during exercise were shown to be linked to serotonergic pathways (Leite et al., 2010). These findings provide evidence that the inhibition of the central angiotensinergic system during exercise causes an increase in serotonin content in the preoptic area and hypothalamus that is directly associated with hyperthermia and a higher body heating rate and that is indirectly related to the time to fatigue. In addition, although losartan did not alter the concentration of dopamine in the analyzed brain areas, it did lead to a high hypothalamic serotonin/dopamine ratio, which was directly correlated with the body heating rate and inversely correlated with the time to fatigue. Thus, serotonin and dopamine interaction in these regions contributes to hyperthermia and premature central fatigue when central angiotensinergic pathways are inhibited. Taken together, the data indicate that central angiotensinergic transmission has important effects on serotonin levels in the brain during exercise and interacts with dopamine-affected central fatigue through a modulation of body temperature control.

There is also the possibility that serotonin interacts with noradrenaline in the establishment of central fatigue, despite results from Piacentini et al. (2002), where the administration of a serotonin/noradrenaline reuptake inhibitor (venlafaxine) had no effect on exercise performance. Evidence indicates that the dorsal raphe serotonin neurons receive noradrenergic projections from the locus coeruleus (Szabo & Blier, 2001, 2002). Conversely, noradrenaline neurons of the locus coeruleus receive dense serotonergic projections mainly from the dorsal raphe (Szabo & Blier, 2001, 2002). These pathways suggest the possible existence of modulation between the activity of serotonin and noradrenaline in the brain nuclei that are responsible for thermoregulation, which could interfere with thermal balance and exercise performance.

A question remains regarding the participation of other neurotransmitters that also influence thermal control, such as GABA and glutamate (Ishiwata et al., 2005; Nikolov & Yakimova, 2011), which could interact with central monoamines in the development of hyperthermic central fatigue. Thus, knowledge of the mechanisms of central fatigue is still limited and presupposes a complex interplay of different neurotransmitter systems that affect thermoregulation and exercise performance; serotonin, dopamine and noradrenaline likely play the most important roles.

8. Predictors of fatigue: Static and dynamic perspectives

The combination of exercise with excessive hyperthermia appears to diminish the central nervous system drive to the working muscles, protecting the brain from thermal damage in detriment of exercise performance (Kay & Marino, 2000; Nielsen & Nybo, 2003; Noakes, 1998). The thermoregulatory-sensed variables that initiate these central inhibitory signals of exercise performance in order to avoid heat stroke are still the subject of debate. Even though it has been stated that central fatigue coincides with the attainment of fixed high body and brain temperatures (Fuller et al., 1998; Gonzalez-Alonso et al., 1999; Nielsen et al., 1993; Walters et al., 2000), there is evidence that dynamic mechanisms are consistent regulators of feelings of fatigue. In support of this hypothesis, the rates of heat storage and body heating that are associated with changes in neurotransmitter content in thermoregulatory centers emerge as important factors in determining fatigue (Cheuvront et al., 2010; Hasegawa et al., 2008; Lacerda et al., 2005, 2006; Leite et al., 2006, 2010, L. O. Rodrigues et al., 2003; A. G. Rodrigues et al., 2004, 2009; Soares et al., 2004, 2007; Wanner et al., 2007).

Reaching critically high and predetermined body and brain temperatures, very close to the level of heat stroke, has been proposed as an ultimate warning sign that causes a reduction in the mental drive for exercise performance (Fuller et al., 1998; Gonzalez-Alonso et al., 1999; Nielsen et al., 1993; Walters et al., 2000). In this light, fatigue would be anticipated by such a static thermal indicator, which would establish a hyperthermic threshold to prevent homeostasis failure. There are a number of reports that have linked the attainment of a decisive high body temperature to the settlement of fatigue in humans and in animals. This was the conclusion of Nielsen et al. (1993), who reported that endurance-trained individuals always stopped exercising until exhaustion (~60% of VO_2 max) when esophageal temperatures reached 39.5°C. In addition, these subjects exhibited a prolonged endurance time after 9-12 consecutive days of exercising at an ambient temperature of 40°C, which was associated with a decreased body temperature rise rate; these changes suggest that the body heating rate could interfere with the physical capacity. To hold Nielsen's hypothesis, results from Fuller et al. (1998) indicate that exercise (~60% of VO2 max) trials that differed in ambient temperature (33.0 and 38.0°C) and initial body temperature (23 and 38°C) promoted fatigue at the same abdominal (~39.9°C) and brain temperatures (~40.2°C). It is important to point out that the exercises were executed under a higher thermal load that induced fatigue earlier, which leaves open the possibility that the rates of body heating and heat storage might have been higher in this circumstance to enable fatigue to be reached at equal abdominal and brain temperatures. This possibility was seen in the case of trained subjects cycling in the heat (60% VO2, 40°C), whose time to fatigue was directly related to the body temperature increase rate, which was controlled at 0.10 or 0.05°C/min-1, and inversely related to the initial level of esophageal temperature (35.9 ± 0.2, 37.4 ± 0.1, or 38.2 ± 0.1) (Gonzalez-Alonso et al., 1999). In both experimental conditions, all subjects reached exhaustion at similar esophageal (40.1–40.2°C) and muscle temperatures (40.7–40.9°C) (Gonzalez-Alonso et al., 1999). However, the manipulation of the body temperature increase rate was restricted to a very narrow range and was possibly not large enough to induce noticeable changes in body temperature. Moreover, individual body temperatures respond differently to heat stimuli and depend on many factors, such as dehydration, nutrition, fitness and motivation, as well as exercise intensity and thermal environmental stress (Kay & Marino, 2000; L. O. Rodrigues et al., 2003). Therefore, in absolute terms, the thermal load imposed would be expected to vary between subjects. Also contributing to the concept that a critical body temperature limits exercise, Walters et al. (2000) demonstrated that running (~60% of VO2max) at an ambient temperature of 35°C establishes both hypothalamic and rectal temperatures at exhaustion of 42.1°C and 42.4°C, respectively, regardless of a manipulation in the initial hypothalamic temperature (41.5°C, 42.5°C or 43.5°C). The hypothalamic and rectal temperatures before exercise correlate negatively with the run-time until exhaustion, which means that the run-time to exhaustion was significantly reduced after preheating. Interestingly, the rectal temperatures at the fatigue point that were observed by the authors were considerably higher than previously seen with exercise at approximately the same intensity (Fuller et al., 1998). Furthermore, the body temperature values at fatigue from the studies mentioned above (Fuller et al., 1998; Walters et al., 2001) also differed from the data from Soares et al. (2004), who demonstrated that increased central serotonin availability with tryptophan treatment before exercise (~66% of VO2max) resulted in the same intraperitoneal temperature at fatigue as in the control group (38.32°C tryptophan vs. 38.03°C saline). It is important to point out that the tryptophan administration elevated the body heating rate and the heat storage rate, and both were negatively correlated with the time to fatigue. Therefore, central serotonergic-activation-induced higher body temperature variations are associated with increased body heating and heat storage rates, which anticipated fatigue (Soares et al., 2004). This detail allows for the possibility that reaching a critically high body temperature by itself may not be the main factor in predicting fatigue. In fact, this result is in agreement with the concept that dynamic variables strongly contribute to the reduction of physical performance (Cheuvront et al., 2010; Hasegawa et al., 2008; Lacerda et al., 2005, 2006; Leite et al., 2006, 2010, L. O. Rodrigues et al., 2003; A. G. Rodrigues et al., 2004, 2009; Soares et al., 2004, 2007; Wanner et al., 2007).

There are many findings that differ from the hypothesis that fatigue is predicted by a defined high body temperature (Cheuvront et al., 2010; Hasegawa et al., 2008; Lacerda et al., 2005, 2006; Leite et al., 2006, 2010, L. O. Rodrigues et al., 2003; A. G. Rodrigues et al., 2004, 2009; Soares et al., 2004, 2007; Wanner et al., 2007). These findings show that the rates of body heating and heat storage play an important role in signaling fatigue development to the brain. Both parameters are characterized by the variation of body temperature as a function of time; the heat storage rate is further corrected for body weight (Lacerda et al.,

2005, 2006; Leite et al., 2006, 2010, L. O. Rodrigues et al., 2003; A. G. Rodrigues et al., 2004, 2009, Soares et al., 2004, 2007; Wanner et al., 2007). Recently, it has been proposed that skin temperature also provides important sensory input to the central nervous system during exercise in the heat and has a negative effect on performance that worsens as the cutaneous temperature progressively increases (Cheuvront et al., 2010).

Considering this dynamic hypothesis, L. O. Rodrigues et al. (2003) demonstrated that exhaustion was inversely correlated with the heat storage rate during running at a speeds of 21 or 24 m/min, without an incline in the treadmill, at three different ambient temperatures (18.0, 23.1 or 29.4°C). The exercise under the higher intensity and thermal load resulted in precipitation of fatigue. More importantly, the intraperitoneal body temperature at the fatigue point was different between the groups and higher after running in the heat. This profile was also seen by Hasegawa et al. (2008), whose data demonstrated that both intraperitoneal and brain temperatures at the point of exhaustion were significantly lower after exercise in a cool condition (18.0°C) compared to a warm environment (30 °C). Therefore, in these two examples, the body temperature at the point of exhaustion in the cool condition did not reach the critical level. Brain manipulations of neurotransmitters/neuromodulators during exercise also give strong evidence of the involvement of dynamic variables on the reduction in exercise time. Central nitric oxide blockade with L-NAME (N-nitro-l-arginine methyl ester, a nitric oxide synthase inhibitor) results in higher intraperitoneal body temperatures at fatigue and lower exercise performances (Lacerda et al., 2005). Due to the increased heat production associated with decreased heat loss, this treatment results in a higher body heating rate that rapidly produces hyperthermia (Lacerda et at., 2005, 2006). It is important to point out that the reduced exercise performance observed after a blockade of nitric oxide pathways is closely associated with the higher body heating rate (Lacerda et al., 2005). This relationship is absent after a stimulation of the central cholinergic transmissions during exercise (~66% of VO_2max). Although this treatment attenuated colonic temperature increases, the time to fatigue was not affected, which was the same as that of controls (A. G. Rodrigues et al., 2004). This evidence emphasizes that even though both groups reached fatigue at the same moment, the body temperature at fatigue was different between groups; that is, body temperatures were lower after central cholinergic stimulation, which is attributable to the activation of heat loss mechanisms (A. G. Rodrigues et al., 2004, 2009). Additionally, this treatment promoted a decrease in the body heating rate (A. G. Rodrigues et al., 2004). On the other hand, a direct relationship between the heat storage rate and the time to fatigue was present when cholinergic transmissions where blocked by a central administration of methylatropine (a muscarinic receptor antagonist) (Wanner et al., 2007). A central cholinergic blockade during running (~80% of VO_2max) increases the heat storage rate, leading to greater exercise-induced hyperthermia and a higher intraperitoneal temperature at fatigue, which is followed by exercise performance impairments. Therefore, the increased heat storage rate, as a consequence of a higher metabolic cost and decreased heat dissipation, contributes significantly to the interruption of exercise (Wanner et al., 2007, 2011). Adding to the hypothesis that fatigue is determined by active variables, Leite et al. (2006) verified that a close correlation between the elevated body heating rate and the reduced time to fatigue (~66% of VO_2max) is seen after central angiotensinergic blockade with losartan. This treatment increases intraperitoneal temperatures at the fatigue point because of an enhanced heat production that is not compensated by a proportional heat loss

(Leite et al., 2006, 2007). Thus, an infusion of losartan induces a significant increase in the body heating rate, and also the heat storage rate, that rapidly produces aggravation of hyperthermia and reduces exercise performance (Leite et al., 2010). In view of the fact that dissimilar values of body temperatures at the fatigue point were seen between groups assessed with distinct approaches, the authors postulated that as the elevated rates of body heating and heat storage progressively exacerbate the exercise-induced hyperthermia, the central nervous system becomes sensitive to such a dynamic event and induces fatigue as a safety mechanism to prevent a dangerously high body temperature that could jeopardize physical integrity.

Recent findings have also associated elevated rates of body heating and heat storage with high levels of serotonin in centers responsible for thermoregulation (Leite et al., 2010; A. G. Rodrigues et al., 2009; Soares et al., 2007). In the case of central angiotensinergic blockade, the augmented body heating rate and reduced exercise performance were directly associated with high levels of serotonin at fatigue in thermoregulatory centers like the preoptic area and hypothalamus (Leite et al., 2010). An elevation of serotonin content in the preoptic area is also related to increased body temperature variations and a reduced time to fatigue shown by central serotonin activation (Soares et al., 2007). In contrast, lower heat storage, which attenuates the exercise-induced hyperthermia as a result of stimulation of the central cholinergic system, is closely associated with decreased serotonin levels in the preoptic area at the moment of fatigue (A. G. Rodrigues et al., 2009). Central dopamine metabolism is also enhanced during exercise (Balthazar et al., 2009; Foley & Fleshner, 2008; Hasegawa et al., 2005), and its interaction with serotonin has been linked with high rates of body heating and precipitation of fatigue (Foley & Fleshner, 2008; Meeusen et al., 2007). A combination of effects is induced by central angiotensinergic blockade, which leads to a higher serotonin/dopamine ratio within the hypothalamus at fatigue that correlates directly with the body heating rate and indirectly with the exercise time to fatigue (Leite et al., 2010). This observation asserts that the high concentrations of serotonin achieved during exercise, in addition to their interactions with dopamine in nuclei responsible for thermoregulation, contribute to the increases in body heating and heat storage rates, thereby adding to exercise-induced hyperthermia and decreasing running performance. Changes in neurotransmitter content in thermoregulatory centers, which are associated with afferent feedback arising from variations in the body heating and heat storage rates during exercise, provide new insights into possible mechanisms by which individuals may terminate exercise.

9. Conclusions

The mechanisms underlying hyperthermic central fatigue include decreased efferent signaling from the central nervous system that protects the brain from thermal damage. There is strong evidence that these mechanisms depend greatly on monoamine traffic, mainly the serotonin/dopamine ratio, in thermoregulatory centers. Hyperthermic central fatigue during exercise should be seen essentially as a defense mechanism. Reaching a critically high body temperature, by itself, may not be the main factor in predicting fatigue. In fact, this is in agreement with the concept that dynamic variables determine physical performance more than static ones.

10. Acknowledgments

We acknowledge CNPq and FAPEMIG for financial support.

11. References

Abdelmalki, A.; Merino, D.; Bonneau, D.; Bigard, A. X. & Guezennec, C. Y. (1997). Administration of a GABAB agonist baclofen before running to exhaustion in the rat: effects on performance and on some indicators of fatigue. *Int J Sports Med*, Vol. 18, No. 2, (Feb, 1997), pp. 75-8, ISSN 0172-4622.

Ament, W. & Verkerke, G. J. (2009). Exercise and fatigue. *Sports Med*, Vol. 39, No. 5, (2009), pp. 389-422, ISSN 0112-1642.

Bailey, S. P.; Davis, J. M. & Ahlborn, E. N. (1993). Neuroendocrine and substrate responses to altered brain 5-HT activity during prolonged exercise to fatigue. *J Appl Physiol*, Vol. 74, No. 6, (Jun, 1993), pp.3006-12, ISSN 8750-7587.

Balthazar, C. H.; Leite, L. H.; Ribeiro, R. M.; Soares, D. D. & Coimbra, C. C. (2010). Effects of blockade of central dopamine D1 and D2 receptors on thermoregulation, metabolic rate and running performance. *Pharmacol Rep*, Vol. 62, No. 1, (Jan-Feb, 2010), pp. 54-61 ISSN 1734-1140.

Balthazar, C. H.; Leite, L. H.; Rodrigues, A. G. & Coimbra, C. C. (2009). Performance-enhancing and thermoregulatory effects of intracerebroventricular dopamine in running rats. *Pharmacol Biochem Behav*, Vol. 93, No. 4, (Oct, 2009), pp.465-9, ISSN 1873-5177.

Barchas, J. D. & Freedman, D. X. (1963). Brain Amines: Response to Physiological Stress. *Biochem Pharmacol*, Vol. 12, No., (Oct, 1963), pp. 1232-5, ISSN 0006-2952.

Baron, B.; Deruelle, F.; Moullan, F.; Dalleau, G.; Verkindt, C. & Noakes, T. D. (2009). The eccentric muscle loading influences the pacing strategies during repeated downhill sprint intervals. *Eur J Appl Physiol*, Vol. 105, No. 5, (Mar, 2009), pp. 749-57, ISSN 1439-6327.

Barros, R. C.; Branco, L. G. & Carnio, E. C. (2004). Evidence for thermoregulation by dopamine D1 and D2 receptors in the anteroventral preoptic region during normoxia and hypoxia. *Brain Res*, Vol. 1030, No. 2, (Dec 31, 2004), pp. 165-71, ISSN 0006-8993.

Bassett, D. R., JR. & Howley, E. T. (2000). Limiting factors for maximum oxygen uptake and determinants of endurance performance. *Med Sci Sports Exerc*, Vol. 32, No. 1, (Jan, 2000), pp.70-84, ISSN 0195-9131.

Bhattacharya, S. K. & Sen, A. P. (1992). Effects of muscarinic receptor agonists and antagonists on rat brain serotonergic activity. *J Neural Transm Gen Sect*, Vol. 90, No. 3, 1992), pp. 241-7, ISSN 0300-9564.

Blomstrand, E. (2006). A role for branched-chain amino acids in reducing central fatigue. *J Nutr*, Vol. 136, No. 2, (Feb, 2006), pp. 544S-547S, ISSN 0022-3166.

Blomstrand, E.; Perrett, D.; Parry-Billings, M. & Newsholme, E. A. (1989). Effect of sustained exercise on plasma amino acid concentrations and on 5-hydroxytryptamine metabolism in six different brain regions in the rat. *Acta Physiol Scand*, Vol. 136, No. 3, (Jul, 1989), pp.473-81, ISSN 0001-6772.

Borg, G. A. (1982). Psychophysical bases of perceived exertion. *Med Sci Sports Exerc*, Vol. 14, No. 5, 1982), pp. 377-81, ISSN 0195-9131.

Bruck, K. & Olschewski, H. (1987). Body temperature related factors diminishing the drive to exercise. *Can J Physiol Pharmacol*, Vol. 65, No. 6, (Jun, 1987), pp. 1274-80, ISSN 0008-4212.

Caperuto, E. C.; Dos Santos, R. V.; Mello, M. T. & Costa Rosa, L. F. (2009). Effect of endurance training on hypothalamic serotonin concentration and performance. *Clin Exp Pharmacol Physiol*, Vol. 36, No. 2, (Feb, 2009), pp. 189-91, ISSN 1440-1681.

Caputa, M.; Feistkorn, G. & Jessen, C. (1986). Effects of brain and trunk temperatures on exercise performance in goats. *Pflugers Arch*, Vol. 406, No. 2, (Feb, 1986), pp. 184-9, ISSN 0031-6768.

Castle, P. C.; MacDonald, A. L.; Philp, A.; Webborn, A.; Watt, P. W. & Maxwell, N. S. (2006). Precooling leg muscle improves intermittent sprint exercise performance in hot, humid conditions. *J Appl Physiol*, Vol. 100, No. 4, (Apr, 2006), pp. 1377-84, ISSN 8750-7587.

Chandler, J. V. & Blair, S. N. (1980). The effect of amphetamines on selected physiological components related to athletic success. *Med Sci Sports Exerc*, Vol. 12, No. 1, (Spring, 1980), pp. 65-9, ISSN 0195-9131.

Chaouloff, F. (1997). Effects of acute physical exercise on central serotonergic systems. *Med Sci Sports Exerc*, Vol. 29, No. 1, (Jan, 1997), pp. 58-62, ISSN 0195-9131.

Chaouloff, F. (2000). Serotonin, stress and corticoids. *J Psychopharmacol*, Vol. 14, No. 2, (Jun, 2000), pp. 139-51, ISSN 0269-8811.

Chaouloff, F.; Laude, D.; Merino, D.; Serrurrier, B.; Guezennec, Y. & Elghozi, J. L. (1987). Amphetamine and alpha-methyl-p-tyrosine affect the exercise-induced imbalance between the availability of tryptophan and synthesis of serotonin in the brain of the rat. *Neuropharmacology*, Vol. 26, No. 8, (Aug, 1987), pp. 1099-106, ISSN 0028-3908.

Chaperon, F.; Tricklebank, M. D.; UNGER, L. & NEIJT, H. C. (2003). Evidence for regulation of body temperature in rats by dopamine D2 receptor and possible influence of D1 but not D3 and D4 receptors. *Neuropharmacology*, Vol. 44, No. 8, (Jun, 2003), pp. 1047-53, ISSN 0028-3908.

Cheung, S. S. (2007). Hyperthermia and voluntary exhaustion: integrating models and future challenges. *Appl Physiol Nutr Metab*, Vol. 32, No. 4, (Aug, 2007), pp. 808-17, ISSN 1715-5312.

Cheung, S. S. & Sleivert, G. G. (2004). Multiple triggers for hyperthermic fatigue and exhaustion. *Exerc Sport Sci Rev*, Vol. 32, No. 3, (Jul, 2004), pp. 100-6, ISSN 0091-6331.

Cheuvront, S. N.; Kenefick, R. W.; Montain, S. J. & Sawka, M. N. (2010). Mechanisms of aerobic performance impairment with heat stress and dehydration. *J Appl Physiol*, Vol. 109, No. 6, (Dec, 2010), pp. 1989-95, ISSN 1522-1601.

Coelho, L. G.; Ferreira-Junior, J. B.; Martini, A. R.; Borba, D. A.; Coelho, D. B.; Passos, R. L.; Fonseca, M. A.; Moura-Lima, F. A.; Prado, L. S. & Rodrigues, L. O. (2010). Head hair reduces sweat rate during exercise under the sun. *Int J Sports Med*, Vol. 31, No. 11, (Nov, 2010), pp. 779-83, ISSN 1439-3964.

Coyle, E. F.; Coggan, A. R.; Hemmert, M. K. & Ivy, J. L. (1986). Muscle glycogen utilization during prolonged strenuous exercise when fed carbohydrate. *J Appl Physiol*, Vol. 61, No. 1, (Jul, 1986), pp. 165-72, ISSN 8750-7587.

Coyle, E. F. & Gonzalez-Alonso, J. (2001). Cardiovascular drift during prolonged exercise: new perspectives. *Exerc Sport Sci Rev*, Vol. 29, No. 2, (Apr, 2001), pp.88-92, ISSN 0091-6331.

Davis, J. M. & Bailey, S. P. (1997). Possible mechanisms of central nervous system fatigue during exercise. *Med Sci Sports Exerc*, Vol. 29, No. 1, (Jan, 1997), pp. 45-57, ISSN 0195-9131.

Denizeau, F. & Sourkes, T. L. (1977). Regional transport of tryptophan in rat brain. *J Neurochem*, Vol. 28, No. 5, (May, 1977), pp. 951-9, ISSN 0022-3042.

Ely, B. R.; Cheuvront, S. N.; Kenefick, R. W. & Sawka, M. N. (2010). Aerobic performance is degraded, despite modest hyperthermia, in hot environments. *Med Sci Sports Exerc*, Vol. 42, No. 1, (Jan, 2010), pp. 135-41, ISSN 1530-0315

Enoka, R. M. & Stuart, D. G. (1992). Neurobiology of muscle fatigue. *J Appl Physiol*, Vol. 72, No. 5, (May, 1992), pp. 1631-48, ISSN 8750-7587.

Evans, W. J. & Lambert, C. P. (2007). Physiological basis of fatigue. *Am J Phys Med Rehabil*, Vol. 86, No. 1 Suppl, (Jan, 2007), pp. S29-46, ISSN 0894-9115.

Febbraio, M. A.; Keenan, J.; Angus, D. J.; Campbell, S. E. & Garnham, A. P. (2000). Preexercise carbohydrate ingestion, glucose kinetics, and muscle glycogen use: effect of the glycemic index. *J Appl Physiol*, Vol. 89, No. 5, (Nov, 2000), pp. 1845-51, ISSN 8750-7587.

Feleder, C.; Perlik, V. & Blatteis, C. M. (2004). Preoptic alpha 1- and alpha 2-noradrenergic agonists induce, respectively, PGE2-independent and PGE2-dependent hyperthermic responses in guinea pigs. *Am J Physiol Regul Integr Comp Physiol*, Vol. 286, No. 6, (Jun, 2004), pp. R1156-66, ISSN 0363-6119.

Fernstrom, J. D. & Fernstrom, M. H. (2006). Exercise, serum free tryptophan, and central fatigue. *J Nutr*, Vol. 136, No. 2, (Feb, 2006), pp. 553S-559S, ISSN 0022-3166.

Fletcher, W. M. & Hopkins, F. G. (1907). Lactic acid in amphibian muscle. *J Physiol*, Vol. 35, No. 4 (Mar, 1907), pp. 247-309.

Flouris, A. D. & Cheung, S. S. (2009). Human conscious response to thermal input is adjusted to changes in mean body temperature. *Br J Sports Med*, Vol. 43, No. 3, (Mar, 2009), pp.199-203, ISSN 1473-0480.

Foley, T. E. & Fleshner, M. (2008). Neuroplasticity of dopamine circuits after exercise: implications for central fatigue. *Neuromolecular Med*, Vol. 10, No. 2, 2008), pp. 67-80, ISSN 1535-1084.

Fregly, M. J. & Rowland, N. E. (1996). Centrally mediated vasodilation of the rat's tail by angiotensin II. *Physiol Behav*, Vol. 60, No. 3, (Sep, 1996), pp. 861-5, ISSN 0031-9384.

Fuller, A.; Carter, R. N. & Mitchell, D. (1998). Brain and abdominal temperatures at fatigue in rats exercising in the heat. *J Appl Physiol*, Vol. 84, No. 3, (Mar, 1998), pp. 877-83, ISSN 8750-7587.

Gandevia, S. C. (2001). Spinal and supraspinal factors in human muscle fatigue. *Physiol Rev*, Vol. 81, No. 4, (Oct, 2001), pp. 1725-89, ISSN 0031-9333.

Garcia, A. M.; Lacerda, M. G.; FOnseca, I. A.; Reis, F. M.; Rodrigues, L. O. & Silami-Garcia, E. (2006). Luteal phase of the menstrual cycle increases sweating rate during exercise. *Braz J Med Biol Res*, Vol. 39, No. 9, (Sep, 2006), pp. 1255-61, ISSN 0100-879X.

Gerald, M. C. (1978). Effects of (+)-amphetamine on the treadmill endurance performance of rats. *Neuropharmacology*, Vol. 17, No. 9, (Sep, 1978), pp. 703-4, ISSN 0028-3908.

Gerin, C. & Privat, A. (1998). Direct evidence for the link between monoaminergic descending pathways and motor activity: II. A study with microdialysis probes implanted in the ventral horn of the spinal cord. *Brain Res*, Vol. 794, No. 1, (May 25, 1998), pp. 169-73, ISSN 0006-8993.

GIsolfi, C. V. & Christman, J. V. (1980). Thermal effects of injecting norepinephrine into hypothalamus of the rat during rest and exercise. *J Appl Physiol*, Vol. 49, No. 6, (Dec, 1980), pp. 937-41, ISSN 0161-7567.

Gomez-Merino, D.; Bequet, F.; Berthelot, M.; Chennaoui, M. & Guezennec, C. Y. (2001). Site-dependent effects of an acute intensive exercise on extracellular 5-HT and 5-HIAA levels in rat brain. *Neurosci Lett*, Vol. 301, No. 2, (Mar 30, 2001), pp. 143-6, ISSN 0304-3940.

Gonzalez-Alonso, J.; Teller, C.; Andersen, S. L.; Jensen, F. B.; HYLDIG, T. & NIELSEN, B. (1999). Influence of body temperature on the development of fatigue during prolonged exercise in the heat. *J Appl Physiol*, Vol. 86, No. 3, (Mar, 1999), pp. 1032-9, ISSN 8750-7587.

Hargreaves, M.; McKenna, M. J.; Jenkins, D. G.; Warmington, S. A.; Li, J. L.; Snow, R. J. & Febbraio, M. A. (1998). Muscle metabolites and performance during high-intensity, intermittent exercise. *J Appl Physiol*, Vol. 84, No. 5, (May, 1998), pp. 1687-91, ISSN 8750-7587.

Hasegawa, H.; Ishiwata, T.; Saito, T.; Yazawa, T.; Aihara, Y. & Meeusen, R. (2005). Inhibition of the preoptic area and anterior hypothalamus by tetrodotoxin alters thermoregulatory functions in exercising rats. *J Appl Physiol*, Vol. 98, No. 4, (Apr, 2005), pp. 1458-62, ISSN 8750-7587.

Hasegawa, H.; Piacentini, M. F.; Sarre, S.; Michotte, Y.; Ishiwata, T. & Meeusen, R. (2008). Influence of brain catecholamines on the development of fatigue in exercising rats in the heat. *J Physiol*, Vol. 586, No. 1, (Jan 1, 2008), pp. 141-, ISSN 0022-3751.

Hill, A.V.; Long, C. N. H. & Lupton, H. (1924). Muscular exercise, lactic acid and the supply and utilization of oxygen. *Proc Royal Soc*, Pt. VII-IX B, pp. 97-155.

Hillegaart, V. & Hjorth, S. (1989). Median raphe, but not dorsal raphe, application of the 5-HT1A agonist 8-OH-DPAT stimulates rat motor activity. *Eur J Pharmacol*, Vol. 160, No. 2, (Jan 31, 1989), pp. 303-7, ISSN 0014-2999.

Holm, K. J. & Spencer, C. M. (2000). Bupropion: a review of its use in the management of smoking cessation. *Drugs*, Vol. 59, No. 4, (Apr, 2000), pp. 1007-24, ISSN 0012-6667.

Hunter, S. K.; Duchateau, J. & Enoka, R. M. (2004). Muscle fatigue and the mechanisms of task failure. *Exerc Sport Sci Rev*, Vol. 32, No. 2, (Apr, 2004), pp. 44-9, ISSN 0091-6331.

Imbery, T. E.; Irdmusa, M. S.; Speidell, A. P.; Streer, M. S. & Griffin, J. D. (2008). The effects of Cirazoline, an alpha-1 adrenoreceptor agonist, on the firing rates of thermally classified anterior hypothalamic neurons in rat brain slices. *Brain Res*, Vol. 1193, No., (Feb 8, 2008), pp. 93-101, ISSN 0006-8993.

Imeri, L.; Mancia, M.; Bianchi, S. & Opp, M. R. (2000). 5-Hydroxytryptophan, but not L-tryptophan, alters sleep and brain temperature in rats. *Neuroscience*, Vol. 95, No. 2, 2000), pp. 445-52, ISSN 0306-4522.

IshiwatA, T.; Saito, T.; Hasegawa, H.; Yazawa, T.; Kotani, Y.; Otokawa, M. & Aihara, Y. (2005). Changes of body temperature and thermoregulatory responses of freely moving rats during GABAergic pharmacological stimulation to the preoptic area and anterior hypothalamus in several ambient temperatures. *Brain Res*, Vol. 1048, No. 1-2, (Jun 28, 2005), pp. 32-40, ISSN 0006-8993.

Kanosue, K.; Crawshaw, L. I.; Nagashima, K. & Yoda, T. (2010). Concepts to utilize in describing thermoregulation and neurophysiological evidence for how the system works. *Eur J Appl Physiol*, Vol. 109, No. 1, (May, 2010), pp. 5-11, ISSN 1439-6327.

Kay, D. & Marino, F. E. (2000). Fluid ingestion and exercise hyperthermia: implications for performance, thermoregulation, metabolism and the development of fatigue. *J Sports Sci*, Vol. 18, No. 2, (Feb, 2000), pp. 71-82, ISSN 0264-0414.

Koob, G. F. & Le Moal, M. (2008). Addiction and the brain antireward system. *Annu Rev Psychol*, Vol. 59, No., 2008), pp.(29-53).0066-4308 (Print) 0066-4308 (Linking).

Korte, S. M.; Van Duin, S.; Bouws, G. A.; Koolhaas, J. M. & Bohus, B. (1991). Involvement of hypothalamic serotonin in activation of the sympathoadrenomedullary system and hypothalamo-pituitary-adrenocortical axis in male Wistar rats. *Eur J Pharmacol*, Vol. 197, No. 2-3, (May 17, 1991), pp. 225-8, ISSN 0014-2999.

Kreider, R. B.; Miriel, V. & Bertun, E. (1993). Amino acid supplementation and exercise performance. Analysis of the proposed ergogenic value. *Sports Med*, Vol. 16, No. 3, (Sep, 1993), pp. 190-209, ISSN 0112-164.

Lacerda, A. C.; Marubayashi, U.; Balthazar, C. H. & Coimbra, C. C. (2006). Evidence that brain nitric oxide inhibition increases metabolic cost of exercise, reducing running performance in rats. *Neurosci Lett*, Vol. 393, No. 2-3, (Jan 30, 2006), pp. 260-3, ISSN 0304-3940.

Lacerda, A. C.; Marubayashi, U. & Coimbra, C. C. (2005). Nitric oxide pathway is an important modulator of heat loss in rats during exercise. *Brain Res Bull*, Vol. 67, No. 1-2, (Sep 30, 2005), pp. 110-6, ISSN 0361-9230.

Leite, L. H.; Lacerda, A. C.; Balthazar, C. H.; Marubayashi, U. & Coimbra, C. C. (2007). Central AT(1) receptor blockade increases metabolic cost during exercise reducing mechanical efficiency and running performance in rats. *Neuropeptides*, Vol. 41, No. 3, (Jun, 2007), pp. 189-94, ISSN 0143-4179.

Leite, L. H.; Lacerda, A. C.; Marubayashi, U. & Coimbra, C. C. (2006). Central angiotensin AT1-receptor blockade affects thermoregulation and running performance in rats. *Am J Physiol Regul Integr Comp Physiol*, Vol. 291, No. 3, (Sep, 2006), pp. R603-7, ISSN 0363-6119.

Leite, L. H.; Rodrigues, A. G.; Soares, D. D.; Marubayashi, U. & Coimbra, C. C. (2010). Central fatigue induced by losartan involves brain serotonin and dopamine content. *Med Sci Sports Exerc*, Vol. 42, No. 8, (Aug, 2010), pp. 1469-76, ISSN 1530-0315.

Lin, M. T.; Tsay, H. J.; Su, W. H. & Chueh, F. Y. (1998). Changes in extracellular serotonin in rat hypothalamus affect thermoregulatory function. *Am J Physiol*, Vol. 274, No. 5 Pt 2, (May, 1998), pp. R1260-7, ISSN 0002-9513.

Lin, M. T.; Wang, H. C. & Chandra, A. (1980). The effects on thermoregulation of intracerebroventricular injections of acetylcholine, pilocarpine, physostigmine, atropine and hemicholinium in the rat. *Neuropharmacology*, Vol. 19, No. 6, (Jun, 1980), pp. 561-5, ISSN 0028-3908.

Magalhaes FDE, C.; Amorim, F. T.; Passos, R. L.; Fonseca, M. A.; Oliveira, K. P.; Lima, M. R.; Guimaraes, J. B.; Ferreira-Junior, J. B.; Martini, A. R.; Lima, N. R.; Soares, D. D.; Oliveira, E. M. & Rodrigues, L. O. (2010). Heat and exercise acclimation increases intracellular levels of Hsp72 and inhibits exercise-induced increase in intracellular and plasma Hsp72 in humans. *Cell Stress Chaperones*, Vol. 15, No. 6, (Nov, 2010), pp. 885-95, ISSN 1466-1268.

Marino, F. E. (2004). Anticipatory regulation and avoidance of catastrophe during exercise-induced hyperthermia. *Comp Biochem Physiol B Biochem Mol Biol*, Vol. 139, No. 4, (Dec, 2004), pp. 561-9. ISSN 1096-4959.

Marino, F. E. (2010). Is it time to retire the 'central Governor'? A philosophical and evolutionary perspective. *Sports Med*, Vol. 40, No. 3, (Mar 1, 2010), pp. 265-8; author reply 268-70, ISSN 0112-1642.

McKenna, M. J. & Hargreaves, M. (2008). Resolving fatigue mechanisms determining exercise performance: integrative physiology at its finest! *J Appl Physiol*, Vol. 104, No. 1, (Jan, 2008), pp. 286-7, ISSN 8750-7587.

Meeusen, R.; Piacentini, M. F.; Van Den Eynde, S.; Magnus, L. & De Meirleir, K. (2001). Exercise performance is not influenced by a 5 HT reuptake inhibitor. *Int J Sports Med*, Vol. 22, No. 5, (Jul, 2001), pp. 329-36, ISSN 0172-4622.

Meeusen, R.; Smolders, I.; Sarre, S.; De Meirleir, K.; Keizer, H.; SErneels, M.; Ebinger, G. & Michotte, Y. (1997). Endurance training effects on neurotransmitter release in rat striatum: an in vivo microdialysis study. *Acta Physiol Scand*, Vol. 159, No. 4, (Apr, 1997), pp. 335-41, ISSN 0001-6772.

Meeusen, R.; Thorre, K.; Chaouloff, F.; Sarre, S.; De Meirleir, K.; Ebinger, G. & Michotte, Y. (1996). Effects of tryptophan and/or acute running on extracellular 5-HT and 5-HIAA levels in the hippocampus of food-deprived rats. *Brain Res*, Vol. 740, No. 1-2, (Nov 18, 1996), pp. 245-52, ISSN 0006-8993.

Meeusen, R.; Watson, P.; Hasegawa, H.; Roelands, B. & Piacentini, M. F. (2006). Central fatigue: the serotonin hypothesis and beyond. *Sports Med*, Vol. 36, No. 10, 2006), pp. 881-909, ISSN 0112-1642.

Meeusen, R.; Watson, P.; Hasegawa, H.; Roelands, B. & Piacentini, M. F. (2007). Brain neurotransmitters in fatigue and overtraining. *Appl Physiol Nutr Metab*, Vol. 32, No. 5, (Oct, 2007), pp. 857-64, ISSN 1715-5312.

Mekjavic, I. B. & Eiken, O. (2006). Contribution of thermal and nonthermal factors to the regulation of body temperature in humans. *J Appl Physiol*, Vol. 100, No. 6, (Jun, 2006), pp. 2065-72, ISSN 8750-7587.

Morrison, S.; Sleivert, G. G. & Cheung, S. S. (2004). Passive hyperthermia reduces voluntary activation and isometric force production. *Eur J Appl Physiol*, Vol. 91, No. 5-6, (May, 2004), pp. 729-36, ISSN 1439-6319.

Myers, R. D. (1981). Serotonin and thermoregulation: old and new views. *J Physiol (Paris)*, Vol. 77, No. 2-3, 1981), pp. 505-13, ISSN 0021-7948.

Myers, R. D.; Beleslin, D. B. & Rezvani, A. H. (1987). Hypothermia: role of alpha 1- and alpha 2-noradrenergic receptors in the hypothalamus of the cat. *Pharmacol Biochem Behav*, Vol. 26, No. 2, (Feb, 1987), pp. 373-9, ISSN 0091-3057.

Nassif, C.; Ferreira, A. P.; Gomes, A. R.; Silva Lde, M.; Garcia, E. S. & Marino, F. E. (2008). Double blind carbohydrate ingestion does not improve exercise duration in warm humid conditions. *J Sci Med Sport*, Vol. 11, No. 1, (Jan, 2008), pp. 72-, ISSN 1440-2440.

Newsholme, E. A.; Blomstrand, E. & Ekblom, B. (1992). Physical and mental fatigue: metabolic mechanisms and importance of plasma amino acids. *Br Med Bull*, Vol. 48, No. 3, (Jul, 1992), pp. 477-95, ISSN 0007-1420.

Nielsen, B.; Hales, J. R.; Strange, S.; Christensen, N. J.; Warberg, J. & Saltin, B. (1993). Human circulatory and thermoregulatory adaptations with heat acclimation and exercise in a hot, dry environment. *J Physiol*, Vol. 460, No., (Jan, 1993), pp.467-85, ISSN 0022-3751.

Nielsen, B.; Hyldig, T.; Bidstrup, F.; Gonzalez-Alonso, J. & Christoffersen, G. R. (2001). Brain activity and fatigue during prolonged exercise in the heat. *Pflugers Arch*, Vol. 442, No. 1, (Apr, 2001), pp. 41-8, ISSN 0031-6768.

Nielsen, B. & Nybo, L. (2003). Cerebral changes during exercise in the heat. *Sports Med*, Vol. 33, No. 1, 2003), pp. 1-11, ISSN 0112-1642.

Nikolov, R. P. & Yakimova, K. S. (2011). Effects of GABA-transaminase inhibitor Vigabatrin on thermoregulation in rats. *Amino Acids*, Vol. 40, No. 5, (May, 2011), pp. 1441-5, ISSN 1438-2199.

Noakes, T. D. (1998). Fluid and electrolyte disturbances in heat illness. *Int J Sports Med*, Vol. 19 Suppl 2, No., (Jun, 1998), pp.S146-9, ISSN 0172-4622.

Noakes, T. D. (2000). Physiological models to understand exercise fatigue and the adaptations that predict or enhance athletic performance. *Scand J Med Sci Sports*, Vol. 10, No. 3, (Jun, 2000), pp.(123-45).0905-7188 (Print) 0905-7188 (Linking).

Noakes, T. D. & St Clair Gibson, A. (2004). Logical limitations to the "catastrophe" models of fatigue during exercise in humans. *Br J Sports Med*, Vol. 38, No. 5, (Oct, 2004), pp. 648-9, ISSN 1473-0480.

Noakes, T. D.; St Clair Gibson, A. & Lambert, E. V. (2005). From catastrophe to complexity: a novel model of integrative central neural regulation of effort and fatigue during exercise in humans: summary and conclusions. *Br J Sports Med*, Vol. 39, No. 2, (Feb, 2005), pp. 120-4, ISSN 1473-0480.

Nunes, J. L.; Sharif, N. A.; Michel, A. D. & Whiting, R. L. (1991). Dopamine D2-receptors mediate hypothermia in mice: ICV and IP effects of agonists and antagonists. *Neurochem Res*, Vol. 16, No. 10, (Oct, 1991), pp. 1167-74, ISSN 0364-3190.

Nybo, L. (2008). Hyperthermia and fatigue. *J Appl Physiol*, Vol. 104, No. 3, (Mar, 2008), pp. 871-8, ISSN 8750-7587.

Nybo, L. & Nielsen, B. (2001). Hyperthermia and central fatigue during prolonged exercise in humans. *J Appl Physiol*, Vol. 91, No. 3, (Sep, 2001), pp. 1055-60, ISSN 8750-7587.

Nybo, L. & Secher, N. H. (2004). Cerebral perturbations provoked by prolonged exercise. *Prog Neurobiol*, Vol. 72, No. 4, (Mar, 2004), pp. 223-61, ISSN 0301-0082.

Pannier, J. L.; Bouckaert, J. J. & Lefebvre, R. A. (1995). The antiserotonin agent pizotifen does not increase endurance performance in humans. *Eur J Appl Physiol Occup Physiol*, Vol. 72, No. 1-2, 1995), pp. 175-, ISSN 0301-5548.

Parise, G.; Bosman, M. J.; Boecker, D. R.; Barry, M. J. & Tarnopolsky, M. A. (2001). Selective serotonin reuptake inhibitors: Their effect on high-intensity exercise performance. *Arch Phys Med Rehabil*, Vol. 82, No. 7, (Jul, 2001), pp. 867-7, ISSN 0003-9993.

Perrey, S. (2010). Predominance of central motor command in the regulation of exercise. *J Appl Physiol*, Vol. 108, No. 2, (Feb, 2010), pp. 458, ISSN 1522-1601.

Piacentini, M. F.; Clinckers, R.; Meeusen, R.; Sarre, S.; Ebinger, G. & Michotte, Y. (2003). Effect of bupropion on hippocampal neurotransmitters and on peripheral hormonal concentrations in the rat. *J Appl Physiol*, Vol. 95, No. 2, (Aug, 2003), pp. 652-6, ISSN 8750-7587.

Piacentini, M. F.; Meeusen, R.; Buyse, L.; DE Schutter, G.; Kempenaers, F.; Van Nijvel, J. & De Meirleir, K. (2002). No effect of a noradrenergic reuptake inhibitor on performance in trained cyclists. *Med Sci Sports Exerc*, Vol. 34, No. 7, (Jul, 2002), pp. 1189-93, ISSN 0195-9131.

Pires, W.; Wanner, S. P.; La Guardia, R. B.; Rodrigues, L. O.; Silveira, S. A.; Coimbra, C. C.; Marubayashi, U. & Lima, N. R. (2007). Intracerebroventricular physostigmine enhances blood pressure and heat loss in running rats. *J Physiol Pharmacol*, Vol. 58, No. 1, (Mar, 2007), pp. 3 17, ISSN 0867-5910.

Prieto-Gomez, B.; Dafny, N. & Reyes-Vazquez, C. (1989). Dorsal raphe stimulation, 5-HT and morphine microiontophoresis effects on noxious and nonnoxious identified neurons in the medial thalamus of the rat. *Brain Res Bull*, Vol. 22, No. 6, (Jun, 1989), pp. 937-43, ISSN 0361-9230.

Primola-Gomes, T. N.; Pires, W.; Rodrigues, L. O.; Coimbra, C. C.; Marubayashi, U. & LIMA, N. R. (2007). Activation of the central cholinergic pathway increases post-exercise tail heat loss in rats. *Neurosci Lett*, Vol. 413, No. 1, (Feb 8, 2007), pp. 1-5, ISSN 0304-3940.

Quan, N.; Xin, L. & Blatteis, C. M. (1991). Microdialysis of norepinephrine into preoptic area of guinea pigs: characteristics of hypothermic effect. *Am J Physiol*, Vol. 261, No. 2 Pt 2, (Aug, 1991), pp. R378-85, ISSN 0002-9513.

Quan, N.; Xin, L.; Ungar, A. L. & Blatteis, C. M. (1992). Preoptic norepinephrine-induced hypothermia is mediated by alpha 2-adrenoceptors. *Am J Physiol*, Vol. 262, No. 3 Pt 2, (Mar, 1992), pp. R407 11, ISSN 0002-9513

Rodrigues, A. G.; Lima, N. R.; Coimbra, C. C. & Marubayashi, U. (2004). Intracerebroventricular physostigmine facilitates heat loss mechanisms in running rats. *J Appl Physiol*, Vol. 97, No. 1, (Jul, 2004), pp. 333-8, ISSN 8750-7587.

Rodrigues, A. G.; Lima, N. R.; Coimbra, C. C. & Marubayashi, U. (2008). Evidence that exercise-induced heat storage is dependent on adrenomedullary secretion. *Physiol Behav*, Vol. 94, No. 3, (Jun 9, 2008), pp. 463-7, ISSN 0031-9384.

Rodrigues, A. G.; Soares, D. D.; Marubayashi, U. & Coimbra, C. C. (2009). Heat loss during exercise is related to serotonin activity in the preoptic area. *Neuroreport*, Vol. 20, No. 8, (May 27, 2009), pp. 804-8, ISSN 1473-558X.

Rodrigues, L. O.; Oliveira, A.; Lima, N. R. & Machado-Moreira, C. A. (2003). Heat storage rate and acute fatigue in rats. *Braz J Med Biol Res*, Vol. 36, No. 1, (Jan, 2003), pp. 131-5, ISSN 0100-879X.

Roelands, B.; Goekint, M.; Buyse, L.; Pauwels, F.; De Schutter, G.; Piacentini, F.; Hasegawa, H.; Watson, P. & Meeusen, R. (2009). Time trial performance in normal and high ambient temperature: is there a role for 5-HT? *Eur J Appl Physiol*, Vol. 107, No. 1, (Sep, 2009), pp. 119-26, ISSN 1439-6327.

Roelands, B.; Goekint, M.; Heyman, E.; Piacentini, M. F.; Watson, P.; Hasegawa, H.; Buyse, L.; Pauwels, F.; De Schutter, G. & Meeusen, R. (2008). Acute norepinephrine reuptake inhibition decreases performance in normal and high ambient temperature. *J Appl Physiol*, Vol. 105, No. 1, (Jul, 2008), pp. 206-12, ISSN 8750-7587.

Roelands, B. & Meeusen, R. (2010). Alterations in central fatigue by pharmacological manipulations of neurotransmitters in normal and high ambient temperature. *Sports Med*, Vol. 40, No. 3, (Mar 1, 2010), pp. 229-46, ISSN 0112-1642.

Romanovsky, A. A. (2007). Thermoregulation: some concepts have changed. Functional architecture of the thermoregulatory system. *Am J Physiol Regul Integr Comp Physiol*, Vol. 292, No. 1, (Jan, 2007), pp. R37-46, ISSN 0363-6119.

Schaechter, J. D. & Wurtman, R. J. (1990). Serotonin release varies with brain tryptophan levels. *Brain Res*, Vol. 532, No. 1-2, (Nov 5, 1990), pp. 203-10, ISSN 0006-8993.

Schlader, Z. J.; Prange, H. D.; Mickleborough, T. D. & Stager, J. M. (2009). Characteristics of the control of human thermoregulatory behavior. *Physiol Behav*, Vol. 98, No. 5, (Dec 7, 2009), pp. 557-62, ISSN 1873-507X.

Schlader, Z. J.; Stannard, S. R. & Mundel, T. (2010). Human thermoregulatory behavior during rest and exercise - a prospective review. *Physiol Behav*, Vol. 99, No. 3, (Mar 3, 2010), pp. 269-75, ISSN 1873-507X.

Sesboue, B. & Guincestre, J. Y. (2006). Muscular fatigue. *Ann Readapt Med Phys*, Vol. 49, No. 6, (Jul, 2006), pp. 257-64, ISSN 348-54.

Shephard, R. J. (2009). Is it time to retire the 'central governor'? *Sports Med*, Vol. 39, No. 9, 2009), pp. 709-21, ISSN 0112-1642.

Soares, D. D.; Coimbra, C. C. & Marubayashi, U. (2007). Tryptophan-induced central fatigue in exercising rats is related to serotonin content in preoptic area. *Neurosci Lett*, Vol. 415, No. 3, (Mar 30, 2007), pp. 274-8, ISSN 0304-3940.

Soares, D. D.; Lima, N. R.; Coimbra, C. C. & Marubayashi, U. (2003). Evidence that tryptophan reduces mechanical efficiency and running performance in rats. *Pharmacol Biochem Behav*, Vol. 74, No. 2, (Jan, 2003), pp. 357-62, ISSN 0091-3057.

Soares, D. D.; Lima, N. R.; Coimbra, C. C. & Marubayashi, U. (2004). Intracerebroventricular tryptophan increases heating and heat storage rate in exercising rats. *Pharmacol Biochem Behav*, Vol. 78, No. 2, (Jun, 2004), pp. 255-61, ISSN 0091-3057.

St Clair-Gibson, A.; Lambert, E. V.; Rauch, L. H.; Tucker, R.; Baden, D. A.; Foster, C. & Noakes, T. D. (2006). The role of information processing between the brain and peripheral physiological systems in pacing and perception of effort. *Sports Med*, Vol. 36, No. 8, 2006), pp. 705-22, ISSN 0112-1642.

Strachan, A. T.; Leiper, J. B. & Maughan, R. J. (2004). Paroxetine administration failed [corrected] to influence human exercise capacity, perceived effort or hormone responses during prolonged exercise in a warm environment. *Exp Physiol*, Vol. 89, No. 6, (Nov, 2004), pp. 657-64, ISSN 0958-0670.

Struder, H. K.; Hollmann, W.; Platen, P.; Donike, M.; Gotzmann, A. & Weber, K. (1998). Influence of paroxetine, branched-chain amino acids and tyrosine on neuroendocrine system responses and fatigue in humans. *Horm Metab Res*, Vol. 30, No. 4, (Apr, 1998), pp. 188-94, ISSN 0018-5043.

Struder, H. K. & Weicker, H. (2001a). Physiology and pathophysiology of the serotonergic system and its implications on mental and physical performance. Part I. *Int J Sports Med*, Vol. 22, No. 7, (Oct, 2001a), pp. 467-81, ISSN 0172-4622.

Struder, H. K. & Weicker, H. (2001b). Physiology and pathophysiology of the serotonergic system and its implications on mental and physical performance. Part II. *Int J Sports Med*, Vol. 22, No. 7, (Oct, 2001b), pp. 482-97, ISSN 0172-4622.

Szabo, S. T. & Blier, P. (2001). Functional and pharmacological characterization of the modulatory role of serotonin on the firing activity of locus coeruleus norepinephrine neurons. *Brain Res*, Vol. 922, No. 1, (Dec 13, 2001), pp. 9-20, ISSN 0006-8993.

Szabo, S. T. & Blier, P. (2002). Effects of serotonin (5-hydroxytryptamine, 5-HT) reuptake inhibition plus 5-HT(2A) receptor antagonism on the firing activity of norepinephrine neurons. *J Pharmacol Exp Ther*, Vol. 302, No. 3, (Sep, 2002), pp. 983-91, ISSN 0022-3565.

Takahashi, H.; Takada, Y.; Nagai, N.; Urano, T. & Takada, A. (2000). Serotonergic neurons projecting to hippocampus activate locomotion. *Brain Res*, Vol. 869, No. 1-2, (Jun 30, 2000), pp. 194-202, ISSN 0006-8993.

Tatterson, A. J.; Hahn, A. G.; Martin, D. T. & Febbraio, M. A. (2000). Effects of heat stress on physiological responses and exercise performance in elite cyclists. *J Sci Med Sport*, Vol. 3, No. 2, (Jun, 2000), pp. 186-93, ISSN 1440-2440.

Taylor, J. L. & Gandevia, S. C. (2008). A comparison of central aspects of fatigue in submaximal and maximal voluntary contractions. *J Appl Physiol*, Vol. 104, No. 2, (Feb, 2008), pp. 542-50, ISSN 8750-7587.

Thomas, C. K.; Johansson, R. S. & Bigland-Ritchie, B. (2006). EMG changes in human thenar motor units with force potentiation and fatigue. *J Neurophysiol*, Vol. 95, No. 3, (Mar, 2006), pp. 1518-26, ISSN 0022-3077.

Todd, G.; Butler, J. E.; Taylor, J. L. & Gandevia, S. C. (2005). Hyperthermia: a failure of the motor cortex and the muscle. *J Physiol*, Vol. 563, No. Pt 2, (Mar 1, 2005), pp. 621-31, ISSN 0022-3751.

Tucker, R. (2009). The anticipatory regulation of performance: the physiological basis for pacing strategies and the development of a perception-based model for exercise performance. *Br J Sports Med*, Vol. 43, No. 6, (Jun, 2009), pp. 392-400, ISSN 1473-0480.

Tucker, R.; Marle, T.; Lambert, E. V. & Noakes, T. D. (2006). The rate of heat storage mediates an anticipatory reduction in exercise intensity during cycling at a fixed rating of perceived exertion. *J Physiol*, Vol. 574, No. Pt 3, (Aug 1, 2006), pp. 905-15, ISSN 0022-3751.

Varty, G. B. & Higgins, G. A. (1998). Dopamine agonist-induced hypothermia and disruption of prepulse inhibition: evidence for a role of D3 receptors? *Behav Pharmacol*, Vol. 9, No. 5-6, (Sep, 1998), pp. 445-55, ISSN 0955-8810.

Walters, T. J.; Ryan, K. L.; Tate, L. M. & Mason, P. A. (2000). Exercise in the heat is limited by a critical internal temperature. *J Appl Physiol*, Vol. 89, No. 2, (Aug, 2000), pp. 799-806, ISSN 8750-7587.

Wanner, S. P.; Guimaraes, J. B.; Pires, W.; Marubayashi, U.; Lima, N. R. & Coimbra, C. C. (2011). Muscarinic receptors within the ventromedial hypothalamic nuclei modulate metabolic rate during physical exercise. *Neurosci Lett*, Vol. 488, No. 2, (Jan 20, 2011), pp. 210-4, ISSN 1872-7972.

Wanner, S. P.; Guimaraes, J. B.; Rodrigues, L. O.; Marubayashi, U.; Coimbra, C. C. & Lima, N. R. (2007). Muscarinic cholinoceptors in the ventromedial hypothalamic nucleus facilitate tail heat loss during physical exercise. *Brain Res Bull*, Vol. 73, No. 1-3, (Jun 15, 2007), pp. 28-33, ISSN 0361-9230.

Waterhouse, J.; Drust, B.; Weinert, D.; Edwards, B.; Gregson, W.; Atkinson, G.; Kao, S.; Aizawa, S. & Reilly, T. (2005). The circadian rhythm of core temperature: origin and some implications for exercise performance. *Chronobiol Int*, Vol. 22, No. 2, 2005), pp. 207-25, 0742-0528.

Watson, P.; Hasegawa, H.; Roelands, B.; Piacentini, M. F.; Looverie, R. & Meeusen, R. (2005). Acute dopamine/noradrenaline reuptake inhibition enhances human exercise performance in warm, but not temperate conditions. *J Physiol*, Vol. 565, No. Pt 3, (Jun 15, 2005), pp. 873-83, ISSN 0022-3751.

Webb, P. (1995). The physiology of heat regulation. *Am J Physiol*, Vol. 268, No. 4 Pt 2, (Apr, 1995), pp. R838-50, ISSN 0002-9513.

Wilson, K. M. & Fregly, M. J. (1985). Factors affecting angiotensin II-induced hypothermia in rats. *Peptides*, Vol. 6, No. 4, (Jul-Aug, 1985), pp. 695-701, ISSN 0196-9781.

Wilson, W. M. & Maughan, R. J. (1992). Evidence for a possible role of 5-hydroxytryptamine in the genesis of fatigue in man: administration of paroxetine, a 5-HT re-uptake inhibitor, reduces the capacity to perform prolonged exercise. *Exp Physiol*, Vol. 77, No. 6, (Nov, 1992), pp. 921-4, ISSN 0958-0670.

15

The Application of Medical Infrared Thermography in Sports Medicine

Carolin Hildebrandt[1], Karlheinz Zeilberger[2],
Edward Francis John Ring[3] and Christian Raschner[1]

[1]University of Innsbruck, Department of Sport Science, Innsbruck,
[2]Medical Practices for Internal and Sports Medicine, Munich,
[3]Medical Imaging Research Group, Faculty of Advanced Technology,
University of Glamorgan,
[1]Austria
[2]Germany
[3]UK

1. Introduction

Medical Infrared Thermography (MIT) is a non-radiating and contact-free technology to monitor physiological functions related to skin temperature control. The efficiency, safety and low cost of MIT make it a useful auxiliary tool for detecting and locating thermal abnormalities characterized by increases or decreases in skin surface temperature. It has been successfully utilized in the field of veterinary medicine to detect locomotion injuries in racehorses and to monitor their health status. However, research on human athletes with modern infrared sensor technology is more rare. Athletes are exposed to physical stress in training and during competition season. Overuse reactions and so-called "minor traumas" are very frequent; therefore, early detection is critical to avoid injuries. Research suggests that the most beneficial application of MIT is the screening of individuals for overuse injuries. In the following chapters, the use of MIT in clinical practice is presented with special focus on sports injuries and exercise-induced physiological functions. Case studies illustrate the clinical applicability.

2. MIT – Quo Vadis?

2.1 History and development

The association between changes in temperature and disease is almost as old as medicine itself. Hippocrates stated, "should one part of the body be hotter or colder than the rest, then disease is present in that part". The first application of thermal imaging was in the early 19th century and did not have any commercial purpose. Following the 2nd World War, infrared imaging systems were used to monitor changes in skin temperature in relation to certain diseases (Ring, 2007). Poor quality imaging systems and a lack of methodological standards in the past has limited quality, resulting in non-acceptance of the technique (Elliot & Head, 1999). Technological advances in infrared cameras within the last few years have promoted MIT as a powerful measurement tool. A new generation of high-resolution cameras, appropriate software and standardized protocols have been developed for medical imaging, resulting in improved diagnostic capability and reliability (Plassmann et al., 2006; Diakides & Bronzino, 2008). In 1987, the American Medical Association recognized MIT as a feasible diagnostic tool. The following worldwide Thermographic organizations promote the proper application of medical thermal imaging.

- International Academy of Clinical Thermology
- International Thermographic Society
- American Academy of Medical Infrared Imaging
- European Association of Thermology
- Northern Norwegian Centre for Medical Thermography
- German Society of Thermography and Regulation Medicine

2.2 Technical principles

Most of the diagnostic imaging modalities in medicine utilize portions of the electromagnetic spectrum (Hildebrandt et al., 2010) (Figure 1). However, in contrast to other medical devices, MIT uses non-ionising radiation, thus allowing an unconstrained and

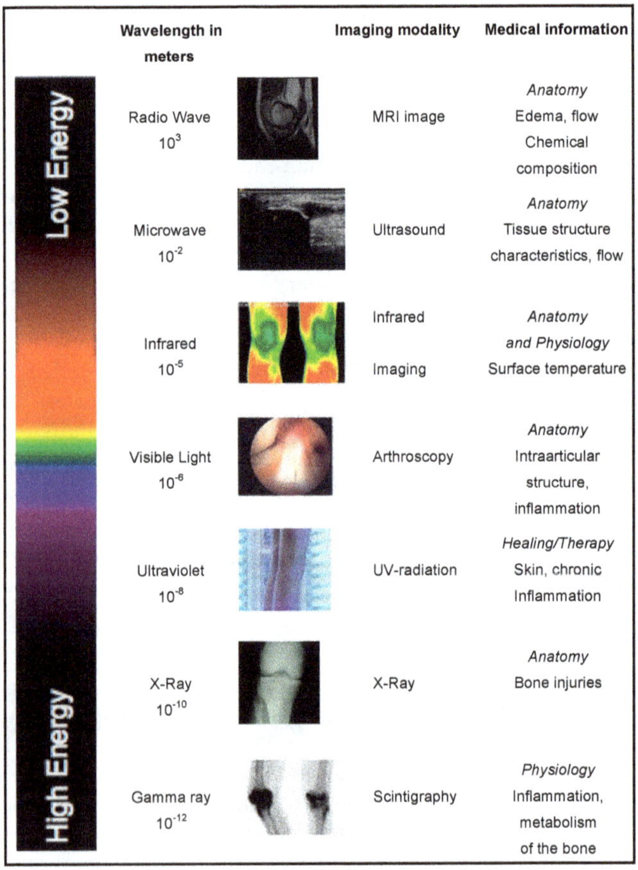

Fig. 1. Medical imaging modalities within the electromagnetic spectrum

harmless application in patients. Using infrared radiation, infrared cameras generate thermal images based on the amount of heat dissipated at the surface. Roughly 80% of the emitted infrared radiation of human skin is in the wavelength range of 8-15μm (Steketee, 1973). The technology operates in the long-wave infrared region and is a sophisticated way of receiving electromagnetic radiation and converting it into electrical signals. These signals are finally displayed and matched to colors on the screen for calculations. Modern focal plane array detectors ensure a stable image with high thermal resolution. Sensitivity and resolution are important parameters for medical devices (Plassmann et al., 2006). High-resolution cameras with focal plane arrays of 320×240 pixels, a thermal sensitivity less than 50mK and a spatial resolution of 25-50μm ensure useful thermal and spatial details (Ring & Ammer, 2000). The resulting information can be used to provide instant feedback on the patient or athlete. Unlike other medical imaging modalities, MIT is not related to morphology. However, to study cutaneous circulation, the non-contact method of MIT was compared with other medical imaging modalities. Merla et al. (2007) calculated blood flow by using MIT and laser Doppler imaging (LDI) and showed that cutaneous blood perfusion values obtained from MIT correlate with those obtained by means of LDI and have the advantage of a better time resolution.

2.3 Biological principles

Human skin, with an emissivity (an object's ability to emit radiation) of 0.98, is almost equal to a black body radiator (Steketee, 1973). The physics of heat radiation and the physiology of thermoregulation in the human body make the reliable and valid interpretation of thermal images difficult. Skin temperature regulation is a complex system that depends on blood-flow rate, local structures of subcutaneous tissues and the activity of the sympathetic nervous system (Kellog & Pergola, 2000). However, there is evidence that the sympathetic nervous system is the primary regulator of blood circulation in the skin and is, therefore, the primary regulator of thermal emission (Charkoudian, 2003). Vasoconstriction and vasodilation of the blood vessels function to regulate blood flow in the skin. Thermoreceptors in the skin, also known as Ruffini corpuscles, recognize the ambient temperature. An increased temperature results in vasodilation, leading to increased blood flow to the skin, whereas vasoconstriction occurs by a decrease in temperature and results in reduced blood flow to the skin (Wallin, 1990). These physiological processes combine with heat transfer and thermoregulation in convection, conduction, radiation and sweat evaporation. Heat transfer by radiation is of great value in medicine (Blatteis, 1998). To date, the mechanism of thermoregulatory adaption to exercise is complex and not entirely understood.

3. MIT – What is its place in medicine?

3.1 Human medicine

MIT is used in a variety of medical applications in the fields of neurology, oncology, orthopedics, and dermatology (Diakides & Bronzino, 2007). The technique has gained widespread use in breast cancer research (Arora et al., 2008; Ng, 2009; Kontos et al., 2011). Tumors are characterized by increased angiogenesis and, therefore, increased metabolic activity, leading to higher temperature gradients compared to surrounding tissue. In addition, MIT is well accepted in surgery. In aortic-coronary bypass surgery, it is possible to monitor the restart of blood flow through the coronary blood vessels (Wild et al., 2003). In plastic surgery, an infrared camera can evaluate the reperfusion of perforator flaps (de Weerd, 2006). For all medical areas, it should be noted that MIT, as an outcome measure, provides a visual map of the skin temperature distribution but cannot quantify absolute temperature values. In addition, MIT alone should not be used as a diagnostic tool; clinical examinations must be included for interpreting thermograms. Several global medical institutions are concerned about scientific work, and the practical application of MIT in medicine has lead to an increased number of publications in peer-reviewed journals. Figure 2 illustrates medical applications including relevant and recent studies.

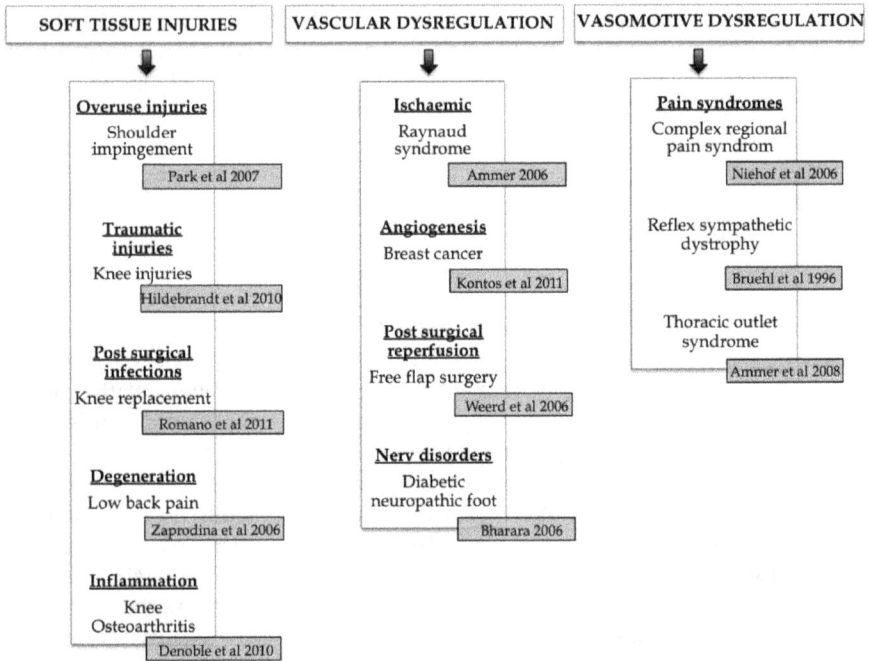

Fig. 2. Recent medical applications of MIT

3.2 Sports medicine

MIT has been successfully utilized in the field of veterinary medicine to detect locomotion injuries in racehorses and to monitor their health status (Turner, 2000; Eddy et al., 2001). By using an infrared camera, Turner et al. (2000) examined tendonitis in race horses and detected hot spots before clinical evidence of swelling and lameness. However, research on human athletes is more rare. Sports medicine must provide high-quality care for athletes, and a modern approach for identifying risk factors and injury prevention should be of primary importance (Bruckner & Khan, 2006). Athletes are exposed to great physical stress in training and during competition. Overuse reactions are frequent; therefore, their early detection is important. Furthermore, early detection and localization of inflammation is a critical step in determining the appropriate treatment. Inflammation will usually cause a localized increase in skin temperature, thereby disturbing the "normal" symmetry. Nerve damage or disturbances to the autonomic nervous system may also cause a change and may lead to a localized cooling of the affected area. Because this is a remote sensing technique, it is possible to monitor body surface temperature during and after movement and thereby detect changes in skin temperature caused by the exercise or therapy (Ring & Ammer, 1998, Hardaker et al., 2007). Within the field of sports medicine, long-time sport specific changes in physiology and therefore thermoregulatory processes, as well as changes in anatomy such as muscle structures, needs to be considered.

3.3 Standardization methods

Modern state-of-the-art technology has made MIT a reliable measurement tool (Jiang et al., 2005). When used as an outcome measure it must satisfy the basic criteria of measurement. The quality of thermal imaging depends on the technical equipment and the experience of the examiner (Plassmann et al., 2006, Ring & Ammer, 2000). Proper care must be taken with standardization of the imaging procedure to avoid misinterpretation of the thermograms. Thermography societies provide protocols including examination recommendations and technical guidelines. The following aspects are considered:

- Control of Examination Room Conditions
- Patient Preparation
- Number of Studies and Views
- Equipment
- Patient Identification
- Thermogram Analysis

A thermogram represents the human skin temperature profile illustrated by a color spectrum. However, false colors do not necessarily represent a particular temperature. To standardize the analyses of medical thermograms used for fever detection, the International Standards Organization (ISO) recommended the use of the "rainbow" temperature scale (Figure 3a) that represents high temperatures with red colors and low temperature with blue colors. To visualize differences within similar tissues or structures, the "rainbow strong-contrast" scale can also be used (Figure 3b). When focusing on the vascular system, a gray color scale is preferred (Figure 3c).

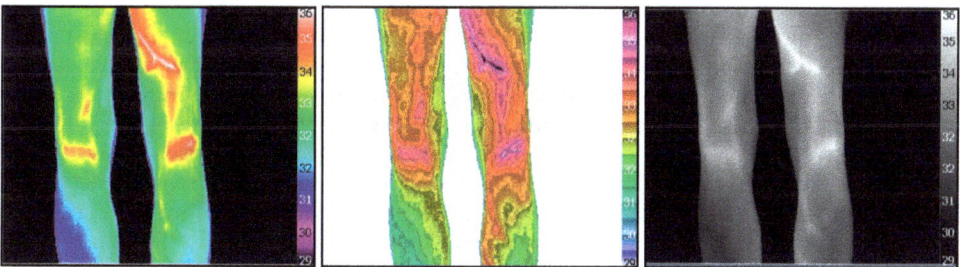

a. "rainbow"   b. "rainbow strong-contrast"   c. "gray color"

Fig. 3. Temperature scales of thermograms

Image fusion (Figure 4a-c), merging the infrared image and a digital image, is another important step for reliable analyses. This technique allows better mapping of anatomical landmarks and therefore provides a precise definition of the region of interest (ROI).

Additional labeling of anatomical landmarks within the ROI provides consistency for repeated measurements.

To provide a standard for size, shape and placement of the ROI, a research group from the University of Glamorgan has proposed a protocol based on anatomical landmarks (Plassmann & Murawski, 2003; Ammer, 2008).

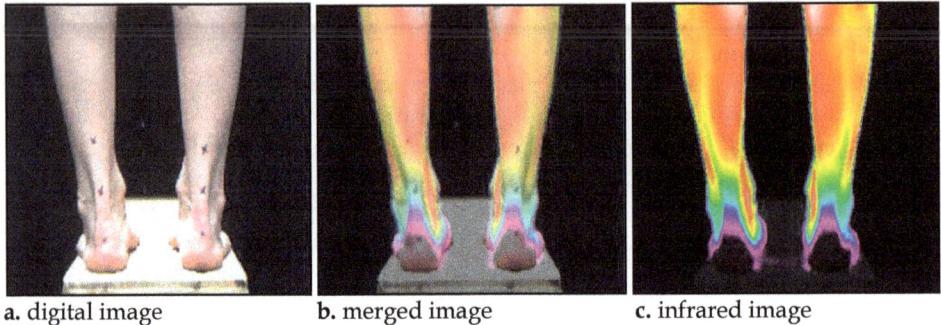

a. digital image   b. merged image   c. infrared image

Fig. 4. Process of image fusion

4. Applicability of MIT in clinical and athletic use

Peripheral circulation plays an important role in tissue healing and thermoregulation. To interpret skin temperature changes following injuries (non-thermal stimuli) and exercise (internal stress stimuli), we need to understand the different physiological responses in the structures involved.

4.1 Non-thermal stimuli / sport-specific case studies of injuries

The following chapter focuses on case reports of specific sport injuries. Thermal images were taken with a modern infrared camera. Further technical details can be found in the article from Hildebrandt et al. (2010). Normal findings in human body skin temperature are a symmetrical distribution (Vardasca 2008; Selfe et al., 2008), and injury can affect this thermal symmetry. Figure 5 represents an example of a symmetrical temperature distribution of the knees from a healthy subject. On the anterior view (Figure 5a), the patella appears as a cold shield due to bony structure. The muscles of the upper and lower leg represent hot areas due to high metabolic activity in the muscles. The posterior aspect of the knee (Figure 5b) shows high temperature in the popliteal fossa because of the popliteal arteries and veins. From a qualitative point of view, side-to-side comparison shows a very symmetrical pattern. To define whether a thermogram is normal, a current project at the University of Glamorgan aimed to create a database of thermal images from different parts of the body from healthy subjects. Previous literature has shown that a difference of more than one degree centigrade between sides of the body may indicate a pathophysiological process (Selfe et al., 2008). However, long-time, observational data from injured and non-injured athletes needs to be investigated to define sports specific thermogrammes. An injury causes blood flow variations that then affect skin temperature. Many medical conditions are associated with regional vasodilation and constriction, hyperperfusion, hypervascularization and hypermetabolism that cause higher temperature profiles of the skin surface. Physicians need a deeper understanding of the biological nature of thermal signals and consistent thermal alterations of sport specific injuries for early intervention and correct treatment. In addition, the natural healing process of traumatic and overuse injuries can be easily monitored by using thermal imaging. However, this requires the comparison of baseline images prior to and following an injury.

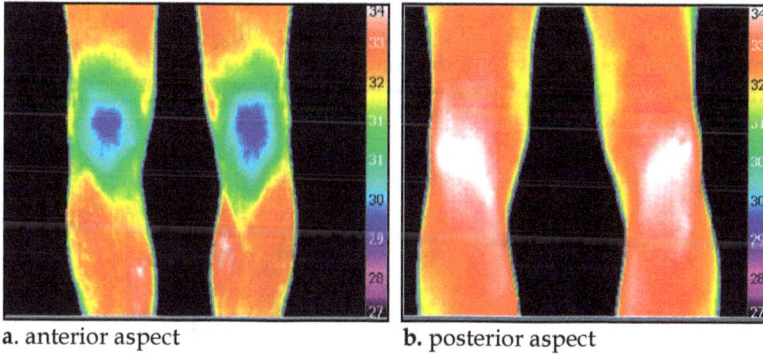

a. anterior aspect b. posterior aspect

Fig. 5. Infrared image of healthy knee

4.1.1 Overuse injuries

FOOTBALL

High-intensity training combined with frequent competition pushes the locomotor system to its anatomical and physiological limits. Woods et al. (2002) stated that young football players are at a greater risk of minor injuries, overuse injuries, lower leg injuries and muscle strains during the preseason period. We conducted preseason measurements of 25 football players (mean age 17.6± 3.9 years, height 176.1± 8.1 cm, mass 67.8±9.1 kg) from a Football Academy. Fifty two percent of the athletes reported no injuries, 28% had an overuse injury and 20% sustained a traumatic injury within the previous 6 months. The following example shows a non-acute overuse injury of a 17-year old football player. He was diagnosed with recurrent medial shin splint on his left leg and was asymptomatic when the baseline images were taken (Figure 6a). However, the area of referred pain on the left leg matches the area of

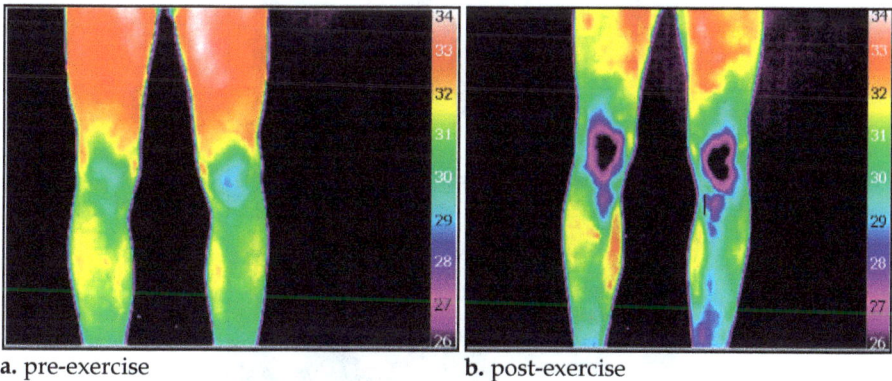

a. pre-exercise b. post-exercise

Fig. 6. Infrared image of the anterior aspect of the knee

cooler skin along the tibiae. This problem became even more visible following a sport-specific warm up program, indicating a low metabolic activity around the affected structures (Figure 6b). In addition, the athlete had a history of osteochondrosis at the tibial tuberosity of both knees. Especially following exercise, the tibial tuberosity on both knees appeared as a cold area.

The following example of a 25-year old professional football player represents an incidental finding. Images were taken within the scope of a team screening. On the injury questionnaire, no acute problems were reported. Upon enquiry no signs of venous disease were reported. However, the subject´s right greater saphenous vein appeared very clearly as an area of increased warmth on the thermogram that may indicate a vascular dilatation with beginning venous insufficiency (Figure 7). Further observational research will determine if this abnormality predict future problems prior to the onset of symptoms.

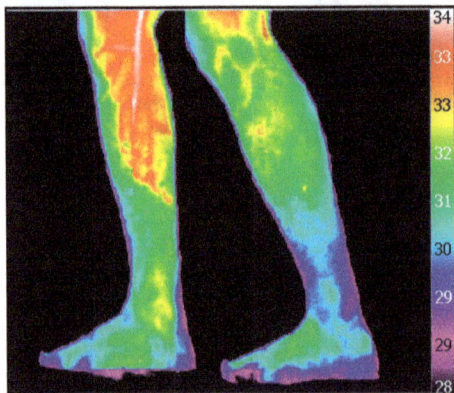

Fig. 7. Infrared image of the medial aspect of the right leg

The thermogram of a 26-year old professional football player represents a problem in the Achilles region (Figure 8). This athlete reported a feeling of morning stiffness on the musculotendinosus junction on his left leg. The thermograms showed a side-to-side difference in the affected area of 1.7° C.

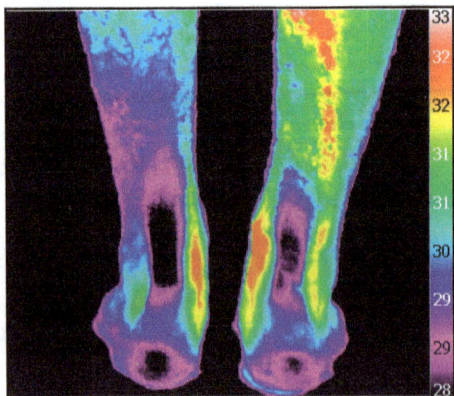

Fig. 8. Infrared image from the dorsal view of the lower leg

RUNNING

Epidemiological studies have shown an alarmingly high incidence of knee, foot, ankle and lower leg injuries in recreational and competitive runners. Most of these injuries were overuse injuries including stress fractures, shin splints, patellar tendinitis and, most prevalently Achilles tendinitis (Hreljac, 2005). The following thermograms were taken of a 22-year old competitive middle distance runner who runs 40-100km a week (Figure 9). He reported pain in his right Achilles tendon that occurs gradually, especially during exercise. The athlete was diagnosed with midportion Achilles tendinopathy with mild morphological abnormalities. At the time the images were taken, there was a small but noticeable pain at rest and no swelling. The average temperature of the ROI on the right side was 1.6° C lower compared to the non-affected side. The lower temperature may indicate lower metabolic activity due to affected tissue with a loss of normal fiber structure.

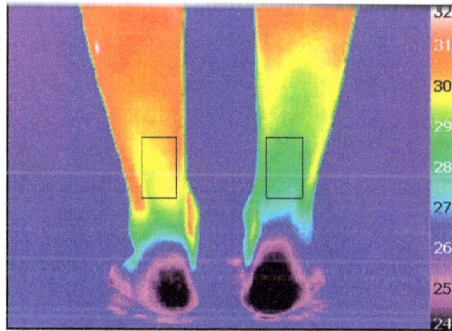

Fig. 9. Infrared image from the dorsal view of the lower legs with ROI

Following a treatment period of 8.5 weeks, including electro-physical and physiotherapeutic treatment, thermograms were taken again under resting conditions (Figure 10a) and following a 45-minute run of low intensity (Figure 10b). The side-to-side temperature difference dropped to 0.6°C before exercise, indicating better metabolic activity of the affected side. Following exercise, the right Achilles tendon junction was colder compared to the left one, with a temperature difference of 1.0°C. The athlete reported no pain at rest or following exercise. The regular treatment seemed to improve the Achilles tendon metabolism. However, the impaired metabolic activity following the sport-specific exercise needs to be further addressed with continuing therapy to prevent recurrent problems.

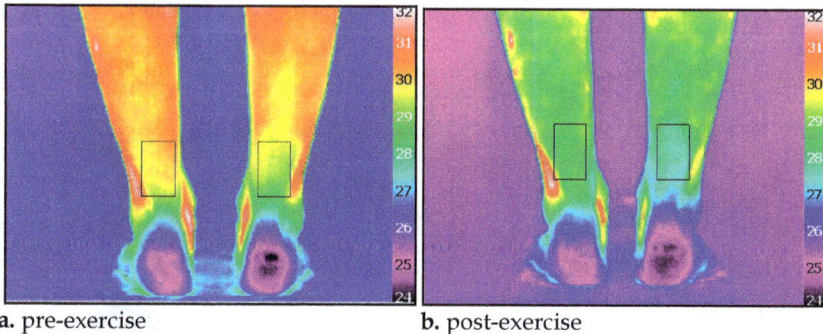

a. pre-exercise   b. post-exercise

Fig. 10. Infrared image of the lower legs with ROI

SWIMMING

A study, by Sein and co-workers in 2008, investigated shoulder pain in elite swimmers and found that 91% of the swimmers reported shoulder pain; moreover, 84% of the athletes demonstrated a positive impingement sign. The following thermal image was taken of a 27-year-old elite female swimmer under resting conditions (Figure 11). Following a high-volume swimming program, she reported pain and stiffness in both shoulders. With her right arm, she had difficulty reaching behind her back. The clinical examination confirmed overloading of the supraspinatus tendon and general stiffness of the shoulder muscles on both sides. The thermal image shows a hot area above the right deltoid muscle and a hot spot on both shoulders in the region of the humeral head, near the insertion of the supraspinatus muscle. Based on healthy baseline thermal images, MIT should be used to further monitor pathophysiological thermal changes during high-volume swim training prior to the onset of symptoms.

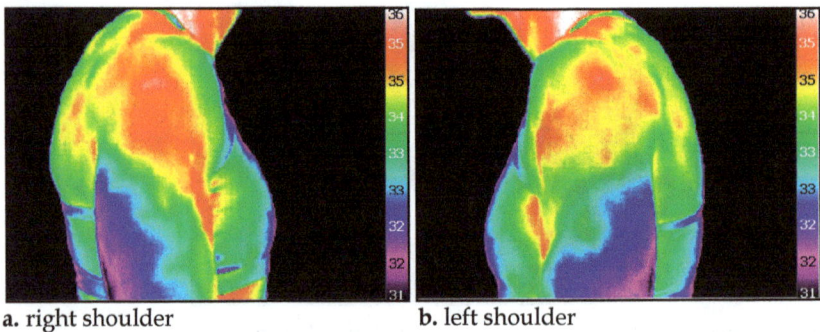

a. right shoulder   **b.** left shoulder

Fig. 11. Infrared image from the lateral view of the shoulder

YOUTH SPORTS

A common problem, predominantly in young, male athletes is the occurrence of enthesopathy of the ligamentum patellae (Gholve et al., 2007). This insertion tendinitis, caused by repetitive mechanical strain of the patella tendon, is characterized by pain, swelling and tenderness above the tibial tuberosity (Brukner & Khan, 2006). Thermal images clearly show a hyperthermic area above the tibial tuberosity (Figure 12). Long term evaluation of affected athletes from alpine skiing (n= 7), football (n=3), running (n=2) and tennis (n=1), who showed acute symptoms in one leg, revealed a side-to-side temperature difference of 1.1°C (± 0.71 °C). The technique provides a quick screening tool and should be used as a first-line detection tool prior to ultrasound or conventional X-rays.

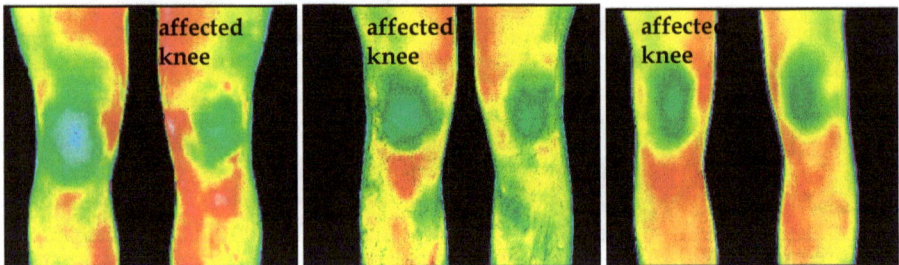

Fig. 12. Infrared images from athletes with enthesopathy of the ligamentum patellae

4.1.2 Traumatic injuries

Traumatic injuries usually involve a long, costly rehabilitation period, and they are challenging for the athlete. An injured athlete is under pressure to return to competition as soon as possible. High-quality treatment can reduce the duration and negative impact of the rehabilitation period. It is well known that richly vascularized areas heal faster compared to poorly vascularized areas (Singer et al., 1999). MIT may give information about the state of vascularization and the on-going healing process to ensure the most effective treatment and provide recovery information to decrease the likelihood of re-injury by returning to the sport too quickly.

ALPINE SKIING

Knee injuries, especially ruptures of the anterior cruciate ligament (ACL), represent a significant problem in professional alpine skiing (Flørenes et al., 2009) as illustrated by the case of a 21-year-old skier. At 16 years the skier ruptured his left anterior cruciate ligament, medial collateral ligament and the medial meniscus. Since that time, he has suffered from periodic pain, predominantly around the patellae. At age 20 years he was diagnosed with articular cartilage, damage grade three. According to the International Cartilage Repair Society, grade three indicates that the lesion affects more than 50% of the cartilage layer. The average temperature difference of the left patellae was found to be 1.6°C lower compared to the right side (Figure 13). The temperature difference from the area above the upper kneecap showed a side difference of 1.2°C, indicating poor metabolic activity of the lower quadriceps muscle under resting conditions.

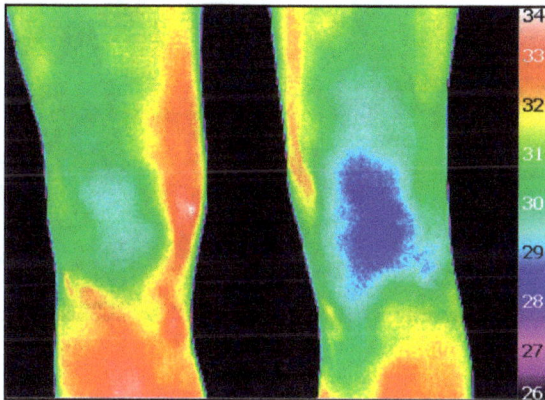

Fig. 13. Infrared image from the anterior view of the knees

TRIATHLON

The incidence of tendon ruptures has increased in recreational sport activities, with the highest incidence in older age groups (Clayton et al., 2008). However, Rettig et al. (2005) stated that the potential risk of re-rupture is highest in athletes younger than 30 years of age. The infrared images below were taken of a 26-year old triathlete, 6 months following a complete rupture and direct operation of his right Achilles tendon (Figure 14). When the images were taken, he was reffered with mild pain that was exercise dependent and a feeling of numbness in the outer toes. The ongoing healing process did not seem to be sufficiently complete. The temperature difference of an area from the upper Achilles tendon to the muscle belly of the musculus triceps surae was found to be 1.6°C, suggesting delayed healing with impaired circulation. In particular the cooler area of the musculotendinous junction should be considered further within physiotherapeutic treatment.

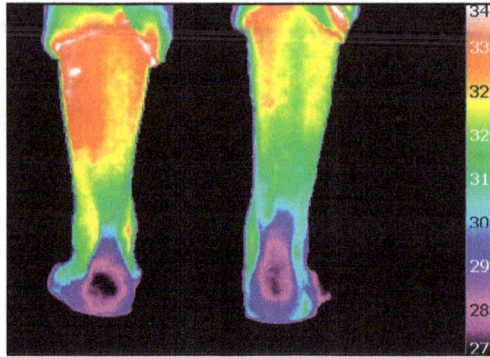

Fig. 14. Infrared image posterior view of lower leg

The area of numbness becomes visible through a clear hypothermia on the affected toes and must be a target of further rehabilitation (Figure 15a,b). Future research will determine if tissue remodeling is still on-going after symptoms disappear.

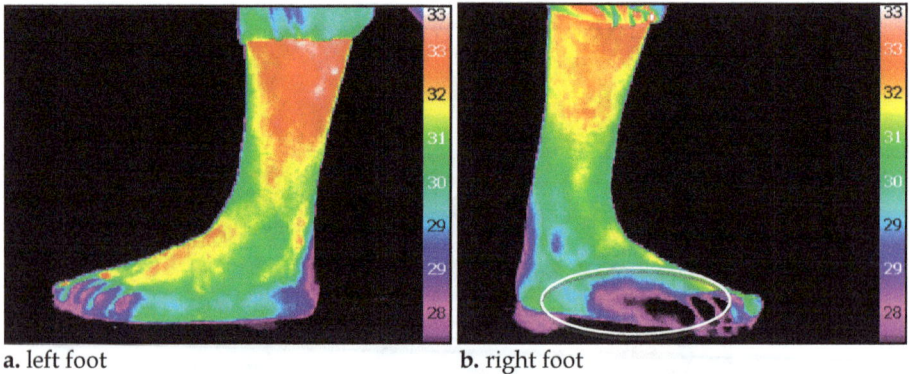

a. left foot   b. right foot

Fig. 15. Infrared image of the lateral view of the foot

4.1.3 Static versus dynamic measurements

Baseline recordings, following a sport-specific strain, should be conducted to visualize thermal regulatory processes. Regarding infrared images of overuse injuries, repeated measurements following sport-specific exercise will clarify if symptom-free asymmetrical temperature distributions are predictive for presymptomatic identification of initiating overuse reactions. The following example of an 18-year old football player indicates a presymptomatic thermal abnormality during pre-season measurement. The thermogram at rest demonstrated symmetrical patterns (Figure 16a). Following sport-specific exercise, local side differences on the knee were visible (Figure 16b). The athlete reported no pain at that time.

However, during the season, he reported a feeling of load-dependent, diffuse knee pain in his left leg. The medical examination confirmed a low threshold for pressure on the medial aspect of the knee. No clear diagnosis could be confirmed, indicating a local overuse reaction. Excessive stress should be administered with caution.

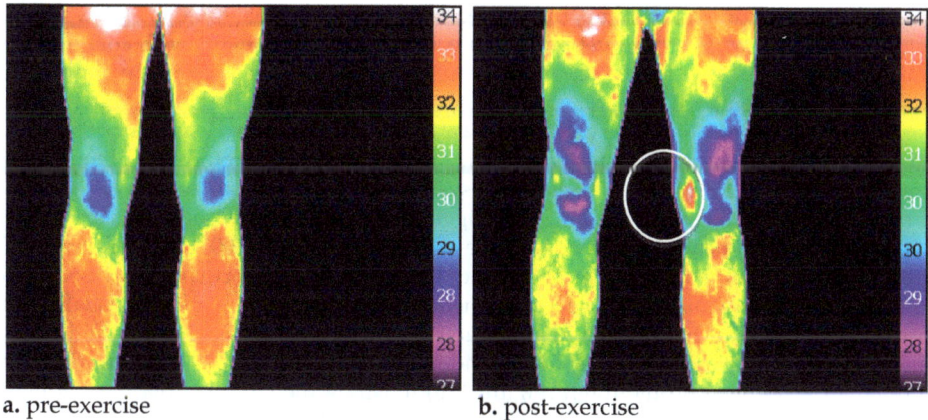

a. pre-exercise   b. post-exercise

Fig. 16. Infrared image of the anterior view of the legs

4.2 Thermal stimuli- time sequential images following different exercise

Physical exercise and repetitive strain is a challenge to thermal homeostasis. During exercise, the thermoregulatory control of blood flow in the skin is important to maintain normal body temperature and leads to changes in hemodynamics, and, therefore, thermal signals (Kenney & Johnson, 1991). Using state-of-the art infrared sensor technology, cutaneous temperature changes during exercise can be evaluated. Skin blood flow is predominantly regulated by neural regulation (Thomas & Segal, 2004). By taking time-sequential images of exercise, the immediate response of the sympathetic nervous system via the somatocutaneous reflex can be visualized. The investigation of infrared images taken before and after sport-specific exercise may further determine the applicability of MIT to investigate the physiology of biological tissue. Furthermore systemic cutaneous blood flow regulation can be monitored as a function of exercise type, duration and intensity.

AEROBIC VERSUS ANAEROBIC EXERCISE

The mechanism of homeostasis during exercise is guaranteed through multiple functions, such as cardiac processes, peripheral circulatory control, blood pressure regulation and temperature control (Berne & Levy, 2000). A better understanding of the cutaneous circulation, and, therefore, the control of blood flow during exercise is a challenge in integrative physiology (Kellog & Pérgola, 2000). We investigated thermal characteristics of aerobic and anaerobic bicycle exercise to predict evidence of altered perfusion. Twelve athletic males (mean age 26.0 ± 2.7 years, height 177.2cm ± 4.3 cm, mass 71.1 ± 8.4 kg) performed both, anaerobic exercise (5 minutes, 80rpm, 90%HRmax) and aerobic exercise (45 minutes, 80rpm, 60%HRmax) under thermo-neutral conditions.

Images were taken prior to (Figure 17a) and immediately following aerobic (Figure 17b) and anaerobic exercise (Figure 17c). The ROI was defined above the middle portion of the M. quadriceps. The temperature above the exercising muscle increased following aerobic exercise (0.7°C, p=0.215) and decreased following anaerobic exercise (-1.5°C, p=0.094). In addition hot colored dots over the thigh occurred after aerobic exercise. To meet the increased metabolic demand of active muscles, short- term, intense exercise leads to a redistribution of blood flow away from inactive tissues such as the skin, to exercising muscles through the vasoconstrictor system (Kenney & Johnson, 1991). This process explained the marginal skin temperature decrease following anaerobic exercise. From a clinical point of view, this observation becomes interesting for patients with compromised cardiac function. As previously reported, these patients showed a higher magnitude of vasoconstriction compared to a healthy group, suggesting that the initial reflex vasoconstriction may be linked to cardiovascular functional capacity (Zelis et al., 1969). With continuing exercise, the body core temperature begins to rise. When internal temperature increases toward a threshold, a regulating system starts to stimulate thermo- sensitive neurons in the central nervous system. This triggering of cutaneous vasodilation ensures the transfer of metabolic heat from the core to the skin (Charkoudian, 2003). The present study showed that the competing system of thermoregulatory drive for cutaneous vasodilation and the non-thermoregulatory drive for cutaneous vasoconstriction could be visualized by using MIT. As previously reported, the interactive control system, as a normal function of dynamic muscular exercise, seems to dependent upon the intensity and duration. The multiple hot spots seen on the thigh (Figure 17b) illustrate the so-called perforating blood vessels that originate in deeper lying tissue. The vasoconstrictor mechanism at the beginning of the exercise is mainly in the skin blood vessels, whereas the perforator vessels are less affected. As exercise duration increases, they contribute to the rewarming of the skin (Merla et al., 2010). The identification of a skin thermographic map of perforator vessels that includes their perfusion area can be important to define individual anatomy of certain tissues (Salmon et al., 1988). Further research should examine the time-course of thermal changes by taking multiple images during and following an exercise. In addition, the relationship between thermal changes, aerobic capacity and performance may further determine different functional states of the body dependent on intensity and duration.

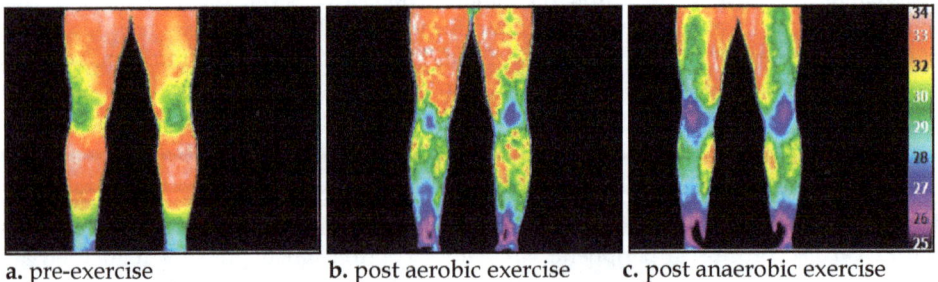

a. pre-exercise   b. post aerobic exercise   c. post anaerobic exercise

Fig. 17. Infrared images of the anterior aspect of lower legs

5. Conclusion

High-quality scientific work with modern 21st-century technology coupled with a better understanding of the regulation of skin blood flow has improved the capability of MIT in medical use. Our research findings suggest that the most beneficial output of MIT seems to be in the screening of athletes for overuse injuries. We suggest combining baseline images with images taken following sport-specific exercise to provoke sufficient thermal alterations in the tissues. A main challenge is to combine the anatomical and physiological information demonstrated by the thermal pattern of the skin. The biological nature of thermal signals and consistent thermal alterations of different sport-specific injuries should be further addressed. Thermal screening of injured and non-injured athletes is the first step to create a sport-specific database with individual thermograms. Repeated follow-up measurements during the sport season will further clarify the link between asymmetrical temperature distributions, pathophysiological changes on the skin surface and the extent of injury. The long-term aim is to create a knowledge-based database of thermograms of overuse and traumatic injuries. However, it should be considered that within a certain time span, different pathologies could alter their patterns of temperature. A deeper understanding of the different time courses of injuries is important to clarify the benefit of MIT in injury management and to define whether a thermogram is "normal" or not. In terms of quantification of side-to side differences within a defined ROI, it is important to use the medical analysis function of image fusion. The main advantage of MIT is its safety, however, the disadvantage of MIT results from its physical limitations. The non-radiating, two-dimensional technique provides information about surface structures. A conclusion of processes in deeper tissues needs to be further investigated by combining different medical imaging modalities. In addition, it must be clearly stated that the aim of MIT use in sports medicine is not to be a substitute for clinical examination, but to enhance and support it. It can be concluded that MIT is a reliable, low-cost detection tool that should be applied for pre-scanning athletes.

6. References

Ammer, K. (2006). Diagnosis of Raynaud´s phenomen by thermography. *Skin Research and Technology*, Vol.2, No.4, pp. 182-185, ISSN 0909-752X

Ammer, K. (2008). The Glamorgan Protocol for recording and evaluation of thermal images of the human body. *Thermology International*, Vol.18, No.4, pp. 125-144, ISSN1560-604X

Ammer, K. (2008). The sensitivity of infrared imaging for diagnosing Raynaud´s phenomenon or Thoracic Outlet Syndrome is dependent on the method of temperature extraction from thermal images. *Thermology International*, Vol.18, No. 3, pp.81-88, ISSN1560-604X

Arora, N.; Martins, D.; Ruggerio, D.; Tousimis, E.; Swistel, A.J.; Osborne, M.P.& Simmons, R.M. (2008). Effectiveness of a noninvasive digital infrared thermal imaging system in the detection of breast cancer. *The American Journal of Surgery*, Vol.196, No.4, pp. 523-526, ISSN 0002- 9610

Berne, R.M. & Levy, M.N. (2000). *Principles of Physiology*. Third Edition, Mosby, ISBN 84-8174-550-2, St. Louis

Bharara, M. (2006). Thermography and Thermometry in the Assessment of Diabetic Neuropathic Foot: A Case for furthering the role of thermal techniques. *The International Journal of Lower Extremity Wounds*, Vol.5, No.4, pp. 250-260, ISSN 1534-7346

Blatteis, C.M. (1998). *Physiology and pathophysiology of temperature regulation*. First edition, World scientific printers, ISBN 981-02-3172-5, Singapore

Bruckner, P. & Khan, K. (2006). Fundamental principals, In: *Clinical Sports Medicine*. Third edition. Bruckner, P; Khan, K pp. 3-7, McGraw-Hill Medical Publishing Division, ISBN 0070278997, Canada

Bruehl, S.; Lubenow, T.; Nath, H. & Ivankovich, O. (1996). Validation of Thermography in the Diagnosis of Reflex Sympathetic Dystrophy. *Clinical Journal of Pain*, Vol.12, No.4, pp. 316-325, ISSN 07498047

Charkoudian, N. (2003). Skin blood flow in adult human thermoregulation: how it works, when it does not and why. *Mayo Clinic Proceedings*, Vol.78, No.5, pp. 603-612, ISSN 0025-6196

Clayton, R.A.E. & Court-Brown, C.M. (2008). The epidemiology of musculoskeletal tendinous and ligamentous injuries. *Injury*, Vol.39, No.12, pp.1338-1344, ISSN 0020-1383

Cochrane, D.J.; Sanard, S.R.; Firth, E.C. & Rittweger, J. (2010). Comparing Muscle Temperature during static and dynamic Squatting with and without Whole- Body Vibration. *Clinical Physiology and Functional Imaging*, Vol.30, No.4, pp. 223-229, ISSN 1475-0961

Denoble, A.E.; Hall, N.; Pieper, C.F. & Kraus, V.P. (2010). Patellar skin surface temperature by thermography reflects knee osteoarthritis. *Clinical medicine insights. Arthritis and musculoskeletal disorders*, Vol.3, No.1, pp. 69-75, ISSN 11795441

Diakides, N.A. & Bronzino J.D. (2008). *Medical Infrared Imaging*, First Edition, CRC Press, ISBN 0849390272, Broken

de Weerd, L.; Mercer J. & Setså, L. (2006). Intraoperative Dynamic Infrared Thermography and Free-Flap Surgery. *Annals of Plastic Surgery*, Vol.57, No.3, pp. 279-284, ISSN 01487043

Eddy, A.L.; Van Hoogmoed, L.M. & Snyder, J.R. (2001). The role of Thermography in the Management of Equine Lameness. *The Veterinary Journal*, Vol.162, No.3, pp. 172-181, ISSN 1090-0233

Elliot, R.L. & Head, J.F. (1999). Medical infrared imaging in the twenty-first century. *Thermology International*, Vol.9., No.4, pp. 111, ISSN 1560-604X

Flørenes, T.W.; Bere, T.; Nordsletten, L. Heir, S. & Bahr, R. (2009). Injuries among male and female world cup alpine skiers. *British Journal of Sports Medicine*, Vol.43, No.13, pp. 973-978, ISSN 0306-3674

Gholve, P.; Scher, D.; Khakharia, S.; Widmann, R. & Green, D. (2007). Osgood Schlatter syndrome. *Current Opinion in Pediatrics*, Vol.19, No.1, pp. 44-50, ISSN 1531-698X

Hardaker, N.J.; Moss, A.D.; Richards, J.; Jarvis, S.; McEwan, C. & Selfe, J. (2007). The relationship between skin surface temperature measured via non-contact thermal imaging and intra-muscular temperature of the rectus femoris muscle. *Thermology International*, Vol.17, No.2; pp. 45-50, ISSN 1560-604X

Hildebrandt, C.; Ammer, K. & Raschner, C. (2010). An Overview of Recent Application of Medical Infrared Thermography in Sports Medicine in Austria. *Sensors*, Vol.10, No.5, pp. 4700-4715, ISSN 1424-8220

Hreljac, A. (2005). Etiology, prevention and early intervention of overuse injuries in runners: a biomechanical perspective. *Physical medicine and rehabilitation clinics of North America*, Vol.16, No.3, pp. 651-667, ISSN 1047-9651

Jiang, L.J.; Ng, E.Y.K.; Yeo, A.C.B.; Wu, S.; Pan, F.; Yau, W.Y.; Chen, J.H. & Yang, Y. (2005). A perspective on medical infrared imaging. *Journal of Medical Engineering and Technology*, Vol.29, No.6, pp. 257-267, ISSN 0309-1902

Kellog D. L. & Pérgola P. (2000). Skin Response to exercise and training. In: *Exercise and Sports Science*, Garrett, W.E.; Kirkendall, D.T. published by Lippincott Williams &Wilkins, pp. 239-250, ISBN 0-683-03421 9, Philadelphia

Kenney W.L. & Johnson J.M. (1992). Control of skin blood flow during exercise. *Medicine and Science in Sports and Exercise*, Vol. 24, No.3, pp. 303-312, ISSN 1530-0315

Kontos, M.; Wilson, R. & Fentiman, I. (2011). Digital infrared thermal imaging (DITI) of breast lesions: sensitivity and specificity of detection of primary breast cancers. *Clinical Radiology*, Vol. 66, No.6, pp. 536-539, ISSN 0033-8419

Merla, A.; DiRomualdo, S.; DiDonato, L.; Proietti, M.; Salsano, F. & Romani, G.L. (2007). Combined thermal and laser Doppler imaging in the assessment of cutaneous tissue perfusion. *Conference Proceedings of the IEEE Engineering Medicine and Biology Society*, pp. 2630-2633, ISSN 1557-170X

Merla, A; Mattei, P.A.; di Donato, L. & Romani, G.L. (2010). Thermal Imaging of Cutaneous Temperature Modifications in Runners During Graded Exercise. *Annals of Biomedical Engineering*, Vol.38, No.1, pp.158-163, ISSN 1573-9686

Ng, E.Y.K. (2009). A review of thermography as promising non-invasive detection modality for breast tumor. *International Journal of Thermal Science*, Vol.48, No.5, pp. 849-859, ISSN 1290-0729

Niehof, S.P.; Huygen, F.; van der Weerd, R.; Westra, M. & Zijlstra, F.J. (2006). Thermography imaging during static and controlled thermoregulation in complex regional pain syndrome type 1. *Biomedical Engineering OnLine*, Vol.5, No.30, pp. 1-13, ISSN 1475-925X

Park, J.Y.; Hyun, J.K. & Seo, J.B. (2007). The effectiveness of digital infrared thermographic imaging in patients with shoulder impingement syndrome. *Journal of Shoulder and Elbow Surgery*, Vol.16, No.5, pp. 548-554, ISSN 1058-2746

Plassmann,P. & Murawski, P. (2003). CTHERM for standardized thermography, *Proceedings of Abstracts the 9th congress of Thermology*, ISBN N/A, Poland

Plassman, P.; Ring, E.F.J. & Jones, C.D. (2006). Quality assurance of thermal imaging systems in medicine. *Thermology International*, Vol.16, No.1, pp.10-15, ISSN 1560-604X

Rettig, A.C.; Liotta, F.J.; Klootwyk, T.E.; Porter, D.A. & Mieling, P. (2005). Potential Risk of Rerupture in Primary Achilles Tendon Repair in Athletes Younger Than 30 Years of Age. *American Journal of Sports Medicine*, Vol.33, No.1, pp.119-123, ISSN 0363-5465

Ring, E.F.J. & Ammer, K. (1998). Thermal imaging in sports medicine. *Sport and Medicine Today*, Vol.1, No.2, pp.108-109, ISSN N/A

Ring, E.F.J. & Ammer, K. (2000). The technique of infrared imaging in medicine. *Thermology international*, Vol.10, No1, pp. 7-14, ISSN 1560-604X

Ring E.F.J. (2007). The Historical development of temperature measurement in medicine. *Infrared Physics and Technology*, Vol.49, No.3, pp. 297-301, ISSN 1350-4495

Romano, C.L.; Logoluso, N.; Dellóro, F.; Elia, A. & Drago, L. (2011) Telethermographic findings after uncomplicated and septic total knee replacement. *Knee*, Epub ahead of print, ISSN 0968-0160

Salmon, M.; Taylor, G.I. & Tempest, M.N. (1988). Arteries of the skin, Churchill Livingstone, ISBN 0443036055, London

Sein, M.L.; Walton, J.; Linklater, J.; Appleyard, R.; Kirkbride, B.; Kuah, D. & Murrell G.A.C. (2010). Shoulder pain in elite swimmers: primarily due to swim-volume-induced supraspinatus tendinopathy. *British Journal of Sports Medicine*, Vol.44, No.2, pp.105-113, ISSN 0306-3674

Selfe, J.; Whitaker, J. & Hardaker, N. (2008). A narrative literature review identifying the minimum clinically important difference for skin temperature asymmetry at the knee. *Thermology International*, Vol.18, No.2, 41-44, ISSN 1560-604X

Singer, A.J. & Clark, R.A.F. (1999). Cutaneous wound healing. *The New England Journal of Medicine*, Vol. 341, No.10, pp. 738-746, ISSN 0028-4793

Steketee, J. (1973). Spectral emissivity of skin and pericardium. *Physics in Medicine and Biology*. Vol. 18, No. 5, pp. 686-694, ISSN 0031-9155

Thomas, G.D. & Segal, S.S. (2004). Neural control of muscle flow during exercise. *Journal of Applied Physiology*, Vol.97, No.2, pp. 731-738, ISSN 8750-7587

Turner, T.A. (2000). Diagnostic thermography. *Veterinary Clinics of North America-Equine Practice*, Vol.17, No.1, pp. 95-113, ISSN 0749-0739

Vardasca, R. (2008). Symmetry of temperature distribution in the upper and lower extremities. *Thermology International*, Vol.18, No.4, pp. 154-155, ISSN 1560-604X

Wallin, B.G. (1990). Neural control of human skin blood flow. *Journal of the autonomic nervous system*, Vol. 30, No.S1, pp.185-190, ISSN 1529-8027

Wild, W.; Schütte, S.R.; Pau, H.W.; Kramp, B. & Just, T. (2003). Infrared thermography as a non invasive application for medical diagnostic. *Proceedings XVII IMEKO World Congress*, June 22-27, 2003, ISBN 0-7803-8493-8, Dubrovnik Croatia

Woods, C.; Hawkins, R.; Hulse, M. & Hodson A. (2002). The Football Association Medical Research Programme: an audit of injuries in professional football — analysis of preseason injuries. *British Journal of Sports Medicine*, Vol.36, No.6, pp. 436-441, ISSN 0306-3674

Zaprodina, N.; Ming, Z. & Hänninen, O.P. (2006). Plantar infrared thermography measurements and low back pain intensity. *Journal of Manipulative Physiological Therapeutics*, Vol.29, No.3, pp.219-223, ISSN 0161-4754

Zelis, R.; Mason, D.T. & Braunwald, D. (1969). Partition of blood flow to the cutaneous and muscular beds of the forearm at rest and during leg exercise in normal subjects and in patients with heart failure. *Circulation Research*, Vol.24, No.6, pp.799-806, ISSN 0009-7330

Permissions

The contributors of this book come from diverse backgrounds, making this book a truly international effort. This book will bring forth new frontiers with its revolutionizing research information and detailed analysis of the nascent developments around the world.

We would like to thank Kenneth R. Zaslav MD, for lending his expertise to make the book truly unique. He has played a crucial role in the development of this book. Without his invaluable contribution this book wouldn't have been possible. He has made vital efforts to compile up to date information on the varied aspects of this subject to make this book a valuable addition to the collection of many professionals and students.

This book was conceptualized with the vision of imparting up-to-date information and advanced data in this field. To ensure the same, a matchless editorial board was set up. Every individual on the board went through rigorous rounds of assessment to prove their worth. After which they invested a large part of their time researching and compiling the most relevant data for our readers. Conferences and sessions were held from time to time between the editorial board and the contributing authors to present the data in the most comprehensible form. The editorial team has worked tirelessly to provide valuable and valid information to help people across the globe.

Every chapter published in this book has been scrutinized by our experts. Their significance has been extensively debated. The topics covered herein carry significant findings which will fuel the growth of the discipline. They may even be implemented as practical applications or may be referred to as a beginning point for another development. Chapters in this book were first published by InTech; hereby published with permission under the Creative Commons Attribution License or equivalent.

The editorial board has been involved in producing this book since its inception. They have spent rigorous hours researching and exploring the diverse topics which have resulted in the successful publishing of this book. They have passed on their knowledge of decades through this book. To expedite this challenging task, the publisher supported the team at every step. A small team of assistant editors was also appointed to further simplify the editing procedure and attain best results for the readers.

Our editorial team has been hand-picked from every corner of the world. Their multi-ethnicity adds dynamic inputs to the discussions which result in innovative outcomes. These outcomes are then further discussed with the researchers and contributors who give their valuable feedback and opinion regarding the same. The feedback is then collaborated with the researches and they are edited in a comprehensive manner to aid the understanding of the subject.

Apart from the editorial board, the designing team has also invested a significant amount of their time in understanding the subject and creating the most relevant covers. They scrutinized every image to scout for the most suitable representation of the subject and create an appropriate cover for the book.

The publishing team has been involved in this book since its early stages. They were actively engaged in every process, be it collecting the data, connecting with the contributors or procuring relevant information. The team has been an ardent support to the editorial, designing and production team. Their endless efforts to recruit the best for this project, has resulted in the accomplishment of this book. They are a veteran in the field of academics and their pool of knowledge is as vast as their experience in printing. Their expertise and guidance has proved useful at every step. Their uncompromising quality standards have made this book an exceptional effort. Their encouragement from time to time has been an inspiration for everyone.

The publisher and the editorial board hope that this book will prove to be a valuable piece of knowledge for researchers, students, practitioners and scholars across the globe.

List of Contributors

Jean-Frédéric Brun and Jacques Mercier
U1046, INSERM, Université de Montpellier 1, Université de Montpellier 2, Montpellier, CHRU Montpellier, Département de Physiologie Clinique, Montpellier, France

Emmanuelle Varlet-Marie
Laboratoire Performance Santé Altitude, Sciences et Techniques des Activités Physiques et Sportives, Université de Perpignan Via Domitia, France

Ahmed Jérôme Romain
Laboratoire EA4556 Epsylon, Dynamique des Capacités Humaines et des Conduites de Santé (Montpellier), France

Juliette Hussey
F.T.C.D. Discipline of Physiotherapy, School of Medicine, Trinity Centre for Health Sciences, St James's Hospital, Dublin, Ireland

Rodrigo Hohl, Lázaro Alessandro Soares Nunes, Rafael Alkmin Reis, René Brenzikofer and Rodrigo Perroni Ferraresso
Laboratory of Exercise Biochemistry (LABEX), Biology Institute, University State of Campinas (UNICAMP), Brazil

Foued Salmen Spindola
Laboratory of Biochemistry and Molecular Biology (LABIBI), Federal University of Uberlândia (UFU), Brazil

Lázaro Alessandro Soares Nunes, Fernanda Lorenzi Lazarim, René Brenzikofer and Denise Vaz Macedo
Laboratory of Exercise Biochemistry (LABEX), Biology Institute, State University of Campinas (UNICAMP), Brazil
Laboratory of Instrumentation for Biomechanics, Physical Education Faculty, State University of Campinas (UNICAMP), Campinas, SP, Brazil

Athanasios Z. Jamurtas
Department of Physical Education and Sport Science, University of Thessaly, Trikala, Greece Institute of Human Performance and Rehabilitation, Center for Research and Technology –Thessaly, Trikala, Greece

Ioannis G. Fatouros
Department of Physical Education and Sport Science, Democritus University of Thrace, Komotini, Greece
Institute of Human Performance and Rehabilitation, Center for Research and Technology –Thessaly, Trikala, Greece

Paul M. Vanderburgh
University of Dayton, Dayton, OH, USA

Monica C. Serra, Shawna L. McMillin and Alice S. Ryan
VA Research Service, Department of Medicine, Division of Gerontology and Geriatric Medicine, University of Maryland School of Medicine, Baltimore VA Medical Center Geriatric Research, Education and Clinical Center (GRECC), VA Maryland Health Care System, Baltimore, USA

Xiaolin Yang
LIKES-Research Center for Sport and Health Sciences, Jyväskylä, Finland

Baruch Wolach
The Sackler School of Medicine, Tel Aviv University, Israel

Bakhtyar Tartibian and Behzad Hajizadeh Maleki
Department of Cellular and Molecular Exercise Physiology, Faculty of Physical Education and Sport Science, Urmia University, Urmia, Iran

Asghar Abbasi
Institute of Sport Science, University of Tuebingen, Germany

Mehdi Eghbali and Siamak Asri-Rezaei
Department of Clinical Science, Faculty of Veterinary Medicine, Urmia University, Urmia, Iran

Hinnak Northoff
Institute of Clinical and Experimental Transfusion Medicine (IKET), University of Tuebingen, Germany

Nicola Scichilone, Laura Chimenti and Roberta Santagata
Biomedical Department of Internal and Specialistic Medicine (DiBiMIS), Section of Pneumology, Italy

Daniele Zangla
Department of Motor Sciences (DISMOT), Italy

Maria R. Bonsignore
Biomedical Department of Internal and Specialistic Medicine (DiBiMIS), Section of Pneumology, Italy
Institute of Biomedicine and Molecular Immunology (IBIM), National Research Council, Palermo, Italy

Giuseppe Morici
Institute of Biomedicine and Molecular Immunology (IBIM), National Research Council, Palermo, Italy
Department of Experiental Biomedicine and Clinical Neurosciences (BIONEC), University of Palermo, Italy

Jonathan S. Leventhal and Brook E. Tlougan
NYU School of Medicine, Department of Dermatology New York, NY, USA

Francisca Galindo-Garre and Sanne I. de Vries
TNO, The Netherlands

Cândido C. Coimbra
Federal University of Minas Gerais, Department of Physiology and Biophysics, Brazil

Danusa D. Soares
Federal University of Minas Gerais, Department of Physical Education, Brazil

Laura H. R. Leite
Federal University of Juiz de Fora, Department of Physiology, Brazil

Carolin Hildebrandt and Christian Raschner
University of Innsbruck, Department of Sport Science, Innsbruck, Austria

Karlheinz Zeilberger
Medical Practices for Internal and Sports Medicine, Munich, Germany

Edward Francis John Ring
Medical Imaging Research Group, Faculty of Advanced Technology, University of Glamorgan, UK